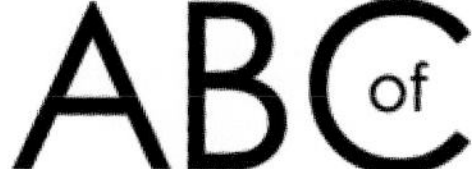

Dermatology

Sixth Edition

EDITED BY

Rachael Morris-Jones, FRCP, PhD, PCME
Dermatology Consultant
Kings College Hospital
Denmark Hill
London, UK

WILEY Blackwell

BMJ | Books

BMJ Books is an imprint of BMJ Publishing Group Limited, used under licence by John Wiley & Sons.

Registered office: John Wiley & Sons, Ltd, The Atrium, Southern Gate, Chichester, West Sussex, PO19 8SQ, UK

Editorial offices: 9600 Garsington Road, Oxford, OX4 2DQ, UK
The Atrium, Southern Gate, Chichester, West Sussex, PO19 8SQ, UK
111 River Street, Hoboken, NJ 07030-5774, USA

For details of our global editorial offices, for customer services and for information about how to apply for permission to reuse the copyright material in this book please see our website at www.wiley.com/wiley-blackwell

Library of Congress Cataloging-in-Publication Data
ABC of dermatology / [edited by] Rachael Morris-Jones. – Sixth edition.
p. ; cm.
Preceded by: ABC of dermatology / edited by Paul K. Buxton, Rachael Morris-Jones. 5th ed. 2009.
Includes bibliographical references and index.
ISBN 978-1-118-52015-4 (pbk.)
I. Morris-Jones, Rachael, editor of compilation.
[DNLM: 1. Skin Diseases. WR 140]
RL74
616.5 – dc23
2013049508

A catalogue record for this book is available from the British Library.

Wiley also publishes its books in a variety of electronic formats. Some content that appears in print may not be available in electronic books.

Cover image: Patient with urticaria – photo supplied by Dr Rachael Morris-Jones.
Cover design by Andy Meaden.

Set in 9.25/12pt MinionPro by Laserwords Private Ltd, Chennai, India
Printed and bound in Malaysia by Vivar Printing Sdn Bhd

1 2014

Contents

List of Contributors

Kapil Bhargava
St. John's Institute of Dermatology, Guy's and St. Thomas' Hospitals, London, UK

Bernadette Byrne
Department of Tissue viability, Kings College Hospital, London, UK

David de Berker
Dermatology Department, United Bristol Healthcare Trust, Bristol, UK

Alun V. Evans
Dermatology Department, Princess of Wales Hospital, Bridgend, UK

David Fenton
St. John's Institute of Dermatology, Guy's and St. Thomas' Hospitals, London, UK

Raj Mallipeddi
Cutaneous Laser and Surgery Unit, St. John's Institute of Dermatology, St. Thomas' Hospital, London, UK

Rachael Morris-Jones
Dermatology Department, Kings College Hospital, London, UK

Sarah Walsh
Kings College Hospital, London, UK

Karen Watson
Dermatology Department, Orpington Hospital, Orpington, Kent, UK

Preface

The Sixth Edition of the *ABC of Dermatology* incorporates all the latest scientific advances in genetics, pathophysiology and management strategies whilst at the same time remaining a practical clinical approach to dermatology. The current editor has striven to uphold the style and emphasis that Paul Buxton brought to the *ABC of Dermatology* to ensure that it is a valuable resource for any medical and nursing practitioner who is diagnosing and managing skin disease.

In addition to a wholly practical approach to clinical dermatology, the Sixth Edition gives insights into the latest thinking around the pathophysiological processes that explain the characteristic features of skin disease and the current approach to its management including the newer biological agents for treating inflammatory disease and tumours.

The fascination of dermatology lies partly in the visual nature of the discipline and also in one's ability to diagnose systemic disease through examination of the skin surface. Manifestations of an underlying disease can form specific patterns in the skin, which in some instances are pathognomonic. Internal physicians need to be aware of the 'signs posting' of skin disorders towards the unifying underlying diagnosis. However, even a highly skilled dermatologist will at times be uncertain of the diagnosis and a simple skin biopsy for histopathology/immunohistochemistry and/or culture is greatly helpful in most cases in the diagnosis and to reach a definitive management plan.

Nonetheless, for those working in poor resource settings, there may be little access to modern investigations for skin disease patients and therefore the clinical diagnosis will be the benchmark on which skin disease is managed. To this end the Sixth Edition is full of clinical photographs eliciting the appearances of skin disease in a multitude of different pigmented skin tones and ethnic groups. Descriptions of skin management include simple and relatively cheap interventions as well as sophisticated cutting edge immunotherapies.

On a global scale, the number of people with access to the internet via computers or mobile devices is increasing at a rapid pace. This enables them to access a multitude of resources including those related to the diagnosis and management of human disease. An informed patient can be hugely beneficial to everyone involved in the provision of healthcare; however, at times this can lead to patients becoming overly anxious or misinformed. There is an increasing use of teledermatology in many parts of the world where populations are a long distance away from a skin specialist from where images of the patient's skin complaints are taken and sent to an expert for a virtual opinion. This can be immensely helpful; however, ultimately the gold standard for accurate diagnosis and management of skin disease is still seeing patients in person preferably by a practitioner with personal knowledge and experience of skin disease.

I sincerely hope the Sixth Edition of the *ABC of Dermatology* will not only introduce the reader to a fascinating clinical discipline but will also help them to diagnose and manage skin disease in whichever part of the world they are working.

We are all hugely grateful to Paul Buxton for all his hard work on the previous editions of the *ABC of Dermatology* and I hope he will be proud of how the Sixth Edition has enhanced what he originally created.

I would like to dedicate the Sixth Edition of the *ABC of Dermatology* to all the unsung heroes of medical education who work enthusiastically with absolute dedication for little recognition or reward other than to know that by sharing their knowledge they ultimately help more patients.

Rachael Morris-Jones

Acknowledgements

I would very much like to sincerely thank all my co-contributors whose expertise in specialist areas of dermatology has been invaluable in ensuring that this Sixth Edition is right up to date and written by experts in their field.

Dr Sarah Walsh has taken over writing the chapter on drug rashes, which is immensely important in modern medicine where more and more patients are receiving an increasing number of medications. Many of these drug rashes can be severe and even life-threatening and are referred to as severe cutaneous adverse reactions (SCAR). Recognising that a medication has triggered a skin disease and stopping the culprit drug can be life-saving and is therefore something that all medical practitioners should be able to diagnose and manage. Dr Sarah Walsh is one of the UK's leading experts on the diagnosis and management of cutaneous drug rashes and her expertise hugely enhances the Sixth Edition of the *ABC of Dermatology*.

Tissue viability clinical nurse specialist Bernadette Byrne has taken over the chapter dedicated to wound management and bandaging. She has an impressive depth of knowledge as well as decades of experience managing literally thousands of complex wounds in patients from the out-patient setting to the intensive care unit. Her clinical practical approach will be an invaluable guide to wound management in any setting.

Dr Raj Mallippeddi has updated his chapter on practical procedures in dermatology, which describes in detail how to perform simple skin surgery and the techniques used by experts in the field of dermatological surgery. He describes Mohs' micrographic surgery that is fast becoming the gold standard in the UK for excision of certain types of skin cancers on the face that ensures tumours are completely excised and at the same time sparing vital normal tissue.

Dr Alun Evans has included in his updated chapter on lasers and photodynamic therapy a description of intense pulsed light, fractional lasers and dermabrasion/chemical peels. What these relatively newer approaches have in common is less potential side effects and 'down-time' for patients when carried out by a highly skilled practitioners compared to some of the more traditional ablative laser treatments.

Dr David de Berker has updated his chapter on the diagnosis and management of nail disorders, which is highly specialised but nonetheless a common and important aspect of dermatology. The expanding practice of nail cosmetics is discussed in the management and cause of nail disorders in this Sixth Edition.

Dr Karen Watson has a background in pharmacology before training as a dermatology consultant and is therefore uniquely placed to update the chapter on cutaneous formulary. There have been rapid and dynamic developments in the range of medications available to treat a multitude of skin diseases and therefore many of us will struggle to keep abreast of all the innovations. Consequently, the updated formulary chapter will be useful for the novice and the experienced dermatology practitioner in this ever expanding field of dermatology.

The management of hair disorders has sadly lagged behind in the many therapeutic advances in other areas of dermatology. Nonetheless, Dr Kapil Bhargava and Dr David Fenton have included an increasing number of management strategies in their updated chapter on hair/scalp disorders to help both practitioners and patients alike. Research into the management of hair loss/excessive hair is making headway and we are all hoping for significant breakthroughs in the future.

A large proportion of the illustrations in the Sixth Edition of the *ABC of Dermatology* comes from Kings College Hospital, London, UK. I am indebted to the medical photography department at Kings for their very professional, high-quality clinical images without which this book would be of little use. Many of the images in the hair and scalp chapter have been provided by the St John's institute of Dermatology, St Thomas' Hospital, London, UK. Dr Stephen Morris-Jones, consultant in Infectious Diseases, University College Hospital, London, UK, provided some of the cutaneous infection images and we have retained some of Dr Barbara Leppard's photographs in the tropical dermatology chapter that she took whilst working in Africa. Bernadette Byrne from Kings College Hospital, London, UK, uses photography on a daily basis for monitoring patients' wounds and she has been able to include these in her wound management chapter. Some of the photographs retained from previous editions come from the Victoria Hospital, Kirkcaldy and Queen Margaret Hospital, Dunfermline, Fife, the Royal Infirmary, Edinburgh and from Paul Buxton's own collection. Dr Jon Salisbury, a consultant histopathologist at Kings College Hospital, London, UK, provided all the histopathology images to demonstrate cutaneous disease at the cellular level and Dr Edward Davies consultant immunologist at Kings College Hospital, London, UK, provided the direct immunofluorescence images of the skin in immunobullous disease.

I owe a huge debt of gratitude to all my Dermatology colleagues at Kings College Hospital who diagnosed and managed many of the patients you will see in the illustrations in this Sixth Edition. I would specifically like to thank Dr Elisabeth Higgins, Dr Daniel Creamer, Dr Sarah Walsh, Dr Saqib Bashir and Prof Roderick Hay and Dr Tanya Basu.

I am especially indebted to all the patients for consenting to include their clinical images in the *ABC of Dermatology* to help us to demonstrate the features presenting in a multitude of skin/nail and hair disorders far better than any written description would do.

Dr Rachael Morris-Jones

CHAPTER 1

Introduction

Rachael Morris-Jones

Dermatology Department, Kings College Hospital, London, UK

> **OVERVIEW**
>
> - The clinical features of skin lesions are related to the underlying pathological processes.
> - Skin conditions broadly fall into three clinical groups: (i) those with a well-defined appearance and distribution; (ii) those with a characteristic pattern but with a variety of underlying clinical conditions; (iii) those with a variable presentation and no constant association with underlying conditions.
> - Skin lesions may be the presenting feature of serious systemic disease, and a significant proportion of skin conditions threaten the health, well-being and even the life of the patient.
> - Clinical descriptive terms such as macule, papule, nodule, plaque, induration, atrophy, bulla and erythema relate to what is observed at the skin surface and reflect the pathological processes underlying the affected skin.
> - The significance of morphology and distribution of skin lesions in different clinical conditions are discussed.

Introduction

The aim of this book is to provide an insight for the non-dermatologist into the pathological processes, diagnosis and management of skin conditions. Dermatology is a broad specialty with over 2000 different skin diseases, the most common of which are introduced here. Pattern recognition is key to successful history-taking and examination of the skin by experts, usually without the need for complex investigations. However, for those with less dermatological experience, working from first principles can go a long way in determining the diagnosis and management of patients with less severe skin disease. Although dermatology is a clinically orientated subject, an understanding of the cellular changes underlying the skin disease can give helpful insights into the pathological processes. This understanding aids the interpretation of clinical signs and overall management of cutaneous disease. Skin biopsies can be a useful adjuvant to reaching a diagnosis; however, clinicopathological correlation is essential in order that interpretation of the clinical and pathological patterns is put into the context of the patient.

Interpretation of clinical signs on the skin in the context of underlying pathological processes is a theme running through the chapters. This helps the reader develop a deeper understanding of the subject and should form some guiding principles that can be used as tools to help assess almost any skin eruption.

Clinically, cutaneous disorders fall into three main groups.

1. Those that generally present with a characteristic distribution and morphology that leads to a specific diagnosis – such as chronic plaque psoriasis, basal cell carcinoma and atopic dermatitis (Figure 1.1).
2. A characteristic pattern of skin lesions with variable underlying causes – such as erythema nodosum (Figure 1.2) and erythema multiforme.
3. Skin rashes that can be variable in their presentation and/or underlying causes – such as lichen planus and urticaria.

A holistic approach in dermatology is essential as cutaneous eruptions may be the first indicator of an underlying internal disease. Patients may, for example, first present with a photosensitive rash on the face, but deeper probing may reveal symptoms of joint pains etc. leading to the diagnosis of systemic lupus erythematosus. Similarly, a patient with underlying coeliac disease may first present with blistering on the elbows (dermatitis herpetiformis). It is therefore important not only to take a thorough history (Box 1.1) of the

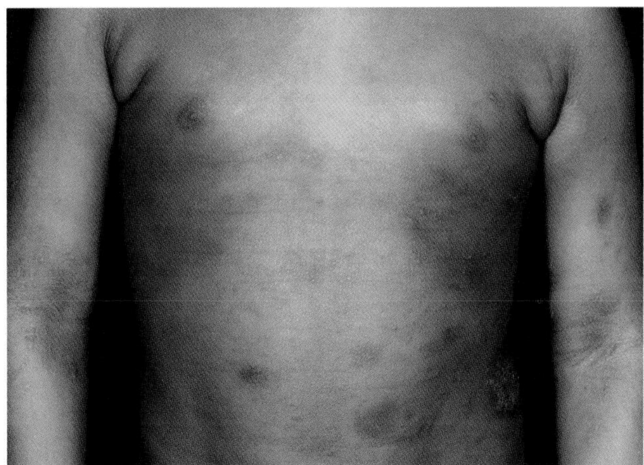

Figure 1.1 Atopic dermatitis.

ABC of Dermatology, Sixth Edition. Edited by Rachael Morris-Jones.

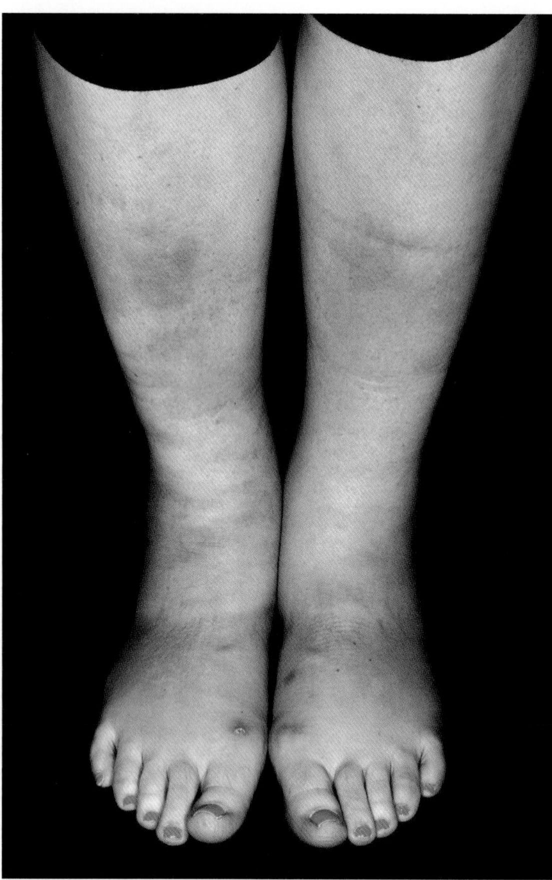

Figure 1.2 Erythema nodosum in pregnancy.

skin complaint but in addition to ask about any other symptoms the patient may have, and examine the entire patient carefully.

Box 1.1 **Dermatology history-taking**

- Where – site of initial lesion(s) and subsequent distribution
- How long – continuous or intermittent?
- Trend – better or worse?
- Previous episodes – timing? Similar/dissimilar? Other skin conditions?
- Who else – Family members/work colleagues/school friends affected?
- Symptoms – Itching, burning, scaling, or blisters? Any medication or other illnesses?
- Treatment – prescription or over the counter? Frequency/time course/compliance?

The significance of skin disease

Seventy per cent of the people living in developing countries suffer skin disease at some point in their lives, but of these, 3 billion people in 127 countries do not have access to even basic skin services. In developed countries the prevalence of skin disease is also high; up to 15% of general practice consultations in the United Kingdom are concerned with skin complaints. Many patients never seek medical advice and self-treat using over-the-counter preparations.

The skin is the largest organ of the body; it provides an essential living biological barrier and is the aspect of ourselves that we present to the outside world. It is therefore not surprising that there is great interest in 'skin care' and 'skin problems', with an associated ever-expanding cosmetics industry. Impairment of the normal functions of the skin can lead to acute and chronic illness with considerable disability and sometimes the need for hospital treatment.

Malignant change can occur in any cell in the skin, resulting in a wide variety of different tumours, the majority of which are benign. Recognition of typical benign tumours saves the patient unnecessary investigations and the anxiety involved in waiting to see a specialist or waiting for biopsy results. Malignant skin cancers are usually only locally invasive, but distant metastases can occur. It is important therefore to recognize the early features of lesions such as melanoma (Figure 1.3) and squamous cell carcinoma before they disseminate.

Underlying systemic disease can be heralded by changes on the skin surface, the significance of which can be easily missed by the unprepared mind. So, in addition to concentrating on the skin changes, the overall health and demeanour of the patient should be assessed. Close inspection of the whole skin, nails and mucous membranes should be the basis of routine skin examination. The general physical condition of the patient should also be determined as indicated.

The majority of skin diseases, however, do not signify any systemic disease and are often considered 'harmless' in medical terms. However, due to the very visual nature of skin disorders, they can cause a great deal of psychological distress, social isolation and occupational difficulties, which should not be underestimated. A validated measure of how much skin disease affects patients' lives can be made using the Dermatology Life Quality Index (DLQI). A holistic approach to the patient both physically and psychologically is therefore highly desirable.

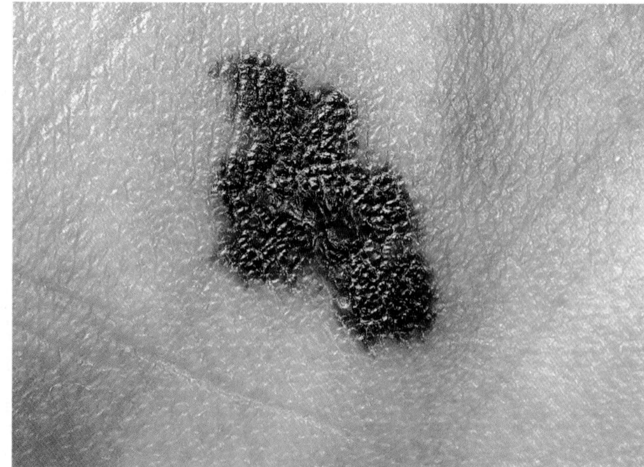

Figure 1.3 Superficial spreading melanoma.

Descriptive terms

All specialties have their own common terms, and familiarity with a few of those used in dermatology is a great help. The most important are defined below.

Macule (Figure 1.4). Derived from the Latin for a stain, the term *macule* is used to describe changes in colour (Figure 1.5) without any elevation above the surface of the surrounding skin. There may be an increase in pigments such as melanin, giving a black or blue colour depending on the depth. Loss of melanin leads to a white macule. Vascular dilatation and inflammation produce erythema. A macule with a diameter greater than 2 cm is called a *patch*.

Papules and nodules (Figure 1.6). A *papule* is a circumscribed, raised lesion, of epidermal or dermal origin, 0.5–1.0 cm in diameter (Figure 1.7). A *nodule* (Figure 1.8) is similar to a papule but greater than 1.0 cm in diameter. A vascular papule or nodule is known as a *haemangioma*.

A plaque (Figure 1.9) is a circumscribed, superficial, elevated plateau area 1.0–2.0 cm in diameter (Figure 1.10).

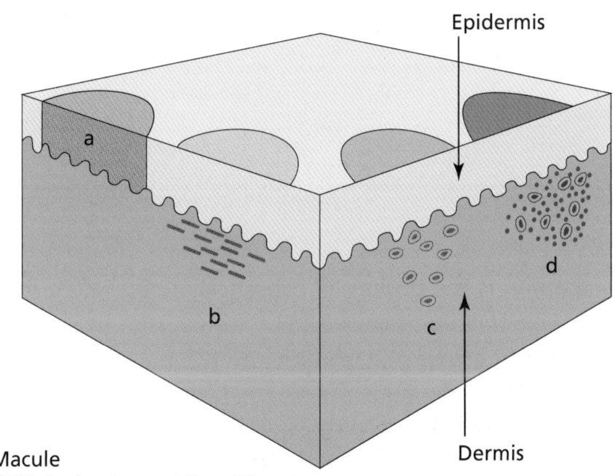

Macule
a) Melanin pigment *in* epidermis
b) Melanin pigment *below* epidermis
c) Erythema due to dilated dermal blood vessels
d) Inflammation in dermis

Figure 1.4 Section through skin.

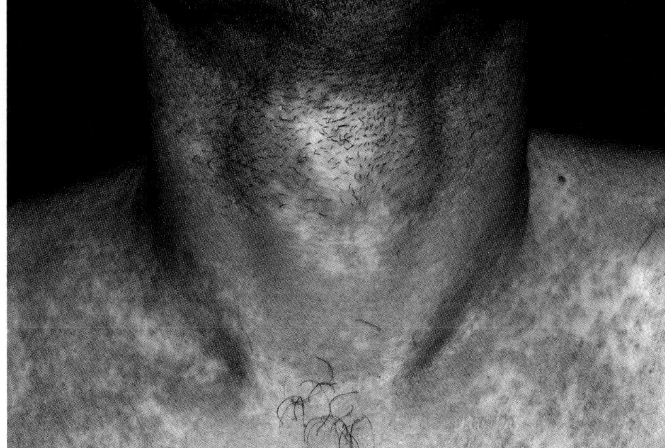

Figure 1.5 Erythema due to a drug reaction.

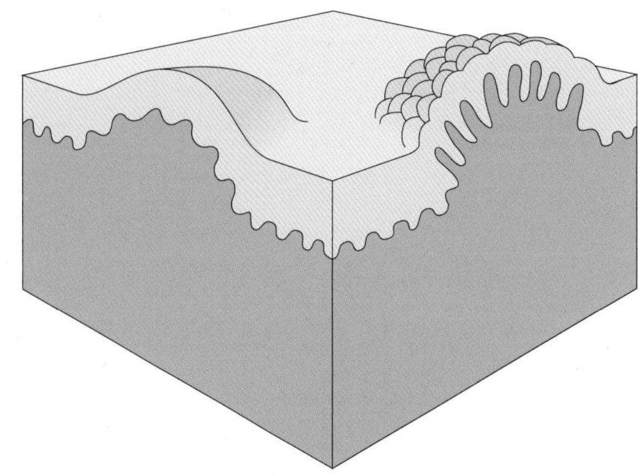

Figure 1.6 Section through skin with a papule.

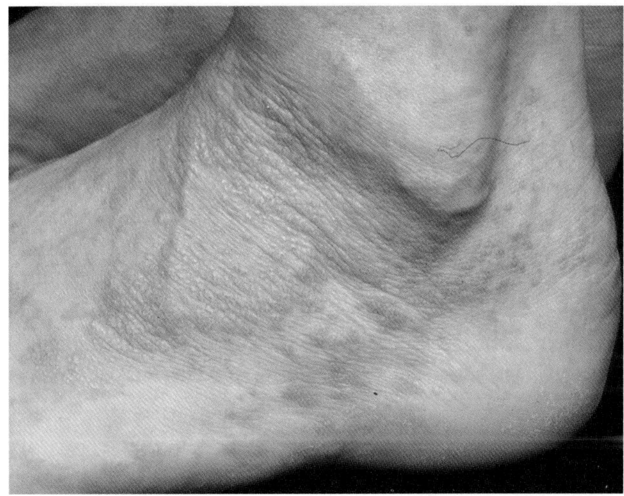

Figure 1.7 Papules in lichen planus.

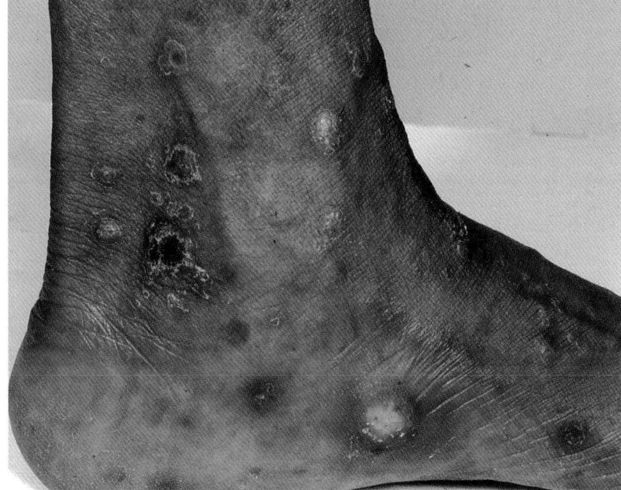

Figure 1.8 Nodules in hypertrophic lichen planus.

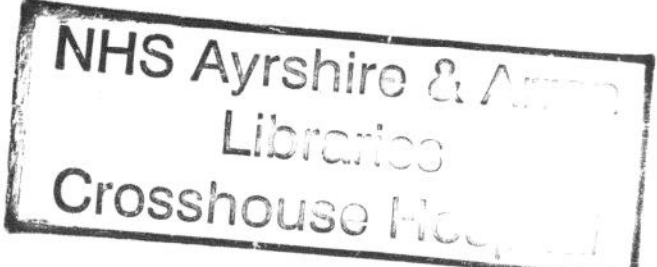

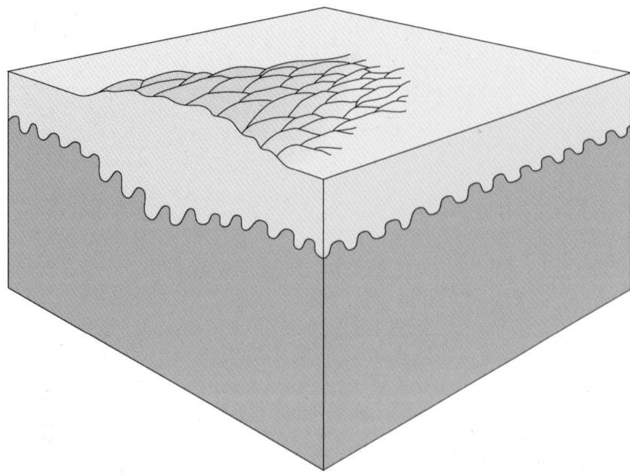

Figure 1.9 Section through skin with plaque.

Vesicles and bullae (Figure 1.11) are raised lesions that contain clear fluid (blisters) (Figure 1.12). A bulla is a vesicle larger than 0.5 cm. They may be superficial within the epidermis or situated in the dermis below it. The more superficial the vesicles/bullae the more likely they are to break open.

Lichenification is a hard thickening of the skin with accentuated skin markings (Figure 1.13). It commonly results from chronic inflammation and rubbing of the skin.

Discoid lesions. These are 'coin-shaped' lesions (Figure 1.14).

Pustules. The term *pustule* is applied to lesions containing purulent material – which may be due to infection – or sterile pustules (inflammatory polymorphs) (Figure 1.15) that are seen in pustular psoriasis and pustular drug reactions.

Atrophy refers to loss of tissue, which may affect the epidermis, dermis or subcutaneous fat. Thinning of the epidermis is characterized by loss of normal skin markings; there may be fine wrinkles, loss of pigment and a translucent appearance (Figure 1.16). In addition, sclerosis of the underlying connective tissue, telangiectasia or evidence of diminished blood supply may be present.

Ulceration results from the loss of the whole thickness of the epidermis and upper dermis (Figure 1.17). Healing results in a scar.

Erosion. An erosion is a superficial loss of epidermis that generally heals without scarring (Figure 1.18).

Excoriation is the partial or complete loss of epidermis as a result of scratching (Figure 1.19).

Fissuring. Fissures are slits through the whole thickness of the skin (Figure 1.20).

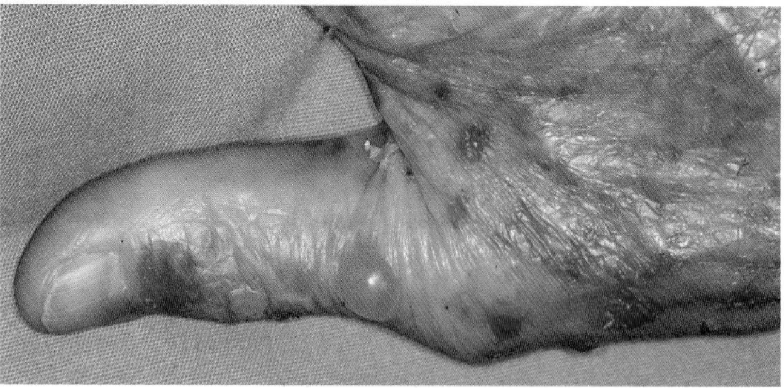

Figure 1.11 Bullae in bullous pemphigoid.

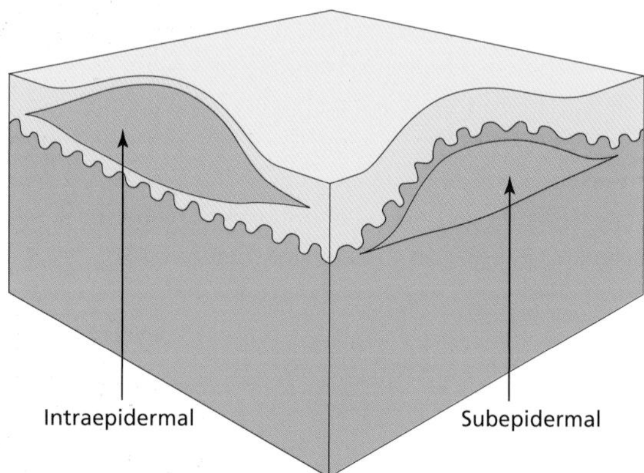

Figure 1.12 Section through skin showing sites of vesicle and bulla.

Desquamation is the peeling of superficial scales, often following acute inflammation (Figure 1.21).

Annular lesions are ring-shaped (Figure 1.22).

Reticulate. The term reticulate means 'net-like'. It is most commonly seen when the pattern of subcutaneous blood vessels becomes visible (Figure 1.23).

Rashes

Approach to diagnosis

A skin rash generally poses more problems in diagnosis than a single, well-defined skin lesion such as a wart or tumour. As in all branches of medicine, a reasonable diagnosis is more likely to be reached by thinking firstly in terms of broad diagnostic categories rather than specific conditions.

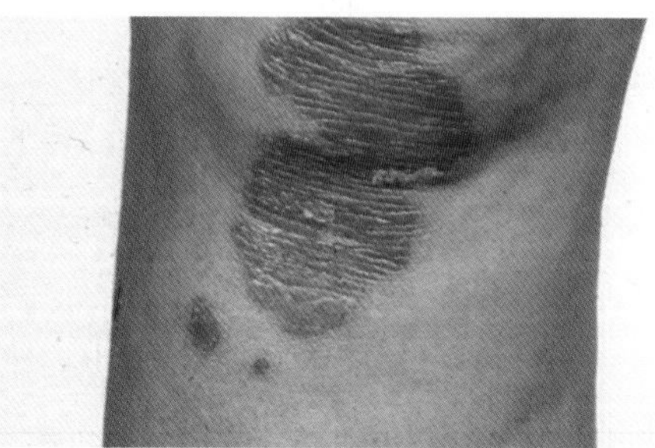

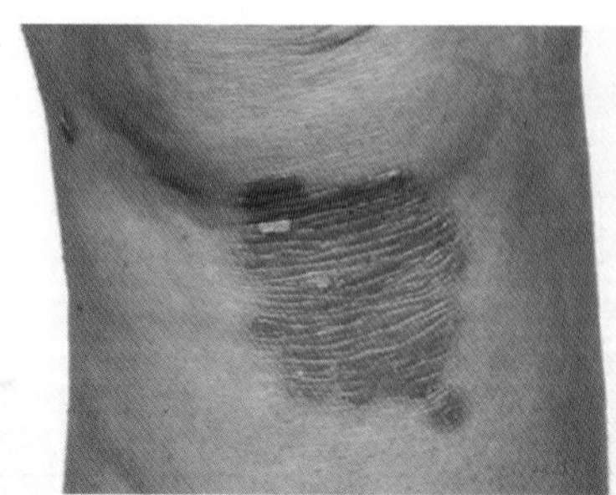

Figure 1.10 Psoriasis plaques on the knees.

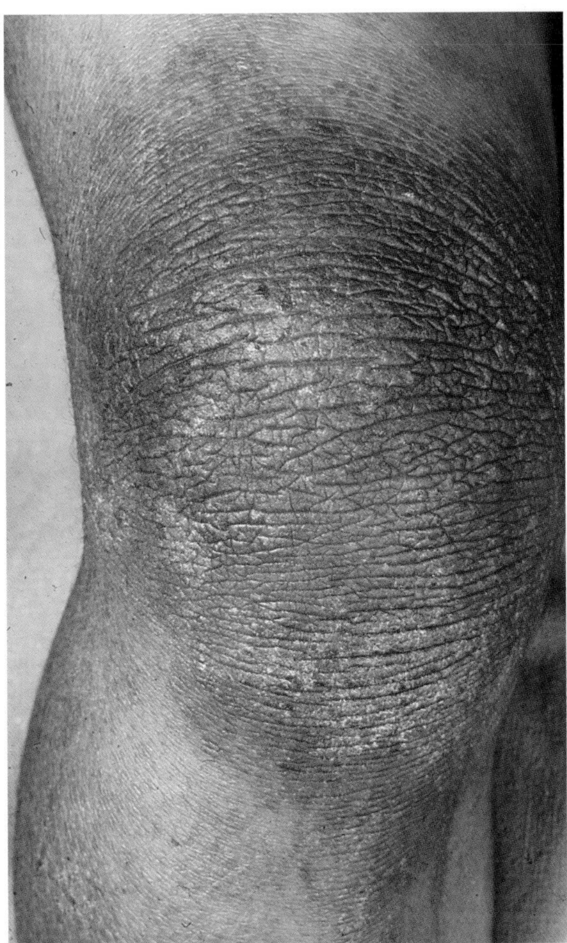

Figure 1.13 Lichenification in chronic eczema.

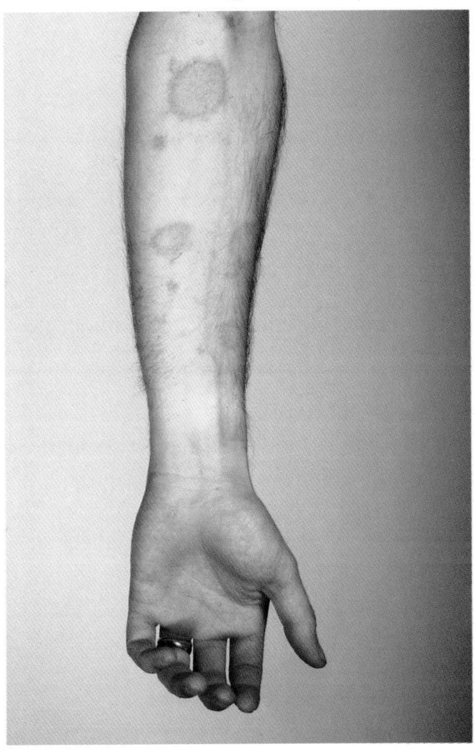

Figure 1.14 Discoid lesions in discoid eczema.

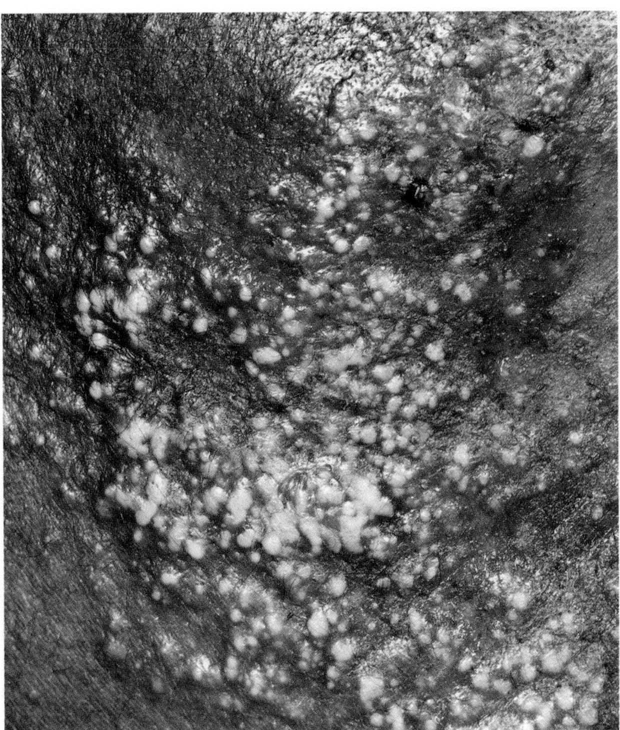

Figure 1.15 Inflammatory sterile pustules in contact dermatitis.

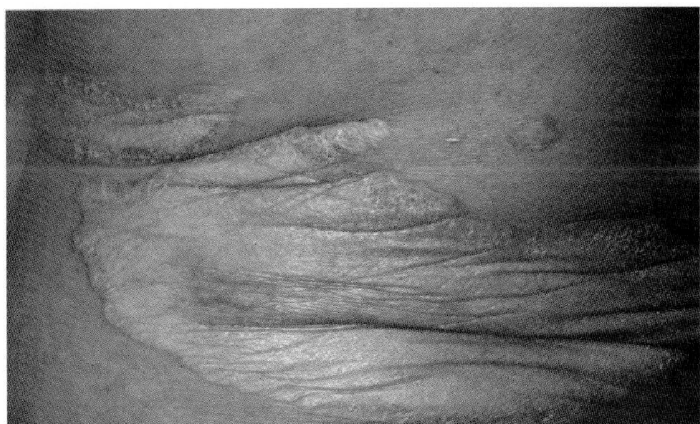

Figure 1.16 Epidermal atrophy in extra-genital lichen sclerosus.

There may be a history of recurrent episodes such as occurs in atopic eczema due to the patient's constitutional tendency. In the case of contact dermatitis, regular exposure to a causative agent leads to recurrences that fit from the history with exposure times. Endogenous conditions such as psoriasis can appear in adults who have had no previous episodes. If several members of the same family are affected by a skin rash simultaneously then a contagious condition, such as scabies, should be considered. A common condition with a familial tendency, such as atopic eczema, may affect several family members at different times.

A simplistic approach to rashes is to classify them as being from the 'inside' or 'outside'. Examples of 'inside' or endogenous rashes are atopic eczema or drug rashes, whereas fungal infection or contact dermatitis are 'outside' or exogenous rashes.

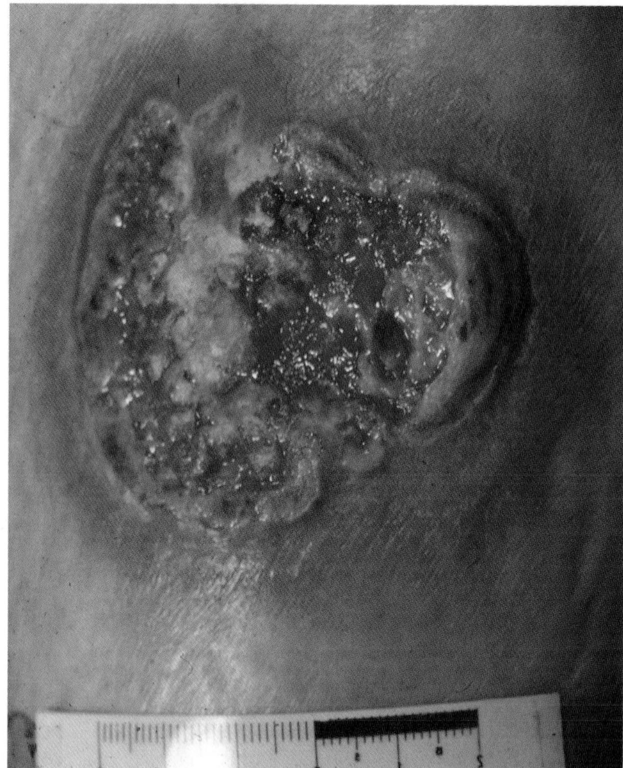

Figure 1.17 Ulceration in pyoderma ganrenosum.

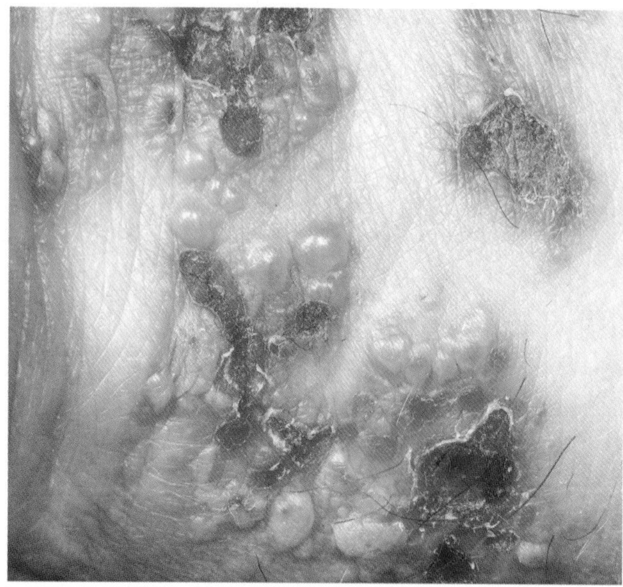

Figure 1.18 Erosions in paraneoplastic bullous pemphigoid.

Symmetry

As a general rule most endogenous rashes affect both sides of the body, as in the atopic child or a patient with psoriasis on the legs (Figure 1.24). Of course, not all exogenous rashes are asymmetrical. Chefs who hold the knife in their dominant hand can have unilateral disease (Figure 1.25) from metal allergy whereas a hairdresser or nurse may develop contact dermatitis on both hands, and a builder bilateral contact dermatitis from kneeling in cement (Figure 1.26).

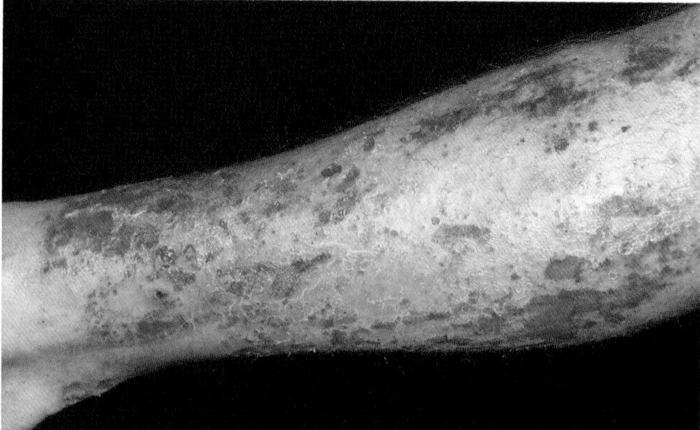

Figure 1.19 Excoriation of epidermis in atopic dermatitis.

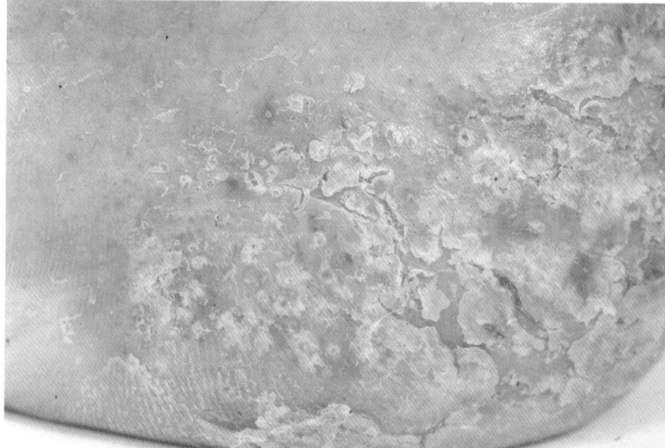

Figure 1.20 Hyperkeratosis with fissures in rubber allergy.

Diagnosis

- Previous episodes of the rash, particularly in childhood, suggest a constitutional condition such as atopic dermatitis.
- Recurrences of the rash, particularly in specific situations, suggest a contact dermatitis. Similarly, a rash that only occurs in the summer months may well have a photosensitive basis (Figure 1.27).
- If other members of the family are affected, particularly without any previous history, there may well be a transmissible condition such as scabies.

Distribution

It is useful to be aware of the usual sites of common skin conditions. These are shown in the appropriate chapters. Eruptions that appear only on areas exposed to sun may be entirely or partially due to sunlight. Some are due to sensitivity to sunlight alone, such as polymorphic light eruption, or a photosensitive allergy to topically applied substances or drugs taken internally.

Morphology

The appearance of the skin lesion may give clues to the underlying pathological process.

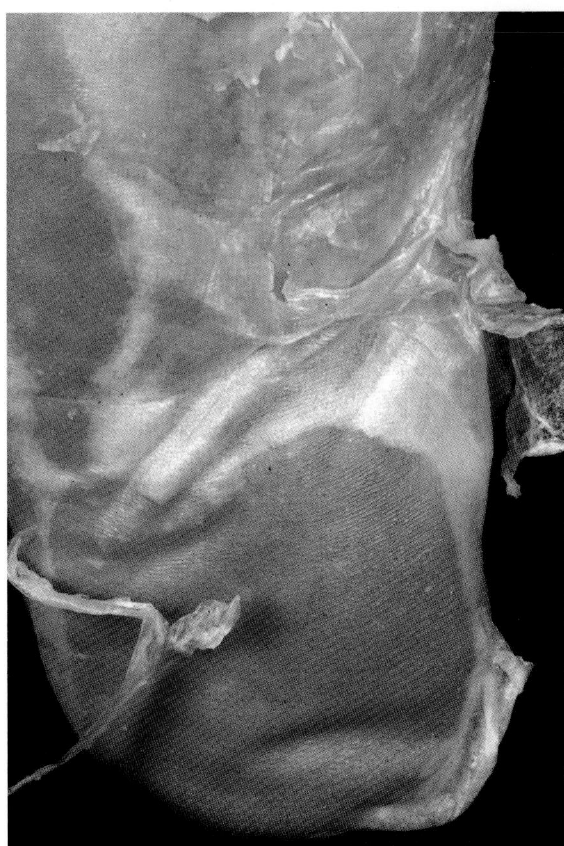

Figure 1.21 Desquamation following a severe drug reaction.

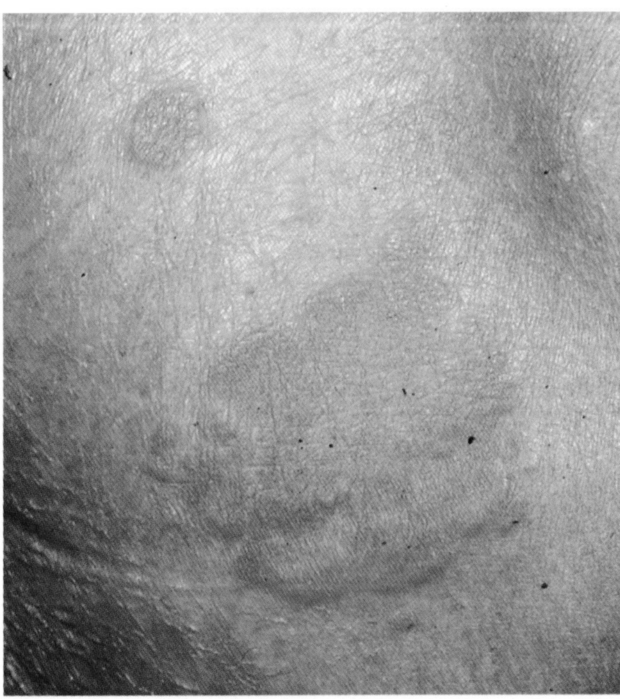

Figure 1.22 Annular (ring-shaped) lesions of granuloma annulare.

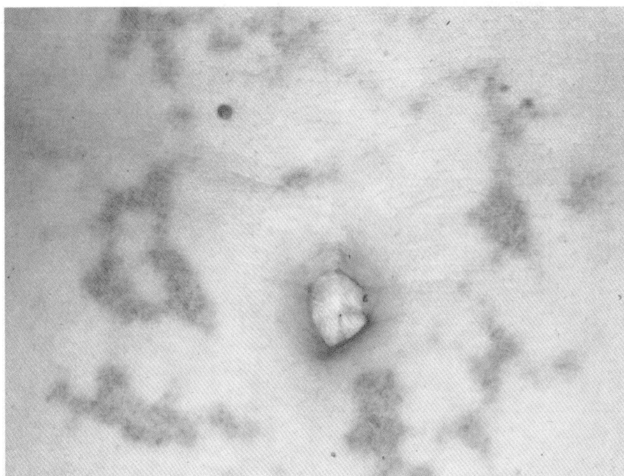

Figure 1.23 Reticulate pattern in vasculitis.

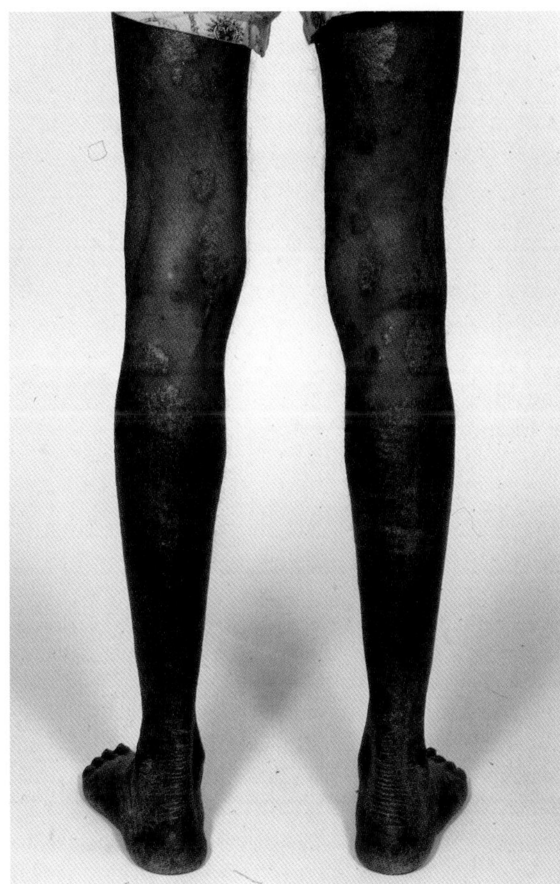

Figure 1.24 Symmetrical chronic plaque psoriasis.

Changes at the *skin surface* (epidermis) are characterized by a change in texture when the skin is palpated. Visually one may see scaling, thickening, increased skin markings, small vesicles, crusting, erosions or desquamation. In contrast, changes in the *deeper tissues* (dermis) can be associated with a normal overlying

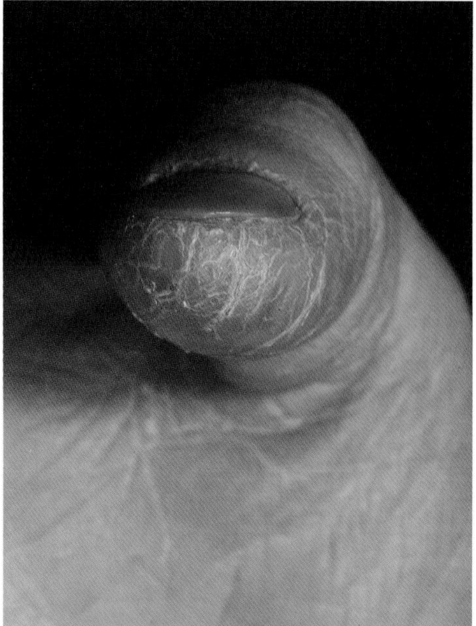

Figure 1.25 Irritant eczema on dominant hand of chef.

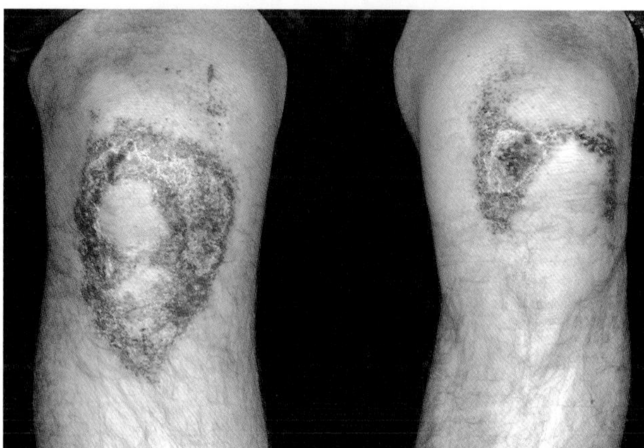

Figure 1.26 Bilateral contact dermatitis to cement.

skin. Examples of changes in the deeper tissues include erythema (dilated blood vessels, or inflammation), induration (an infiltrated firm area under the skin surface), ulceration (that involves surface and deeper tissues), hot tender skin (such as in cellulitis or abscess formation), changes in adnexal structures and adipose tissue.

The *margin* or border of some lesions is very well defined, as in psoriasis or lichen planus, but in eczema it is ill-defined and merges into normal skin.

Blisters or vesicles occur as a result of

- oedema (fluid) between the epidermal cells (Figure 1.28)
- destruction/death of epidermal cells
- separation of the epidermis from the deeper tissues.

There may be more than one mechanism involved simultaneously.

Blisters or vesicles (Figures 1.29–1.33) occur in

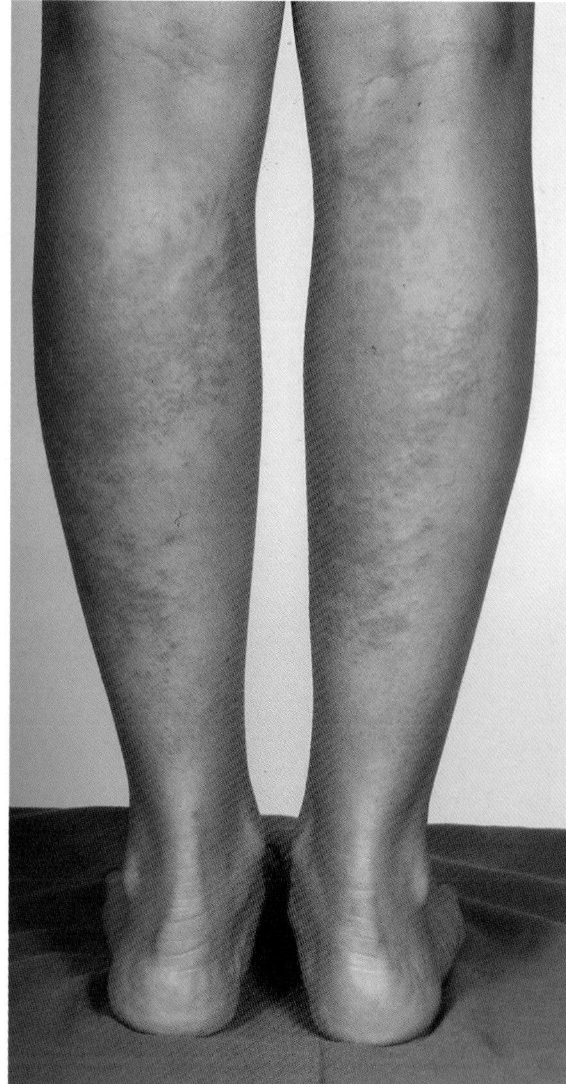

Figure 1.27 Polymorphous light eruption.

- *viral* diseases such as chicken pox, hand, foot and mouth disease, and herpes simplex
- *bacterial infections* such as impetigo or acute cellulitis
- *inflammatory disorders* such as eczema, contact dermatitis and insect bite reactions
- *immunological disorders* such as dermatitis herpetiformis, pemphigus and pemphigoid and erythema multiforme
- *metabolic disorders* such as porphyria.

Bullae (blisters more than 0.5 cm in diameter) may occur in congenital conditions (such as epidermolysis bullosa), in trauma and as a result of oedema without much inflammation. However, those forming as a result of vasculitis, sunburn or an allergic reaction may be associated with pronounced inflammation. Adverse reactions to medications can also result in a bullous eruption.

Induration is the thickening of the dermis due to infiltration of cells, granuloma formation or deposits of mucin, fat or amyloid.

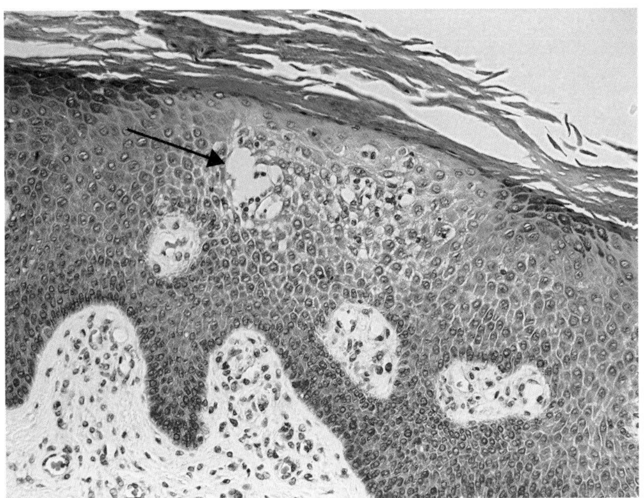

Figure 1.28 Eczema: intraepidermal vesicle (arrow).

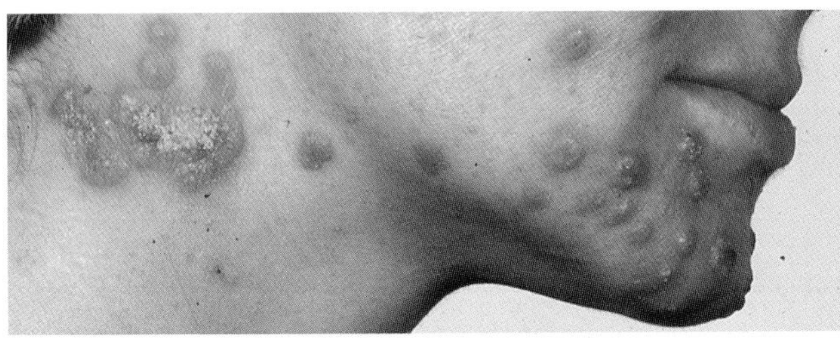

Figure 1.29 Vesicles and bullae in erythema multiforme.

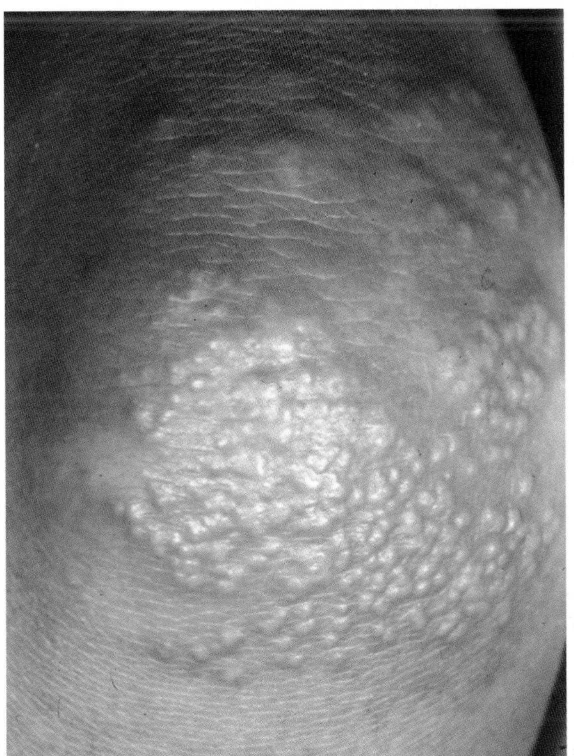

Figure 1.30 Vesicles in herpes simplex.

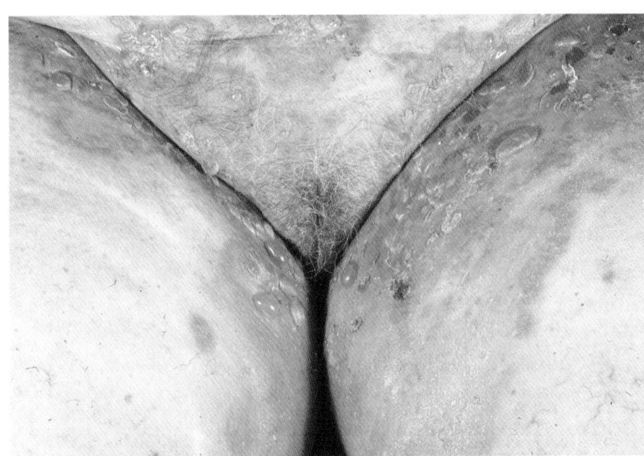

Figure 1.31 Vesicles and bullae in bullous pemphigoid.

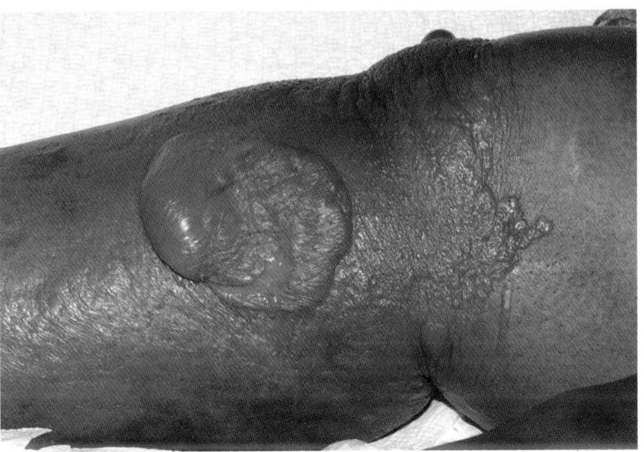

Figure 1.32 Bullae in cellulitis on lower leg.

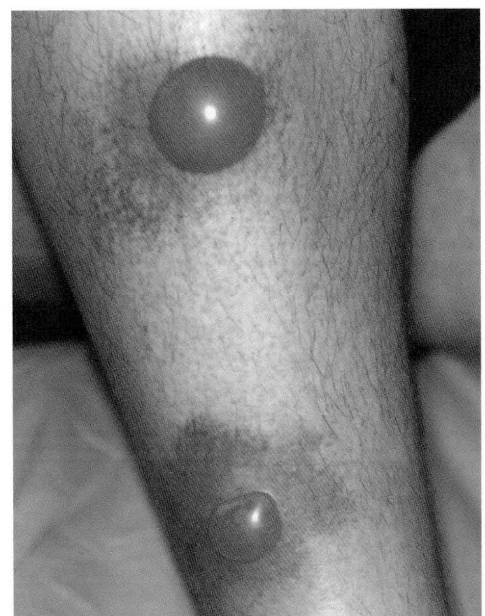

Figure 1.33 Bullae from insect bite reactions.

Inflammation is indicated by erythema, and can be acute or chronic. Acute inflammation can be associated with increased skin temperature such as occurs in cellulitis and erythema nodosum. Chronic inflammatory cell infiltrates occur in conditions such as lichen planus and lupus erythematosus.

Assessment of the patient

A full assessment should include not only the effect the skin condition has on the patients lives but also their attitude to it. For example, some patients with quite extensive psoriasis are unbothered whilst others with very mild localized disease just on the elbows may be very distressed. Management of the skin disease should take into account the patients' expectation as to what would be acceptable to them.

Fear that a skin condition may be due to cancer or infection is often present and reassurance should always be given to allay any hidden fears. If there is the possibility of a serious underlying disease that requires further investigation, then it is important to explain fully to the patient that the skin problems may be a sign of an internal disease.

The significance of occupational factors must be taken into account. In some cases, such as an allergy to hair dyes in a hairdresser, it may be impossible for the patient to continue his or her job. In other situations, the allergen can be easily avoided.

Patients often want to know why they have developed a particular skin problem and whether it can be cured. In many skin diseases these questions are difficult to answer. Patients with psoriasis, for example, can be told that it is part of their inherent constitution but that additional factors can trigger clinical lesions (Figure 1.34). Known trigger factors for psoriasis include emotional stress, local trauma to the skin (Koebner's phenomenon), infection (guttate psoriasis) and drugs (β-blockers, lithium, antimalarials).

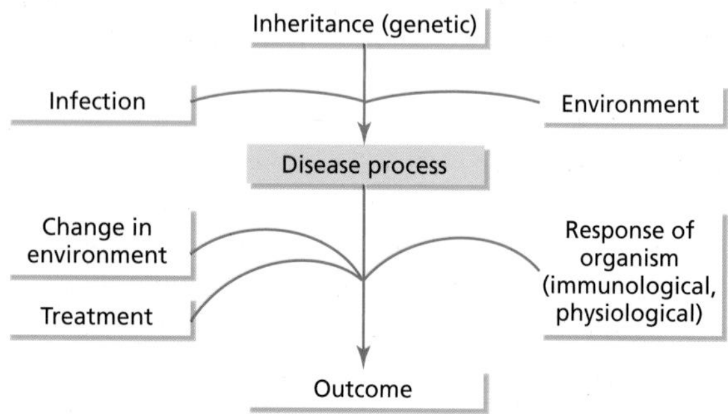

Figure 1.34 Possible precipitating factors in psoriasis.

Skill in recognition of skin conditions will evolve and develop with increased clinical experience. Seeing and feeling skin rashes 'in the flesh' is the best way to improve clinical dermatological acumen (Box 1.2).

> Box 1.2 **Examination of skin lesions – key points**
>
> *Distribution*
>
> Examine all the skin for clues. For example, there are many possible causes for dry thickened skin on the palms, and finding typical psoriasis on the elbows, knees, and soles may give the diagnosis.
>
> *Morphology*
>
> Are the lesions dermal or epidermal? Macular (flat) or forming papules? Indurated or forming plaques? Well defined or indistinct? Forming crusts, scabs or vesicles?
>
> *Pattern*
>
> The overall morphology and distribution of the rash – for example, an indeterminate rash may be revealed as pityriasis rosea when the 'herald patch' is found.

Further Reading

Graham-Brown R and Burns T. *Lecture Notes: Dermatology*, 10th Edition, Wiley Blackwell, New York, 2011.

Wolff K and WolffJohnson RA. *Fitzpatrick's Colour Atlas and Clinical Synopsis of Dermatology*, 6th Edition, McGraw-Hill Medical, Oxford, 2009.

CHAPTER 2

Psoriasis

Rachael Morris-Jones

Dermatology Department, Kings College Hospital, London, UK

> **OVERVIEW**
> - Psoriasis is a chronic inflammatory condition of the skin thought to be autoimmune mediated.
> - Psoriasis has been shown to be an independent risk factor for cardiovascular disease.
> - Specific biological therapies are transforming the management of psoriasis and psoriatic arthropathy.
> - Clinical presentations can be variable from chronic stable plaques, to pustules on the hands and feet, to unstable erythroderma.

Psoriasis is now considered to be a genetically determined inflammatory systemic autoimmune disease. It is characterised by plaques of diseased skin often at sites of minor trauma (elbows/knees), which occur next to areas of clear 'normal' skin. Plaques of psoriasis are clinically well-demarcated and are erythematous (dilated dermal blood vessels) with white surface scale (rapid keratinocyte proliferation). Psoriasis not only affects the skin but can also lead to seronegative arthritis in approximately 8–30% of patients. However, there is an increasing body of evidence that psoriasis is also associated with other important comorbidities such as type 2 diabetes (1.4-fold increased risk), cardiovascular disease, metabolic syndrome, obesity, depression and reduced quality of life.

The pathogenesis of psoriasis is complex; nonetheless, it is largely accepted that the disease is mediated by the dysregulation of T-helper lymphocytes (Th1/Th17). The development of psoriasis is multifactorial, with multiple potential susceptibility factors in a genetically at-risk individual. This combination of susceptibility factors and genetic predisposition results in an interactive web of immune cells/chemical cytokines impacting on skin cells and leading to disease. Increased understanding of these complex cellular changes has led to the introduction of multiple targeted biological therapies that are now used to manage severe psoriasis and psoriatic arthritis (PA).

Globally 1–2% of the population is affected by psoriasis (125 million people in UK/USA/Japan alone). A child who has one parent with psoriasis has a 1 in 4 chance of developing the disease. If one identical twin has psoriasis, there is a 70% chance that the other will also be affected; however, only a 20% chance exists in dizygotic twins. Linkage and genome-wide association studies have started identifying some of the important susceptibility factors leading to the inheritance of psoriasis and psoriatic arthropathy. The first and arguably one of the most important psoriasis susceptibility loci identified is the so-called *PSORS1* found on chromosome 6p21.3. This region of the chromosome contains several genes which may be important in the inheritance of psoriasis including HLA-C (human leukocyte antigen-C), CCHCR1 (coiled-coil α-helical rod protein 1) and CDSN (corneodesmosin). Subsequently, multiple susceptibility loci on several chromosomes have now been identified including 1q21, 3q21, 4q, 7p, 8, 11, 16q, 17q, and 20p. Recently, a loss of function mutation in a gene encoding an IL-36 receptor antagonist has been shown to be associated with the development of palmo-plantar pustular psoriasis.

Plaques of psoriasis are highly infiltrated with CD3+ T-cells and CD11c+ dendritic cells which produce pro-inflammatory cytokines including tumour necrosis factor alpha (TNF-α), interferon gamma (INF-γ) and interleukin 17 (IL-17), IL-22/23/12/1β, which activate keratinocytes and other skin cells. Keratinocytes are the skin cells that predominate in the epidermis; they grow from the basal layer and slowly migrate to the surface (Figures 2.1 and 2.2). In normal skin, this process of cell turnover takes about 23 days; however, in psoriasis cell turnover is rapidly accelerated, taking only 3–5 days for cells to reach the surface and accumulate in large numbers (hyperkeratosis). Keratinocytes normally lose their nuclei as they move to the skin surface; however, in psoriasis they move so quickly that the cells retain their nuclei throughout the epidermis, seen as parakeratosis histologically. This rapid turnover and failure of proper maturation result in defective keratinocytes, which are poorly adherent and easily scraped off ('Auspitz sign') revealing underlying dilated blood vessels.

In addition, inflammatory polymorphs infiltrating the epidermis lead to swelling (oedema), inflammation and erythema. These inflammatory cells may occur in such large numbers that they form collections of sterile pustules at the skin surface. These are most commonly seen in palmo-plantar pustulosis, a variant of psoriasis affecting the palms and soles.

The cellular abnormalities in the skin of patients with psoriasis can occur in the nails, and many patients will therefore have additional nail changes.

ABC of Dermatology, Sixth Edition. Edited by Rachael Morris-Jones.

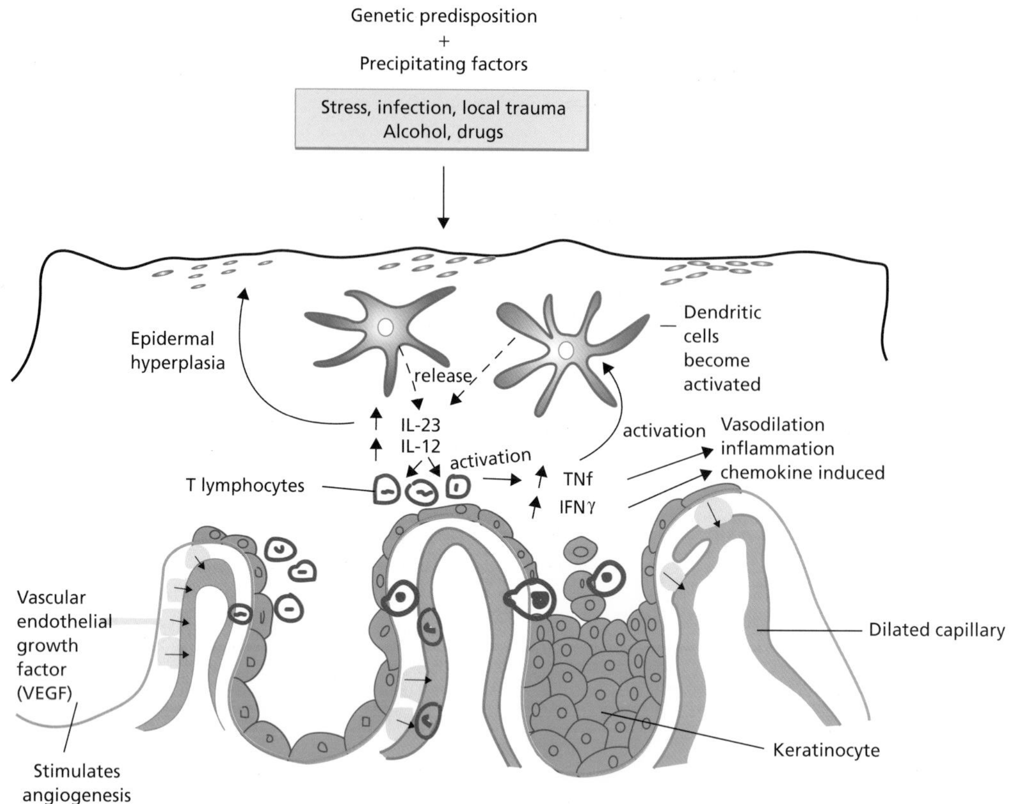

Figure 2.1 Pathophysiological mechanisms involved in the development of psoriasis.

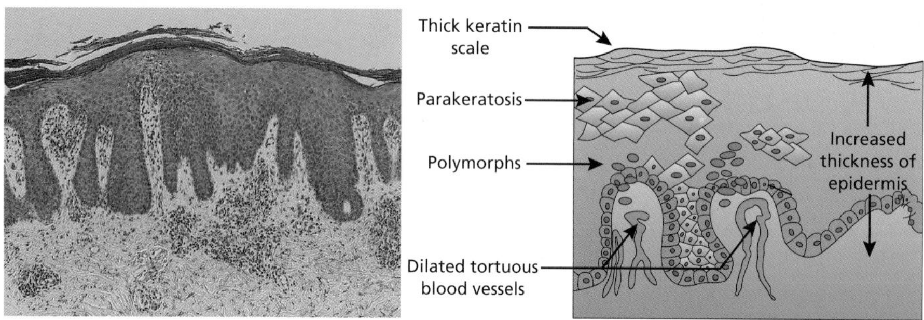

Figure 2.2 (diagram/histology composite) Increased epidermal proliferation.

Psoriatic nail dystrophy is characterised by

- *onycholysis* (lifting of the nail plate off the nail bed) due to abnormal cell adhesion; this usually manifests as a white or salmon patch on the nail plate (Figure 2.3 pitting and onycholysis of nails);
- *subungal hyperkeratosis* (accumulation of chalky looking material under the nail) due to excessive proliferation of the nail bed that can ultimately lead to onycholysis;
- *pitting* (very small depressions in the nail plate) which result from parakeratotic (nucleated) cells being lost from the nail surface;
- *Beau's lines* (transverse lines on the nail plate) due to intermittent inflammation of the nail bed leading to transient arrest in nail growth;
- *splinter haemorrhages* (which clinically look like minute longitudinal black lines) due to leakage of blood from dilated tortuous capillaries.

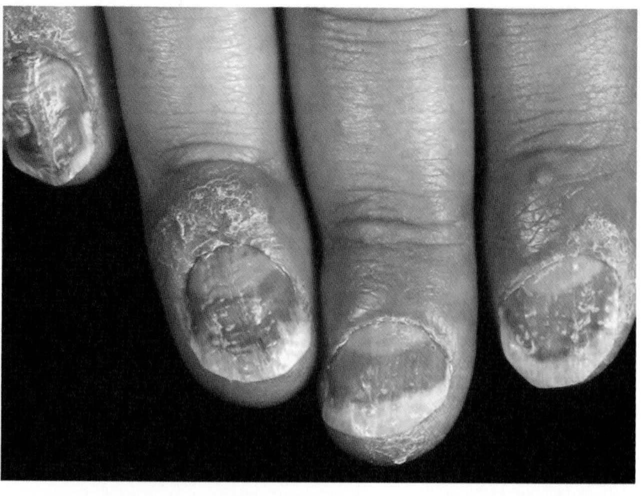

Figure 2.3 Pitting and onycholysis of the nails.

Clinical appearance

The main clinical features of psoriasis reflect the underlying pathological processes (as described above). Patients characteristically have the following:

Plaques which are well-defined raised areas of psoriasis. These may be large or small, few or numerous and scattered over the trunk and limbs (Figures 2.4 and 2.5).

Scaling may be very prominent causing plaques to appear thickened with masses of adherent and shedding white scales. Scratching the surface produces a waxy appearance – the 'tache de bougie' (literally 'a line of candle wax').

Erythema or redness of the affected skin may be very marked especially in the flexures. Erythema is a prominent feature in patients with erythrodermic psoriasis (who have >90% of their body surface involved).

Pustules are commonly seen in *palmo-plantar pustulosis* where deep-seated yellowish sterile pustules are often the dominant feature of this chronic condition. However, if pustules develop around the periphery of chronic plaques of psoriasis or sheets of monomorphic pustules appear more generally in the context of psoriasis, this is a sign of unstable disease – a dermatological emergency.

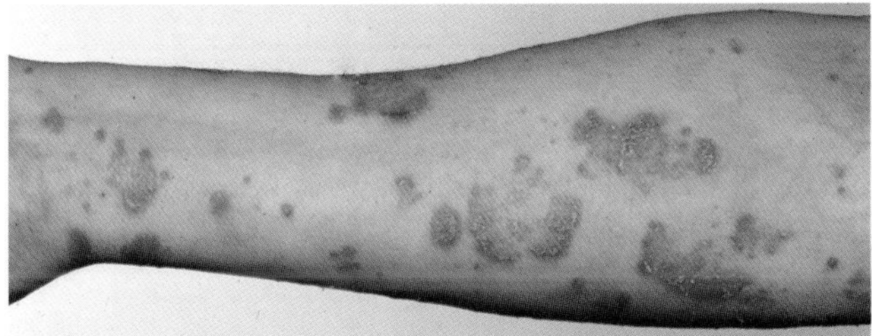

Figure 2.4 Multiple small plaques.

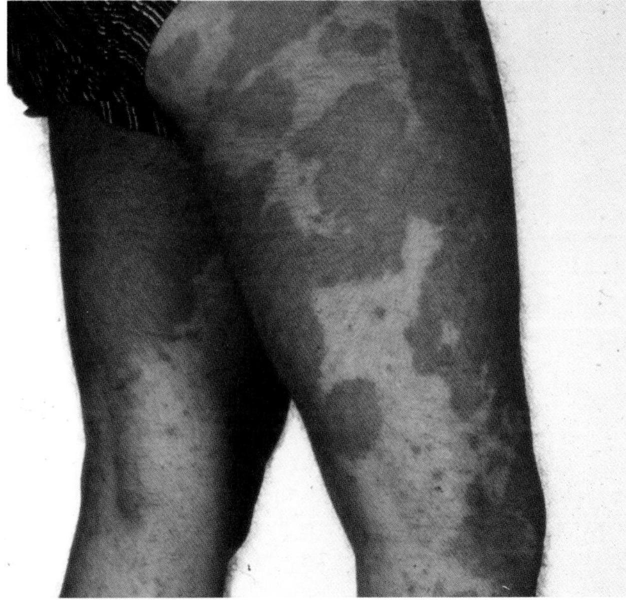

Figure 2.5 Large chronic plaques.

The typical patient

Psoriasis is reported to affect approximately 2% of the US population. The median age of onset is 28 years however it can present from infancy to old age, when the appearance may be atypical.

The following factors in the history may help in making a diagnosis:

- Family history of psoriasis. 16% of the children will have psoriasis if a single parent is affected and 50% if both parents are affected.
- Trigger factors include stress, infections, trauma, or childbirth.
- Lesions may first appear at sites of minor skin trauma – Koebner's phenomenon.
- Lesions usually improve in the sun.
- Psoriasis is usually only mildly itchy.
- Arthropathy may be associated.

Clinical presentation

Classically psoriasis patients present with plaques on the elbows, knees and scalp (Figure 2.6). Lesions on the trunk are variable in size and are often annular (Figure 2.7–2.9). Psoriasis may develop in scars and areas of minor skin trauma – the so-called Koebner's phenomenon (Figure 2.10). This may manifest as hyperkeratosis on the palms, associated with repetitive trauma from manual labour (Figure 2.11). Scalp scaling which affects 50% of patients can be very thick, especially around the hairline, but may be more confluent forming a virtual 'skull cap' (Figure 2.12). Erythema often extends beyond the hair margin. The nails show 'pits' and also thickening with separation of the nail from the nail bed (onycholysis) (Figure 2.13).

Guttate psoriasis – from the Latin *gutta*, a drop – consists of widespread small plaques scattered on the trunk and limbs (Figure 2.14). Adolescents are most commonly affected and there is often a preceding sore throat with associated group β-haemolytic streptococcus. There is frequently a family history of psoriasis. The sudden onset and widespread nature of guttate psoriasis can be very

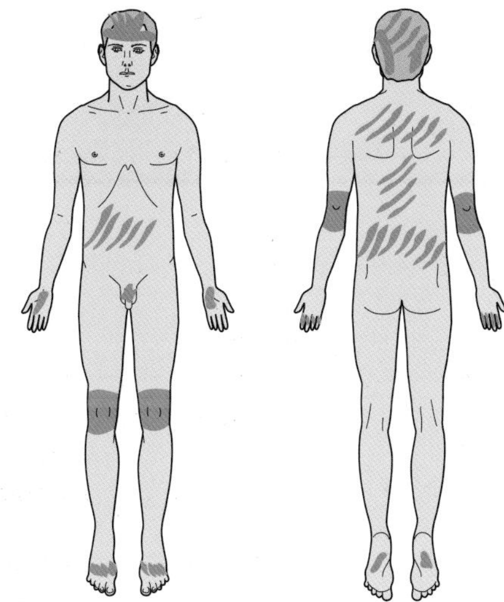

Figure 2.6 Common patterns of distribution of psoriasis.

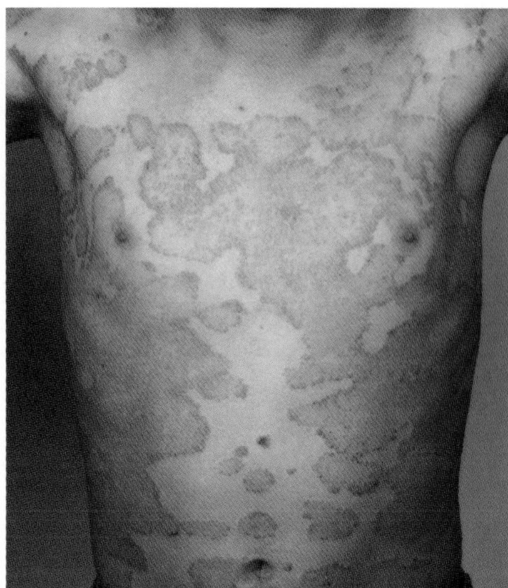

Figure 2.7 Generalised plaques.

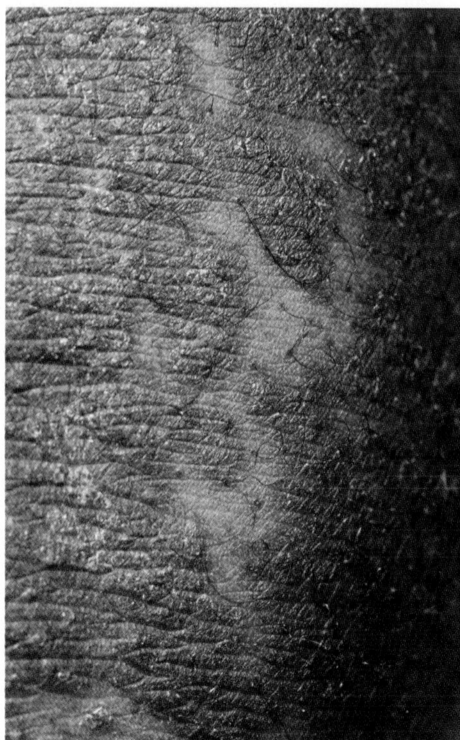

Figure 2.8 Psoriatic plaques on the trunk.

alarming for patients, fortunately it usually resolves completely, but can be recurrent or herald the onset of chronic plaque psoriasis.

Palmo-plantar pustular psoriasis (PPPP) is characterised by multiple sterile pustules on the palms and soles. Pustules first appear as yellowish monomorphic lesions that turn a brown colour with chronicity (Figure 2.15) and associated scaling. Most patients with PPPP are smokers.

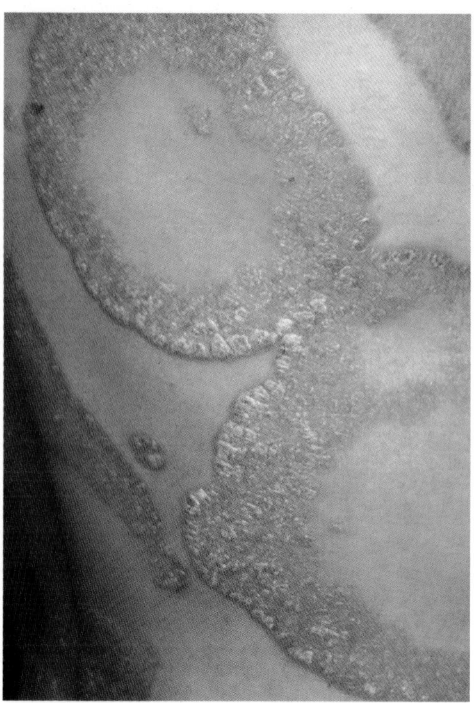

Figure 2.9 Annular plaques.

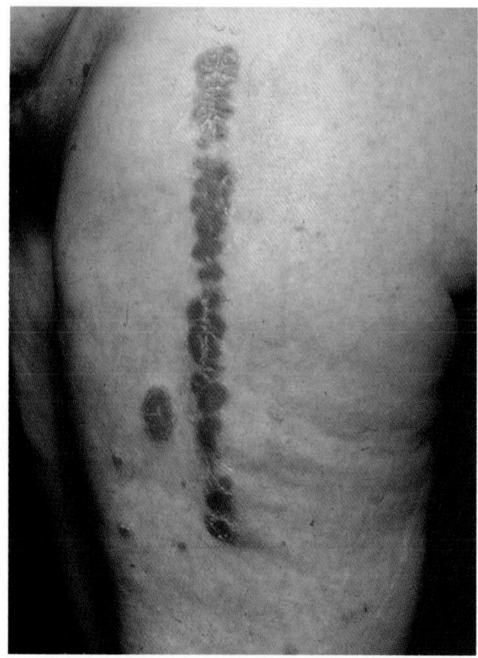

Figure 2.10 Koebner's phenomenon: psoriasis in surgical scar.

Acute generalised pustular psoriasis (Von zumbush) is thankfully uncommon as it is usually an indicator of severe and unstable psoriasis (Figure 2.16). Clinically the skin is erythematous and tender with sheets of monomorphic sterile pustules, which can develop over a few hours/days. It may be precipitated by the patient

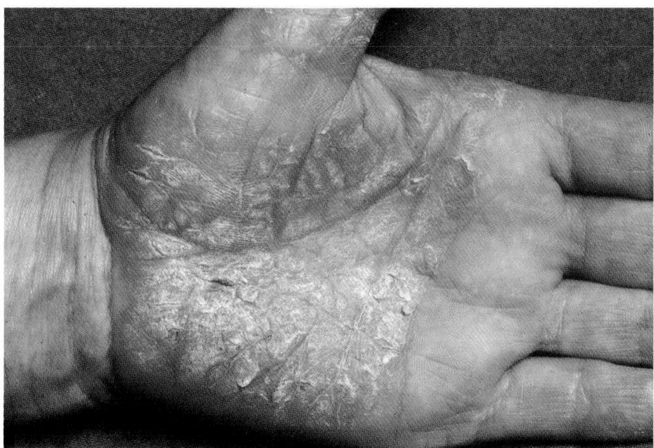

Figure 2.11 Hyperkeratotic palmar psoriasis.

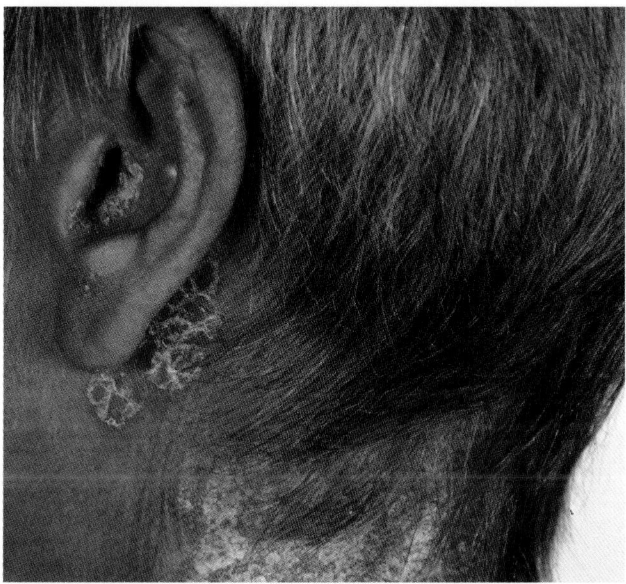

Figure 2.12 Scalp psoriasis.

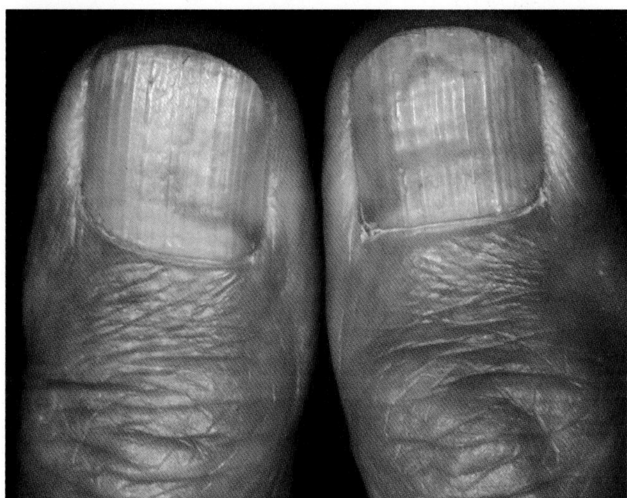

Figure 2.13 Onycholysis in nail psoriasis.

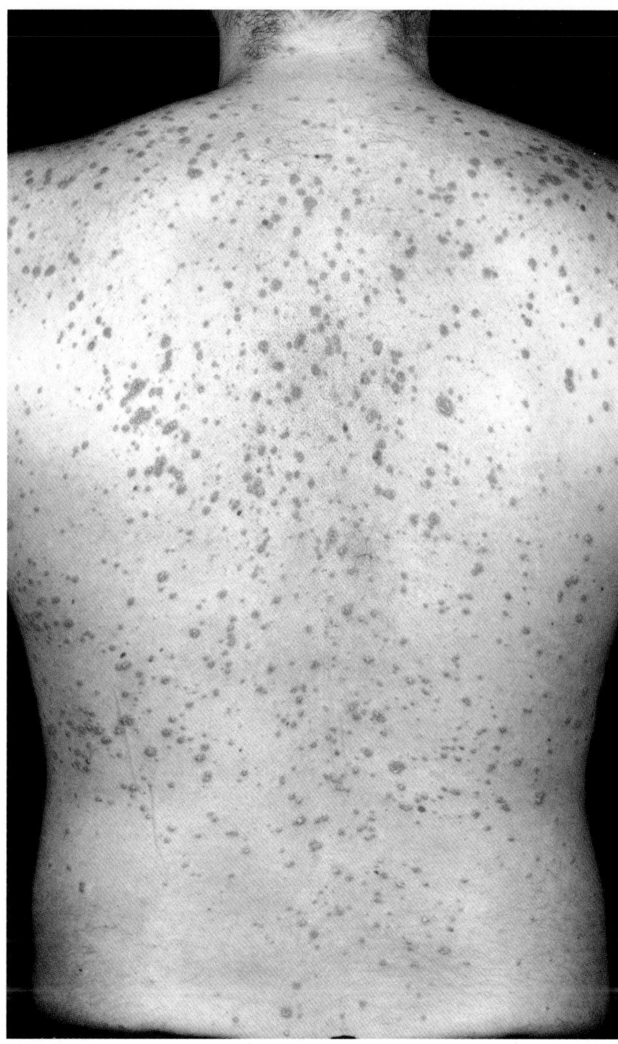

Figure 2.14 Guttate psoriasis.

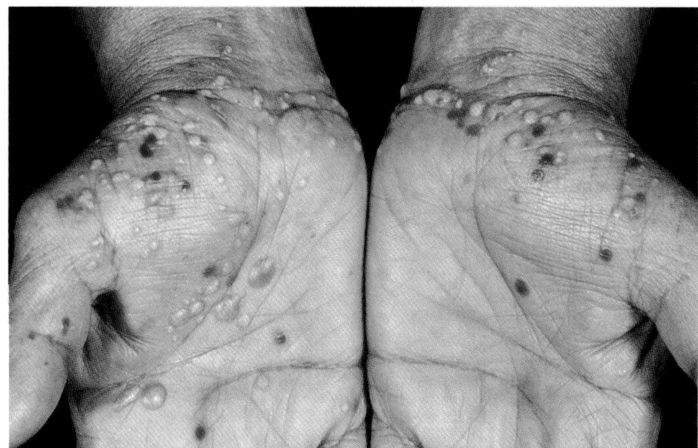

Figure 2.15 Palmar pustular psoriasis.

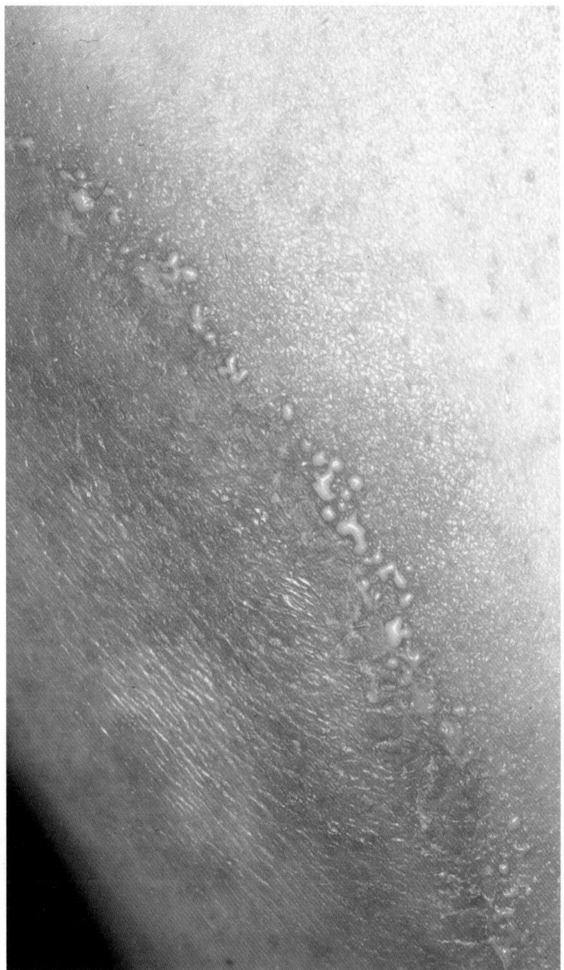

Figure 2.16 Acute unstable pustular psoriasis.

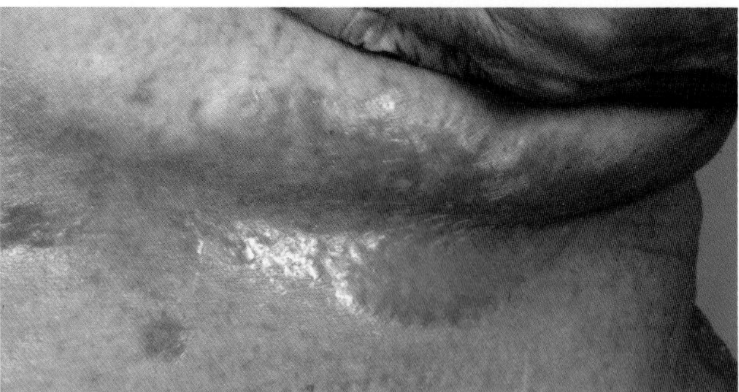

Figure 2.17 Flexural psoriasis.

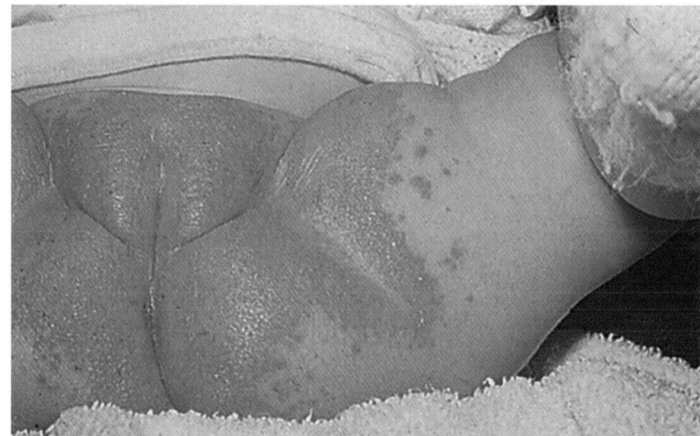

Figure 2.18 Napkin psoriasis.

taking systemic steroids, or using potent topical steroids. The pustules usually occur initially at the peripheral margin of plaques which are often sore and erythematous. Pustules eventually dry and the skin desquamates.

Acropustulosis is a rare variant of psoriasis that usually occurs in young children. Here pustules appear around the nails and the fingertips associated with brisk inflammation.

Flexural psoriasis produces well-defined erythematous areas in the axillae, groin, natal cleft, beneath the breasts and in skin folds. Scaling is minimal or absent (Figure 2.17). It should be distinguished from a fungal infection and if there is any doubt a specimen for mycology should be taken.

Napkin psoriasis in children may present with typical psoriatic lesions or a more diffuse erythematous eruption with exudative rather than scaling lesions (Figure 2.18).

Erythrodermic psoriasis is a serious, even life threatening condition with confluent erythema affecting nearly all of the skin (Figure 2.19). Diagnosis may not be easy as the characteristic scaling of psoriasis is absent. Chronic plaque psoriasis usually, but not always, precedes the erythroderma. Triggers for erythrodermic psoriasis include withdrawal of systemic steroids, infections, excessive alcohol intake, antimalarials, lithium and low calcium. Complications of erythrodermic psoriasis result from increased cutaneous blood flow and fluid loss, including heart failure, hypothermia, dehydration, low protein and consequent oedema, secondary infection and death. Patients should be managed in hospital under the care of a dermatology specialist.

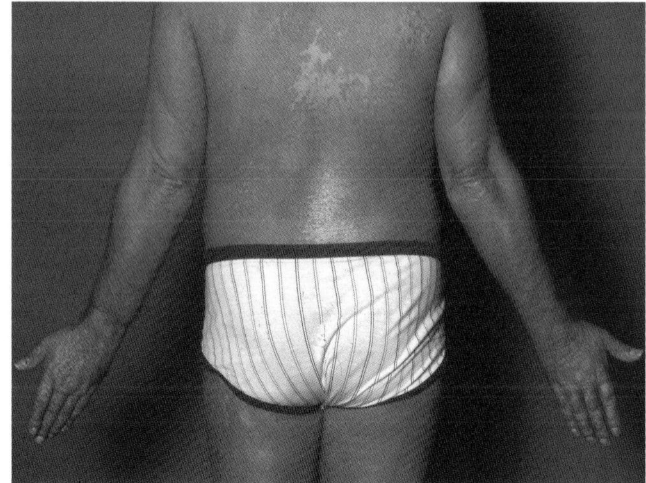

Figure 2.19 Erythrodermic psoriasis.

Psoriatic arthritis – pathophysiology

PA is thought to be an autoimmune joint disease with an inherited genetic predisposition plus immunological/environmental triggers. PA is primarily a disease involving activated CD8 T-memory cells. Genetic susceptibility loci identified as playing a role in PA include HLA-B7,-B27,-B17, -CW6, -DR4 and -DR7, and linkage studies point to the short arm of chromosome 6. Recent studies have shown that gene polymorphisms associated with TNF-α are also important in the development of PA. Immunological stimuli are thought to include complement activation and an increase in T-helper cell cytokine activity including TNF-α, IL-10 and IL-1β, which in turn stimulates increased fibroblast proliferation and activity in the synovium of affected joints. Environmental factors such as infections, super-antigens and trauma have also been associated with the onset of PA but the exact mechanisms are poorly understood. Examination of the affected joints at the cellular level shows an increase in tortuous blood vessels within the synovium, which is thought to result from over-expression of angiogenic growth factors (vascular endothelial growth factor (VEGF) and transforming growth factor beta (TGF-β)). Erosions and osteolysis result from osteoclast proliferation and activation which is triggered by cytokine activity.

Psoriatic arthritis – clinical presentation

Psoriatic arthropathy is reported to affect 5–10% of patients with psoriasis (Figure 2.20), and of these 40% have a family history of psoriasis. Seronegative arthritis in the context of psoriasis is thought to be human leukocyte antigen (HLA) linked. Characteristically, patients develop skin manifestations of psoriasis prior to joint involvement, but in 15% of patients this is reversed. There are five recognised patterns of arthropathy associated with psoriasis. The distal interphalangeal (DIP) joints are most commonly affected (metacarpophalangeal joints are spared), which helps distinguish PA from rheumatoid arthritis. The arthropathy is usually asymmetrical. The sex ratio is equal; however, there is male predominance in the spondylitic form and female predominance in the rheumatoid form. Arthritis mutilans is a rarer form where there is considerable bone resorption leading to 'telescoping' of the fingers. Radiological changes include a destructive arthropathy with deformity (Figure 2.21). Recent MRI imaging studies have shown that the joint inflammation in PA results from extensor tendon enthesitis (sites where tendons insert into bones) at the nail bed in DIP joint disease rather than intra-articular joint synovitis.

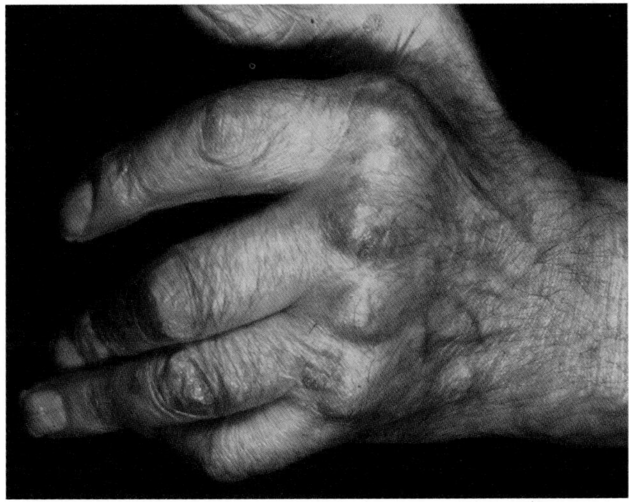

Figure 2.20 Chronic psoriatic arthropathy.

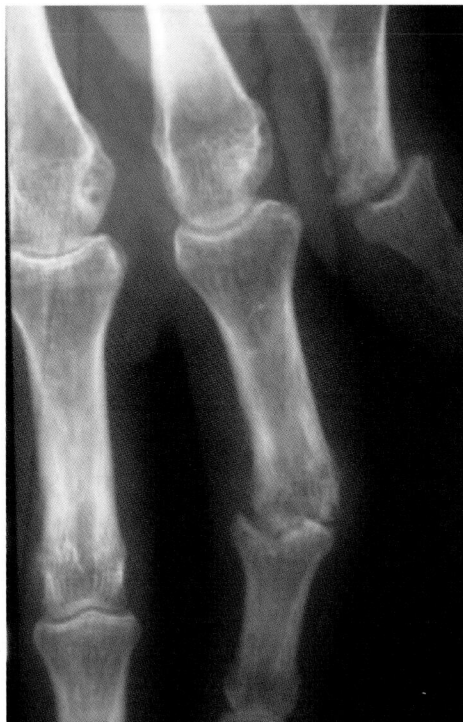

Figure 2.21 Acute arthropathy X-ray signs.

Psoriatic arthropathy usually waxes and wanes but can be severe enough to cause significant functional disabilities. Stiffness, pain and joint deformity are the most common manifestations.

Five types of psoriatic arthropathy:

- *DIP joints* (80% have associated nail changes)
- *Asymmetrical oligoarticular* arthropathy (hands and feet, 'sausage-shaped' digits)
- *Symmetrical polyarthritis* (hands, wrists, ankles, 'rheumatoid pattern')
- *Arthritis mutilans* (digits, resorption of bone, resultant 'telescoping' of redundant skin)
- *Spondylitis* (asymmetrical vertebral involvement, male preponderance) HLA-B27 associated

Further reading

www.bad.org.uk/heathcare/guidelines

Menter MA and Stoff B. *Psoriasis*, Manson Publishing Ltd, 2012.

Gordon KB and Ruderman EM. *Psoriasis and Psoriatic Arthritis – An Integrated Approach*, Springer, 2005.

CHAPTER 3

Management of Psoriasis

Rachael Morris-Jones

Dermatology Department, Kings College Hospital, London, UK

OVERVIEW

- Management of psoriasis is related not only to the severity of the disease but also to patient expectation.
- The treatment ladder starts with topical therapy, then phototherapy and finally systemic medication.
- New biological agents are transforming the management of patients with severe disease who have failed on conventional therapies.
- Encouraging patients to stop smoking, lose weight and reduce alcohol consumption are important to reduce their risk of cardiovascular disease associated with psoriasis.

An essential aspect of managing psoriasis is managing the patient's expectation of the disease and the outcome of any treatment offered. It is also important that medical practitioners understand on an individual level the impact the disease is having on a patient's life. Indeed, managing psoriasis is as much a challenge for patients as it is for medical practitioners. The appearance of the scaly plaques may cause social embarrassment; time needs to be set aside for the application of creams, and even if the skin is cleared recurrence is the rule. Assessing the impact of any skin disease on a patients' quality of life can be undertaken using the validated dermatology life quality index (DLQI) score based on a questionnaire. A more specific survey for psoriasis patients is the psoriasis disability index (PDI) which can also be used to assess the impact of the disease on the patients' life. The questionnaires embrace all aspects of life including work, personal relationships, domestic situation and recreational activities.

Patients often wish to know what has caused their psoriasis and are keen for a cure. However, our current understanding of psoriasis is that it is an inherited autoimmune disease that can be suppressed by current therapies rather than cured. Management comprises avoidance of known exacerbating factors (smoking, alcohol), using topical preparations, undertaking phototherapy or photochemotherapy and taking systemic therapy (tablet, S/C, IV). Selection of the most appropriate treatment for each patient should be tailored to the type of psoriasis, their age, comorbidities, social and occupational factors, their level of motivation, quality of life and patient acceptability. As a general rule, there is a treatment ladder that patients may climb as the disease becomes more severe or recalcitrant to treatments. Patients may start initially using simple topical therapy and/or ultraviolet treatment before switching to the stronger systemic agents if their disease is poorly controlled.

Management of psoriasis

Type of psoriasis	Standard therapy	Alternatives
Localised stable plaques	Tar preparations Vitamin D analogues Salicylic acid preparations Topical steroids	Dithranol/ ichthammol TL01 (UVB)
Extensive stable plaques	TL01 (UVB) PUVA Acitretin PUVA + Acitretin	Methotrexate Ciclosporin A Hydroxyurea Biological agents
Widespread small plaque	TL01 (UVB)	Steroid with LPC
Guttate psoriasis	Moderate-potency topical steroids TL01 (UVB)	Steroid with LPC
Facial psoriasis	Mild-moderate potency topical steroid	Steroid with LPC
Flexural psoriasis	Mild-moderate potency topical steroid + antifungal	Methotrexate
Pustular psoriasis of hands and feet	Moderate-potency topical steroids Potent topical steroid + propylene glycol +/− occlusion	Acitretin Methotrexate Hand and foot PUVA
Acute erythrodermic, unstable/ generalised pustular psoriasis	In-patient management Short-term mild topical steroids	Methotrexate Ciclosporin Biological therapy

Key: PUVA, psoralen with ultraviolet A; TL01, narrow band ultraviolet B; UVB broad band ultraviolet B; LPC, Liquor Picis Carbis.

ABC of Dermatology, Sixth Edition. Edited by Rachael Morris-Jones.

Dermatology Day Treatment Units

Dermatology day treatment units (DDTUs) facilitate the management of psoriasis, particularly in relation to topical therapy, phototherapy and administration of intravenous or subcutaneous injections. Benefits of the DDTU include compliance, monitoring, education, counselling/support and an overall reduction in the patients' stress levels. Treatments not possible at home including short-contact dithranol and crude coal tar that can be applied to psoriatic plaques by specialist nurses, phototherapy can be delivered in custom-built cabinets and regular administration of biological therapy can be given by specialist dermatology nurses. These units have helped reduce the number and frequency of in-patient admissions of patients with severe psoriasis.

Rationalisation of skincare services and a shift in the emphasis away from specialist units to primary care settings however mean DDTUs may become less commonly available and therefore less local and accessible for patients.

Topical treatment

Topical treatments are those applied directly to the skin surface, including ointments, creams, gels, tars, lotions, pastes and shampoo. The topical approach to therapy results in changes at and just below the skin surface (epidermis and dermis). Conventionally, topical medicaments are applied directly to the diseased skin only, in contrast to moisturisers (emollients), which are usually applied more freely. In general, combination therapy is more effective than monotherapy, and change of therapy is superior to continuous usage. The following are the *advantages* of topical treatments:

- local effects only
- self-application
- safe for long-term use
- relatively cheap.

The following are the *disadvantages* of topical treatments:

- time consuming in extensive disease
- poor compliance (insufficient amounts and frequency)
- messy and may affect clothing/bedding/hair
- no benefit for associated joint disease
- tachyphylaxis (become less effective with continuous use).

The majority of psoriasis patients with mild to moderate disease can be managed in the community by their general practitioner, with guidance from local GPwSIs (General Practitioners with a Special Interest) in dermatology. Patients with very extensive, recalcitrant or unstable psoriasis and associated severe arthritis are usually managed in specialist dermatology centres.

Emollients act as a barrier to cutaneous fluid loss, relieve itching and help replace water and lipids and therefore restore the barrier function of dry skin. Patients are able to purchase these over the counter, and personal preference and acceptability usually guide their choice. Regular application of emollients should be encouraged in all patients with dry/flaky skin.

Coal tar obtained by distillation of bituminous coal. Many coal tar preparations are available for purchase over the counter and include ointments, pastes, paints, soaps, solutions and shampoo. Coal tar is keratoplastic (normalises keratinocyte growth patterns), antipruritic (reduces itch) and antimicrobial. It can be used on stable chronic plaque psoriasis but will irritate acute, inflamed skin. Coal tar in combination with salicylic acid may be more effective for very thick plaques.

Ichthammol (ammonium bituminosulfonate) is a distillation of sulfur-rich oil shale. It has anti-inflammatory properties and is therefore suitable to be used on 'unstable' or inflamed psoriasis. Various preparations can be purchased over the counter including ichthammol ointment.

Dithranol (anthralin, Goa powder), originally derived from araroba trees, is now produced synthetically. Irritation and burning can occur if it comes into contact with normal skin; therefore, careful application to psoriatic plaques is needed (Figure 3.1). Normal skin can be protected with petroleum. Dithranol temporarily stains the skin/hair a purple-brown colour. Short/long contact dithranol can be applied by dermatology nurses to chronic stable plaques in specialist units. Dithranol creams can be applied by the patients themselves, left on for 30 min and then washed off. The strength is gradually increased from 0.1% to 3% as necessary. Strengths up to 1% can be purchased over the counter, whereas higher concentrations are available by prescription only.

Calcipotriol and *tacalcitol*, vitamin D analogues, are calmodulin inhibitors used topically for mild or moderate plaque psoriasis. Mild

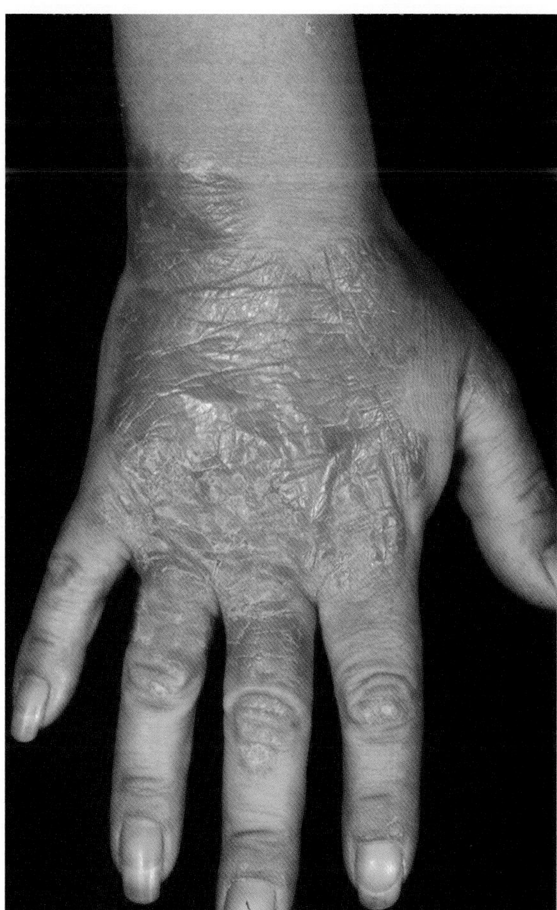

Figure 3.1 Psoriasis suitable for topical dithranol treatment.

irritation can be experienced and after continuous use, a plateau effect may be encountered with the treatment becoming less effective after an initial response. These preparations are therefore best used in combination with other topical agents. It is important not to exceed the maximum recommended dose as there is a risk of altering calcium metabolism.

Corticosteroids in topical formulations are an important adjuvant to the management of patients with psoriasis; these are prescription-only preparations (except very mild steroids) and can be supervised by the general medical practitioner. Corticosteroids help reduce the superficial inflammation within the plaques. However, relapse usually occurs on cessation and tachyphylaxis is observed. Tachyphylaxis is thought to result from tolerance to the vasoconstrictive action of corticosteroids on cutaneous capillaries. Topical steroids should be applied to the affected areas of skin only once or twice daily. Manufacturers suggest topical steroids should be applied sparingly but this is difficult for patients to quantify; therefore, practitioners advise the use of finger tip units (FTUs) as a guide. When the steroid ointment/cream is squeezed out from a tube, it comes out in a line, and the quantity between the finger tip and the first skin crease is 1 FTU (approximately 500 mg) enough to cover a hand-sized area of skin (back and front of the hand).

The strength of topical steroids is graded from mild to very potent. Prolonged use of very potent topical steroids should generally be avoided in the treatment of chronic skin diseases such as psoriasis. Mild/moderate topical steroids are safe to use on the face and flexural skin, and in erythrodermic disease. Moderate or potent preparations can be used on chronic stable plaques on the body. Combination products seem to be among the most effective in the treatment of psoriasis, especially those containing salicylic acid, vitamin D, tar and antibiotics. Systemic corticosteroids should not be used to treat psoriasis.

Scalp psoriasis

Scalp psoriasis affects approximately 50% of patients; it can be one of the earliest skin sites affected. Scalp psoriasis is often difficult to treat because of the thick nature of the scales, inaccessibility of the skin (owing to hair getting in the way) and the difficulty of self-application of treatment (Figure 3.2). Most patients need to treat the scalp regularly. Initially, products are rubbed into the affected scalp skin and left on overnight (combinations of tar, salicylic acid, sulphur and emollient are used), and then washed out with tar-based shampoos; then steroid/salicylic acid/vitamin D-containing scalp applications/gels are applied to the underlying inflamed skin. This sequential and combination approach to scalp treatment is often successful if maintained. Treatment in the DDTU can be immensely helpful in the management of difficult scalp psoriasis for patients who find it difficult to undertake this treatment themselves at home.

Ultraviolet treatment – phototherapy and photochemotherapy

The mechanisms of action of phototherapy are complex. Evidence suggests that phototherapy reduces the antigen-presenting capacity of dendritic cells, induces apoptosis of immune cells and inhibits synthesis and release of pro-inflammatory cytokines. The resultant cutaneous effects are those of topical immunosuppression and a reduction in dermal inflammation and epidermal cell turnover.

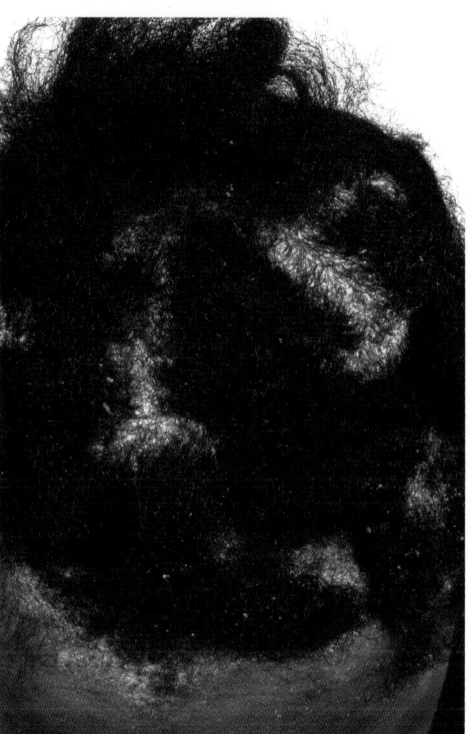

Figure 3.2 Scalp psoriasis.

Phototherapy and photochemotherapy should be delivered in specialist dermatology units. It is suitable for psoriasis patients with extensive disease that has not cleared with topical therapy (Figure 3.3). Patients must be able to attend the phototherapy suite 2–3 times weekly on a regular basis for approximately 6–8 weeks. Contraindications to treatment include a history of previous skin malignancy and photosensitive diseases such as lupus, porphyria, albinism and xeroderma pigmentosum. A full drug history should be taken to ascertain whether the patient is taking any photosensitising medication.

Phototherapy is usually delivered in vertical irradiation units (Figure 3.4). The dose and time of exposure to light is gradually increased as the treatment progresses. Patients apply a layer of emollient to their skin before standing inside the cabinet (this helps remove surface scale and aids UV penetration), they wear UV protective goggles (to protect against corneal keratitis and cataract formation) and 'sanctuary sites' (genitals) are covered.

There is an increased risk of developing cutaneous malignancies with increasing cumulative doses of phototherapy. How much phototherapy can be given safely will depend on the patient's skin type and cumulative dose of UV received. In addition to the increased risk of cutaneous malignancy, premature ageing of the skin and multiple lentigenes can result.

Current estimates suggest that patients can be given approximately 200 individual treatments (<1000 Joules) of light safely within their lifetime. Consequently, an individual patient's light

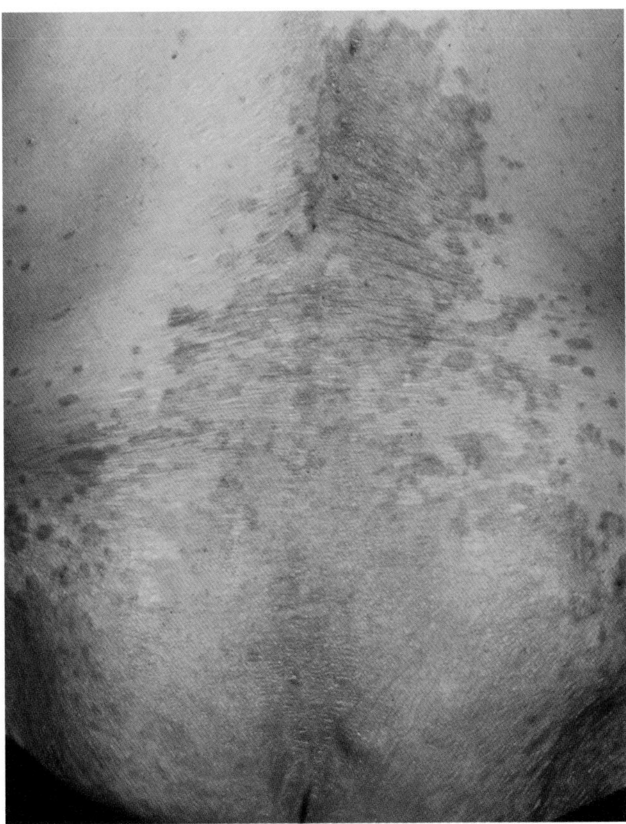

Figure 3.3 Thin plaques of psoriasis suitable for TL01.

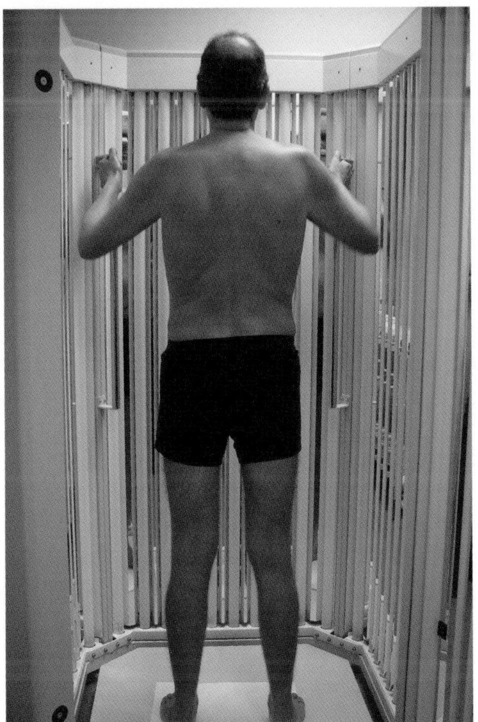

Figure 3.4 Psoralen with ultraviolet A (PUVA) cabinet.

'quota' can soon be used up with a standard course comprising 20–30 treatments (Figures 3.5 and 3.6). Maintenance treatment with phototherapy is no longer recommended and is rarely given for psoriasis. The total cumulative dosage is carefully monitored and kept as low as possible to reduce the risk of side effects.

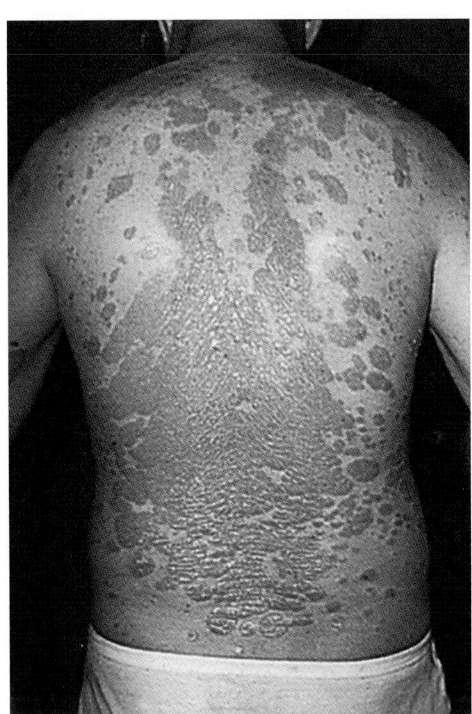

Figure 3.5 Psoriasis before phototherapy.

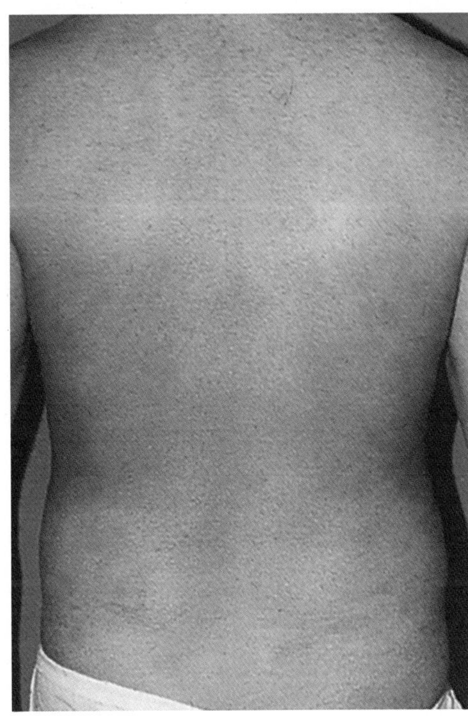

Figure 3.6 Skin after phototherapy.

Two main types of phototherapy are currently available, broadband ultraviolet B (UVB) and narrowband ultraviolet B (TL01) and photochemotherapy ultraviolet A plus psoralen (PUVA). UVB phototherapy has advantages over PUVA as it can be used in children, during pregnancy and does not require the wearing of UV-blocking glasses post-treatment.

Ultraviolet B (UVB)

UVB is short wavelength ultraviolet light and is administered three times weekly, (20–30 treatments) for widespread psoriasis. Conventional broadband UVB lamps emit wavelengths from 280–330 nm; these machines are largely being superseded by TL01 devices which emit ultraviolet light at 311 nm. TL01 is more effective than broadband UVB and there is a reduced risk of burning. The starting dose and subsequent increments (mJ/cm^2) for patients are based either on measuring the MED (minimal erythema dose), which is the dose of UVB just sufficient to cause erythema (the patients starting dose will then commence at 70% of the MED for psoriasis). Alternatively, the patient's skin phototype (I–VI) can be used to guide the starting dose. The patient's phototype reflects the skin's tolerance to sunlight, (type I – very fair skin through to type VI – black skin). UVB can be given in combination with tar (Goeckerman regimen) or dithranol (Ingram regimen) for chronic thick plaques of psoriasis. UVB in combination with oral acitretin can also increase the efficacy.

Ultraviolet A (UVA)

UVA is long wavelength ultraviolet light (320–400 nm) and is given in combination with oral or topical psoralen (PUVA) twice weekly (20–30 treatments) for recalcitrant widespread thick plaque psoriasis. There are two types of psoralen tablets: 8-methoxypsoralen (8MOP) 0.6 mg/kg body weight and 5-methoxypsoralen (5MOP) 1.2 mg/kg taken 2 h before treatment. 8-MOP is associated with a higher incidence of side effects such as nausea, vomiting, pruritus and erythema and is consequently less commonly used than 5MOP. The MPD (minimum phototoxic dose) or skin phototype is used to determine the starting dose of UVA and the subsequent increments used (J/cm^2). Protective goggles are worn during UVA exposure and sunglasses for 24 h post oral psoralen ingestion. Localised PUVA can be given to palmo-plantar psoriasis (Figure 3.7).

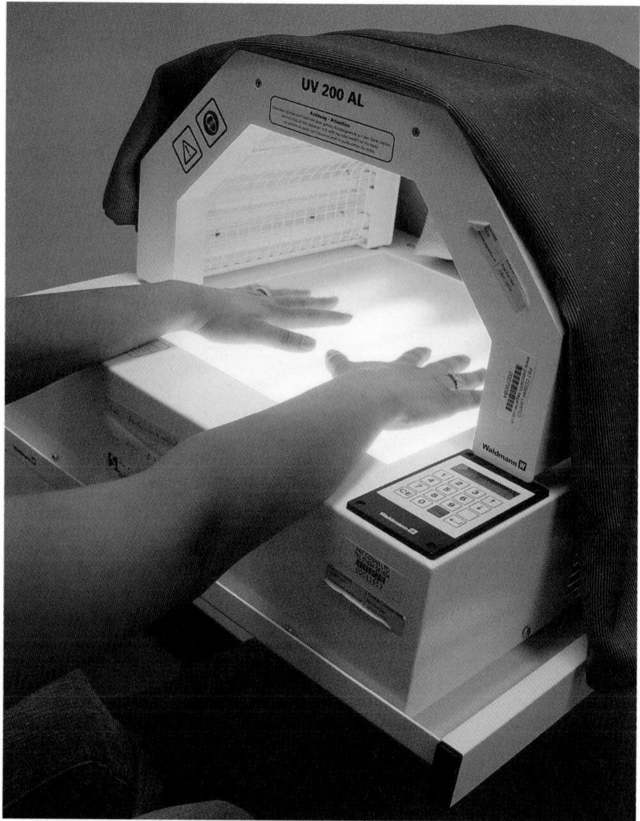

(a)

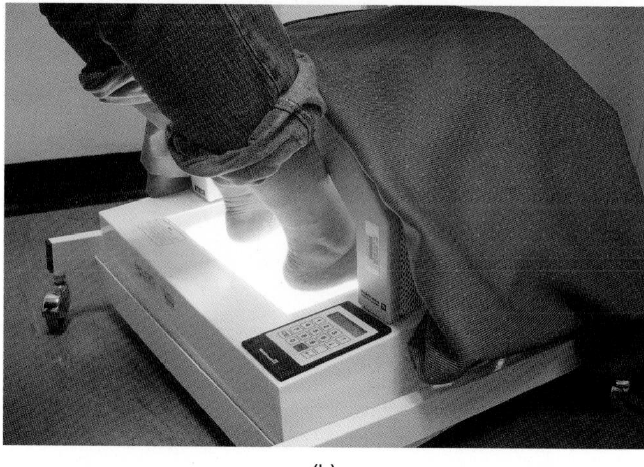

(b)

Figure 3.7 (a, b) Hand and foot PUVA.

Systemic treatment

Systemic therapy for severe psoriasis should ideally be managed by experienced specialist dermatologists. Candidates for systemic therapy include patients with unstable inflamed psoriasis, those with widespread disease (Figure 3.8) that have failed to respond to topical/phototherapy regimens and concomitant psoriatic arthropathy. The first-line systemic agents in most dermatology centres are acitretin, ciclosporin and methotrexate. Alternatives include hydroxyurea, azathioprine and mycophenolate mofetil (MMF). Biological therapies (infliximab, etanercept, ustekinumab and adalimumab) can be considered if patients have failed to respond to first-line agents or suffered side effects precluding the continued use of at least two systemic agents.

Methotrexate

Methotrexate is suitable to treat unstable erythrodermic/pustular psoriasis in the acute setting as well as maintenance for chronic plaque disease and psoriatic arthritis. Methotrexate reduces epidermal cell turnover by the inhibition of folic acid synthesis during the S phase of mitosis. Methotrexate is given once weekly as a tablet or injection. Conventionally, patients are given low doses initially that gradually increase until the psoriasis is 'sufficiently controlled' rather than cleared. Maintenance doses of 7.5–20 mg weekly are usually adequate.

Adverse effects – Methotrexate is hepatotoxic; therefore, liver function tests must be done prior to and during therapy. Routine liver biopsies for monitoring potential liver fibrosis are no longer indicated. Over the past decade, most dermatologists have measured patient's baseline and ongoing serum levels of procollagen III (an indirect marker of liver fibrosis), and if these are persistently

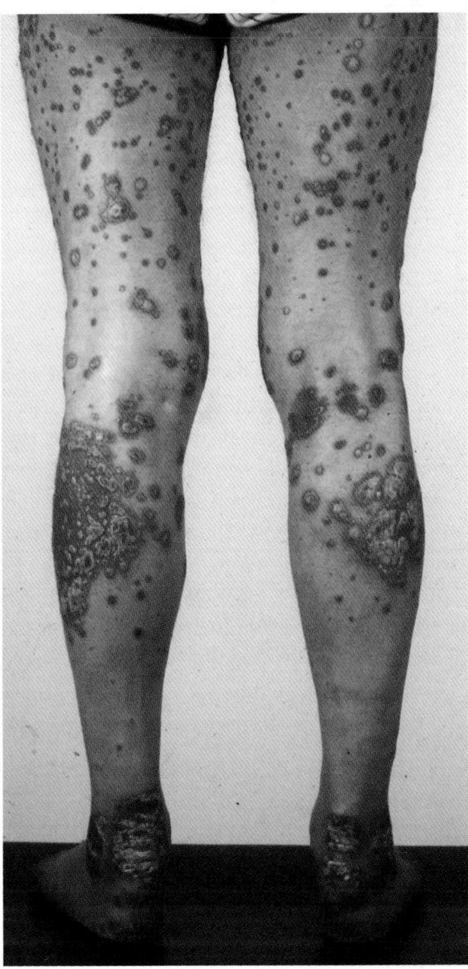

Figure 3.8 Severe psoriasis suitable for systemic therapy.

raised then a liver biopsy may be considered. This approach is however being superseded by a non-invasive transient elastography (FibroScan®) of the liver which assesses hepatic stiffness and hence the degree of liver fibrosis. Good correlation has been shown between liver function tests, liver biopsy and FibroScan results in patients taking methotrexate for monitoring purposes. It is likely that FibroScan will become more widely available and used routinely in the future.

Myelosuppression can occur in patients taking methotrexate, and its onset may be rapid or insidious. Patients should be monitored with regular full blood counts (FBCs). An initial test dose of 5 mg should be given on commencement of methotrexate followed by a FBC 1 week later to ensure there is no idiosyncratic marrow suppression. Folic acid supplements should be given (at least 5 mg weekly, taken on a different day to the methotrexate). Methotrexate is excreted in the urine; therefore, the dose must be reduced in renal impairment. Aspirin and sulphonamides diminish plasma binding. Interactions occur with several drugs including barbiturates, phenytoin, oral contraceptives and colchicine.

Acitretin

Acitretin is a vitamin A derivative that is effective in treating chronic plaque psoriasis with approximately 70% clearance in 8 weeks. A synergistic effect has been observed with concomitant PUVA, when patients require less UV exposure to clear their psoriasis.

Adverse effects – most patients experience mucocutaneous symptoms including drying of the mucous membranes, crusting in the nose, itching, thinning of the hair, and erythema of the palms and nail folds. These are usually not severe and settle when treatment stops.

Hepatotoxicity and raised lipid concentrations occur in 20–30% of patients. Liver function tests and cholesterol/triglyceride concentrations should be carefully monitored. Acitretin can be metabolised to etretinate (half-life 70–100 days) which is teratogenic and therefore women during reproductive years must use effective contraception during treatment and for 3 years afterwards.

Ciclosporin A

Ciclosporin A is an immunosuppressant widely used following organ transplantation. It is effective and suitable for the treatment of inflammatory types of psoriasis because of its rapid onset of action. Patients are given 3–5 mg/kg/day in two divided doses either for short courses or continuous use up to 2 years maximum. The minimum dose required to control the psoriasis should be used.

Adverse effects – include renal impairment and hypertension. Baseline blood tests should include serum creatinine, urea, electrolytes and glomerular filtration rate. Hypertension may be managed by reducing the dose of ciclosporin or by giving the patient nifedipine. Transient nausea, headaches, gum hypertrophy and hypertrichosis may also be observed. Hepatic metabolism of ciclosporin (via cytochrome P450) can be inhibited or induced by many different drugs. Medications inhibiting ciclosporin metabolism include erythromycin, itraconazole, verapamil and diltiazem. Medications increasing ciclosporin metabolism include rifampicin, phenytoin and carbamazepine.

Mycophenolate mofetil (MMF)

MMF is usually used as a second line systemic agent for treating psoriasis and psoriatic arthritis. It is an immunosuppressant medication that selectively inhibits activated lymphocytes. Studies have shown that about two-thirds of patients taking MMF (2–3 g/day for 12 weeks) have a significant reduction (50%) in their PASI (psoriasis area and severity index) score by 12 weeks.

Adverse effects include gastrointestinal upset and myelosuppression, haematological malignancies and opportunistic infections.

Biological therapy

Biological therapy refers to substances originally derived from living organisms such as proteins or antibodies that are designed to block particular molecular steps in the biological pathway that leads to psoriasis. Our greater understanding of the pathophysiology of psoriasis has been exploited to direct treatments against specific cytokine/cell pathways dysregulated in disease. Psoriasis is a T-cell mediated disease and cytokines such as tumour necrosis factor alpha (TNF-α) and interferon gamma (INF-γ) play a role.

Biological therapies are currently directed against T-cells or specific inflammatory mediators such as TNF.

The main biological agents currently used to treat severe psoriasis are infliximab, etanercept and adalimumab and ustekinumab. Clinical guidelines (NICE – National Institute of Clinical Excellence (UK)) exist in most countries to direct the usage of biological agents in patients with psoriasis. These novel agents are expensive and can result in chronic immunosuppression leading to fatal infections or tumours and therefore their usage should be managed in specialist units by experienced practitioners. Biological agents are usually administered S/C or IV by injection/infusions, with frequencies varying from twice weekly to once per month, in either continuous or intermittent regimes. Biological treatments are delivered either at home by the patients themselves/visiting practitioner or are delivered in IV-suites based in the community/local hospitals.

NICE guidelines (UK) for the use of biological agents for psoriasis indicate that biological therapies can only be considered in patients with a PASI score of greater than 10 (or significant localised disease at high-impact sites – hands/genitals/scalp) **and** a DLQI score >10, **plus** the patient has failed to respond to two conventional systemic agents/phototherapy (contraindicated, non-response or stopped due to unacceptable side effects) or have severe/unstable/life-threatening disease.

NICE guidelines (UK) for use of biological agents for psoriatic arthritis indicate that they can be used in severe active disease in patients with at least three tender joints and three swollen joints who have not responded sufficiently to two other disease-modifying drugs.

Many patients starting biological therapy have experienced significant, extensive and recalcitrant psoriasis/psoriatic arthritis for many years prior to their disease being controlled with a biological agent, and consequently they find disease relapse on stopping biologics more unacceptable than ever, as their expectation has now shifted to virtually clear skin and no joint pains.

Etanercept

Etanercept (Enbrel®) is a genetically engineered anti-tumour necrosis factor receptor (anti-sTNF) biological agent. Dosing is twice weekly with either 25 mg or 50 mg given by S/C injection. The higher dose seems to be more effective than lower doses, especially in patients who weigh more than 70 kg. Onset of action is relatively slow, with clinical improvement being observed in the majority of patients between 4 and 8 weeks. Patients may initially have courses of treatment lasting 12 weeks; at that stage an assessment of efficacy should be made (as judged by a reduction in the patient's PASI and DLQI scores); however, continuous therapy may ultimately be needed due to significant disease relapse within 3 months of stopping treatment. The cost of twice weekly 25 mg or once weekly 50 mg etanercept per patient per year is about £9500 (2013).

Adverse effects associated with etanercept include an increased risk of infections, particularly latent TB and hepatitis B and septicaemia, gastrointestinal symptoms, hypersensitivity and injection site reactions, blood disorders and a lupus-like antibody driven syndrome.

Infliximab

Infliximab (Remicade®) is an anti-TNF human-murine monoclonal antibody for the treatment of severe psoriasis/psoriatic arthritis. Infliximab has a rapid onset of action – usually within 2 weeks in the majority of patients. Doses are calculated according to the patient's weight, 5 mg/kg given by an intravenous infusion at weeks 0, 2, 6 and then every 8 weeks. Nearly 80% of patients experience significant improvement in the extent and severity of their disease (reduced PASI and DLQI scores) by 10 weeks, which is usually maintained for at least 6 months. There is evidence from studies (data up to 1 year) that continuous therapy is superior to intermittent treatment. Almost 20% of patients develop antibodies to infliximab (possibly due to the presence of murine proteins), which is clinically associated with reduced efficacy. However, the risk of antibody development seems to be reduced when infliximab is given continuously and when it is given with methotrexate in patients with psoriatic arthritis. The total cost of infliximab maintenance treatment for 1 year per patient in the United Kingdom is about £12,500 (2013).

Adverse effects – as above for etanercept; however, in addition, chest pain, dyspnoea, arrhythmias, demyelinating disorders, sleep disturbance, skin pigmentation, gastrointestinal haemorrhage, seizures and transverse myelitis have been reported, among others.

Adalimumab

Adalimumab (Humira®) is a human anti-TNF monoclonal antibody used to treat severe psoriasis and psoriatic arthritis. It has a fast onset of activity, usually within 2 weeks and is highly effective in 60–70% of patients. The majority of patients receive 40 mg of adalimumab fortnightly by S/C injection (following a loading dose of 80 mg at week 0). Efficacy is assessed at 16 weeks before deciding whether to continue with the treatment; however, a small cohort of patients with slow/partial response may receive weekly injections, rather than discontinuation. There is some evidence to suggest that continuous therapy is more effective than intermittent therapy. Anti-adalimumab antibodies develop in about 8% of patients, which correlates with reduced efficacy. Some patients with psoriatic arthritis take methotrexate plus adalimumab, which seems to be more effective than adalimumab alone. The cost of fortnightly adalimumab per patient/year is about £9,300 in the United Kingdom (2013).

Adverse effects – as for etanercept, plus stomatitis, cough, paraesthesia, rash/pruritus, arrhythmias, chest pain, flushing, flu-like symptoms, sleep disturbance, electrolyte disturbances, alopecia and demyelinating disorders among others.

Ustekinumab

Ustekinumab (Stelara®) is a human monoclonal antibody that targets the p40 subunit of interleukin-12 (IL-12) and IL-23, which prevents them from binding to T-cells and therefore impairs the inflammatory cascade in psoriasis. Because Ustekinumab has only been in clinical use for a few years there is less long-term safety and efficacy data than the other biologic agents. The recommended dose of Ustekinumab is 45 mg (patient weighs <100 kg) or 90 mg (patient weighs >100 kg) by S/C injection at weeks 0, 4, and then every 12 weeks. Efficacy should be assessed at 16 weeks and only continued in those who have achieved a 75% reduction in their PASI score or 50% reduction in PASI plus 5 point reduction in DLQI scores. The cost of 45 mg or 90 mg for any individual patient is the same in the United Kingdom as supplied by the manufacturer. Nonetheless, the total cost of Ustekinumab per patient/year in the United Kingdom is around £11,000 (based on 4.3 injections/year in 2013).

Adverse effects – as for etanercept, plus allergic reactions (urticarial, angiooedema, difficulty breathing), infections, mouth ulcers, haematuria, gastrointestinal symptoms, cough, chest pains, seizures and visual disturbance.

Further reading

www.bad.org.uk/healthcare/guidelines London, UK.

Menter A and Griffiths CE. Current and future management of psoriasis. *Lancet* **370**:272–284, 2007.

Weinberg JM. *Treatment of Psoriasis (Milestones in Drug Therapy)*, Birkhauser Verlag AG, 2007.

CHAPTER 4

Eczema (Dermatitis)

Rachael Morris-Jones

Dermatology Department, Kings College Hospital, London, UK

OVERVIEW

- Eczema describes a pattern of inflammation in the skin caused by a multitude of causes.
- Eczema includes atopic dermatitis, contact allergy, varicose eczema, pompholyx and discoid eczema.
- Atopic dermatitis affects about 3% of infants and can lead to considerable morbidity to the child and the family.
- Management relies heavily on regular applications of emollients and topical steroids.

Eczema and dermatitis are terms used to describe the characteristic clinical appearance of inflamed, dry, occasionally scaly and vesicular skin rashes associated with divergent underlying causes. The word *eczema* is derived from Greek, meaning 'to boil over', which aptly describes the microscopic blisters occurring in the epidermis at the cellular level. *Dermatitis*, as the term suggests, implies inflammation of the skin which relates to the underlying pathophysiology. The terms *eczema* and *dermatitis* encompass a wide variety of skin conditions usually classified by their characteristic distribution, morphology and any trigger factors involved.

Clinical features

Eczema is an inflammatory condition that may be acute or chronic. Acute eruptions are characterised by erythema, vesicular/bullous lesions and exudates. Secondary bacterial infection (staphylococcus and streptococcus) heralded by golden crusting may exacerbate acute eczema. Chronicity of inflammation leads to increased scaling, xerosis (dryness) and lichenification (thickening of the skin where surface markings become more prominent). Eczema is characteristically itchy and subsequent scratching may also modify the clinical appearance leading to excoriation marks, loss of skin surface, secondary infection, exudates and ultimately marked lichenification (Figure 4.1). Inflammation in the skin can result in disruption of skin pigmentation causing post-inflammatory hyper/hypopigmentation. Patients often fear that loss of pigment is due to the application of topical steroids but in the majority of cases it is due to chronic inflammation.

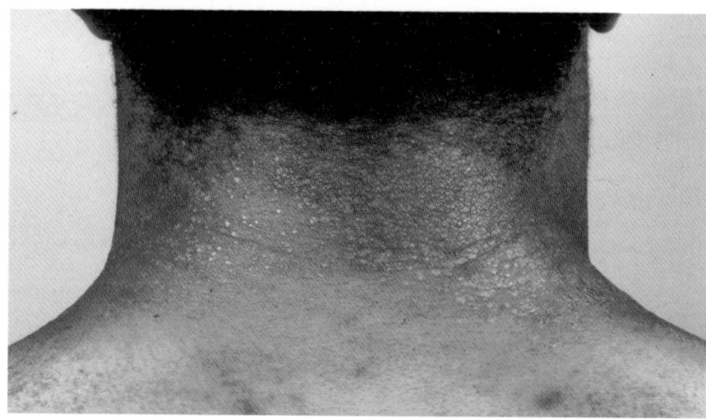

Figure 4.1 Chronic atopic dermatitis.

Pathophysiology

The underling causes of endogenous dermatitis are poorly defined; however, genetic predisposition is common in patients with atopic dermatitis. In these patients there is an abnormality in the balance of T-helper lymphocytes, leading to increasing numbers of Th-2 cells compared to Th-1 and Th-17. The abnormal Th-2 cells interact with Langerhans cells, causing raised levels of interleukins/IgE and a reduction in gamma interferon with resultant upregulation of pro-inflammatory cells. In addition to this, immune dysregulation gene defects have been identified in large cohorts of patients with atopic dermatitis (AD) including filaggrin gene defects which lead to impaired skin barrier function. This impaired barrier leads to increased transepidermal water loss and increased risk of antigens and infective organisms entering the skin.

Pathology

The clinical changes associated with dermatitis are reflected accurately at the cellular level. There is oedema in the epidermis leading to spongiosis (separation of keratinocytes) and vesicle formation. The epidermis is hyperkeratotic (thickened) with dilated blood vessels and an inflammatory (eosinophil) cell infiltrate in the dermis (Figure 4.2).

ABC of Dermatology, Sixth Edition. Edited by Rachael Morris-Jones.

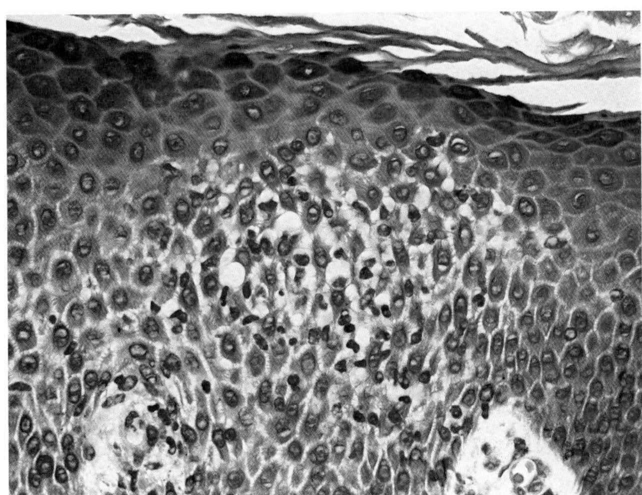

Figure 4.2 Histology of eczema.

Types of eczema

Eczema is classified broadly into endogenous (constitutional) and exogenous (induced by an external factor).

Endogenous eczema

AD typically presents in infancy or early childhood, initially with facial (Figure 4.3) and subsequently flexural limb involvement (Figures 4.4 and 4.5). AD is intensely itchy, and even young babies become highly proficient at scratching, which can lead to disrupted sleep (both patient and family), poor feeding and irritability. The usual pattern is one of flare-ups followed by remissions, exacerbations being associated with inter-current infections, teething, and food allergies. In severely affected babies failure to thrive may result. In older children or adults, AD may become chronic and widespread and is frequently exacerbated by stress. AD is common, affecting 3% of infants; nonetheless, 90% of the patients spontaneously remit by puberty. Patients likely to suffer from chronic AD in adult life are those who have a strong family history of eczema, present at a very young age with extensive disease and have associated asthma/multiple food allergies (Figure 4.6).

Pityriasis alba is a variant of atopic eczema in which pale patches of hypopigmentation develop on the face of children. Juvenile plantar dermatosis is another variant of atopic eczema in which there is dry cracked skin on the forefoot in children (Figure 4.7).

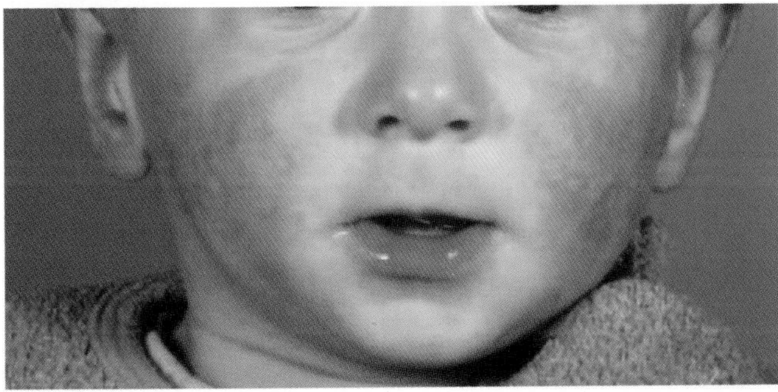

Figure 4.3 Facial atopic dermatitis.

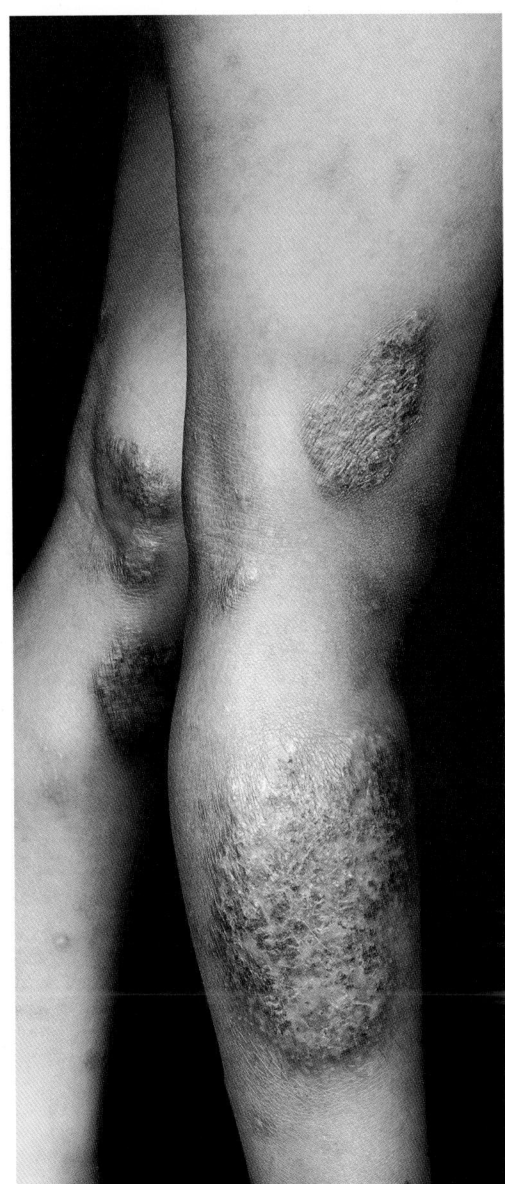

Figure 4.4 Chronic lichenified eczema on the legs.

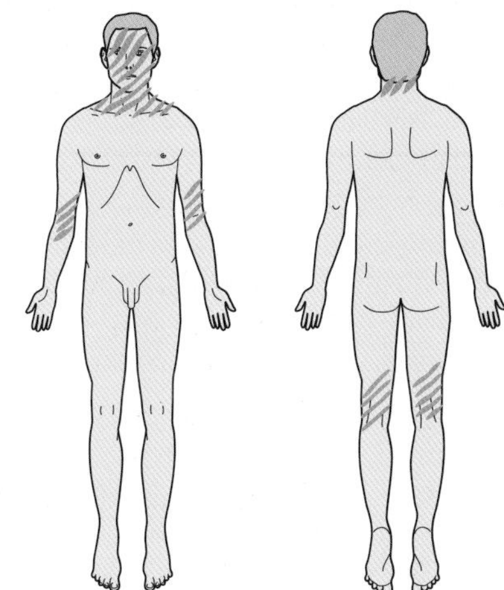

Figure 4.5 Distribution of atopic dermatitis.

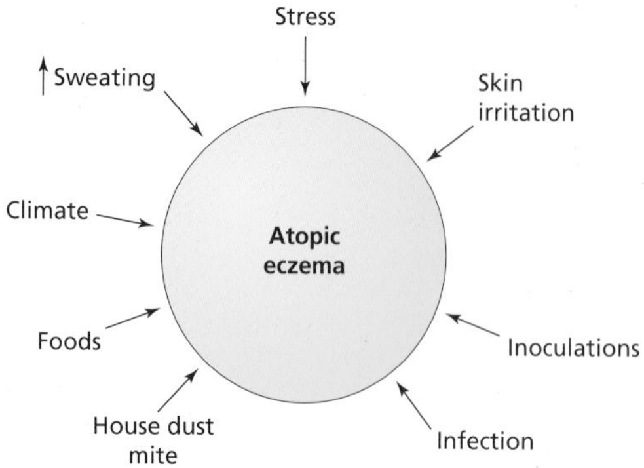

Figure 4.6 Factors leading to the development of atopic dermatitis.

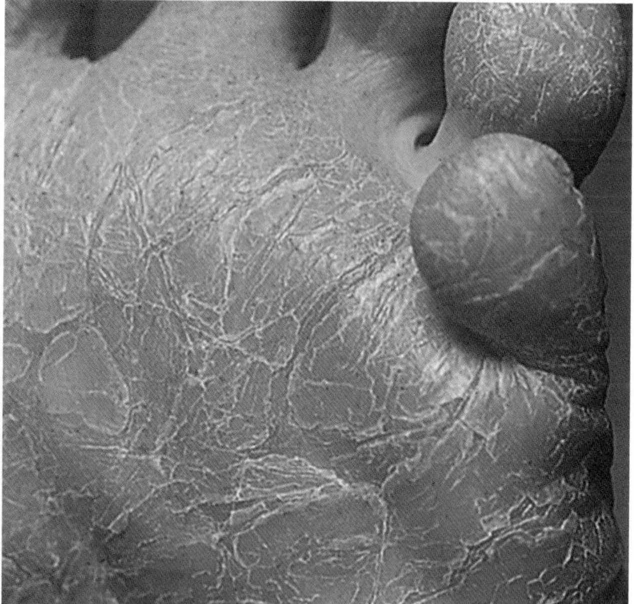

Figure 4.7 Plantar dermatitis.

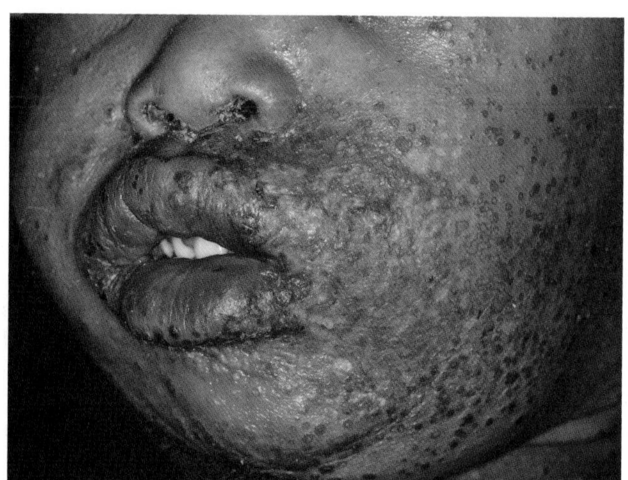

Figure 4.8 Eczema herpeticum.

Eczema herpeticum is herpes simplex viral infection superimposed onto the skin affected by eczema (usually in atopics). There is frequently a history of close contact with an adult with herpes labialis (cold sore). Clinically, there are multiple small 'punched-out' looking ulcers, especially around the neck and eyes (Figure 4.8). Eczema herpeticum is a serious complication of eczema that may be life threatening, and therefore early intervention with systemic aciclovir is essential under the guidance of a dermatology specialist.

Lichen simplex is a localised area of lichenification produced by rubbing (Figure 4.9).

Asteatotic eczema occurs in older people with dry skin, particularly on the lower legs. The pattern on the skin resembles a dry river-bed or 'crazy-paving' (Figure 4.10).

Discoid eczema appears as intensely pruritic coin shaped lesions most commonly on the limbs (Figure 4.11). Lesions may be vesicular and are frequently colonised by *Staphylococcus aureus*. Males are more frequently affected than females.

Pompholyx eczema is itching vesicles on the fingers, palms and soles. The blisters are small, firm, intensely itchy and occasionally painful (Figure 4.12). The condition is more common in patients with nickel allergy.

Venous (stasis) eczema is a common insidious dermatitis that occurs on the lower legs of patients with venous insufficiency. These patients have back flow of blood from the deep to the superficial veins leading to venous hypertension. In the early stages, there is brown haemosiderin pigmentation of the skin, especially on the medial ankle, but as the disease progresses skin changes can extend up to the knee (Figure 4.13). Patients typically have peripheral

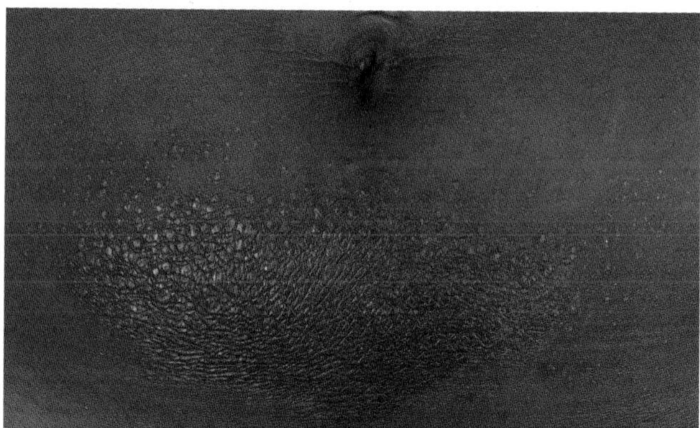

Figure 4.9 Lichen simplex.

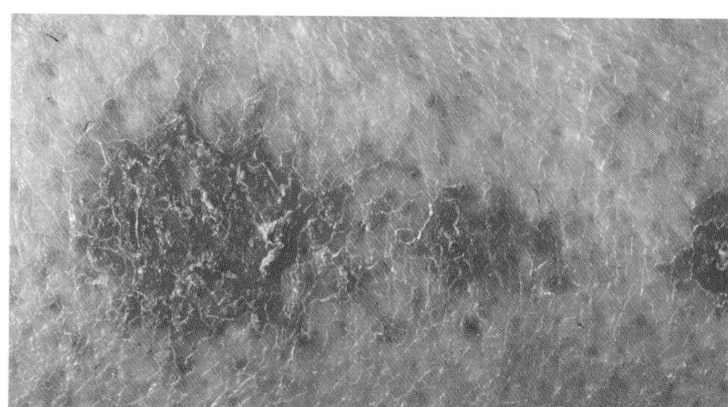

Figure 4.10 Asteatotic eczema.

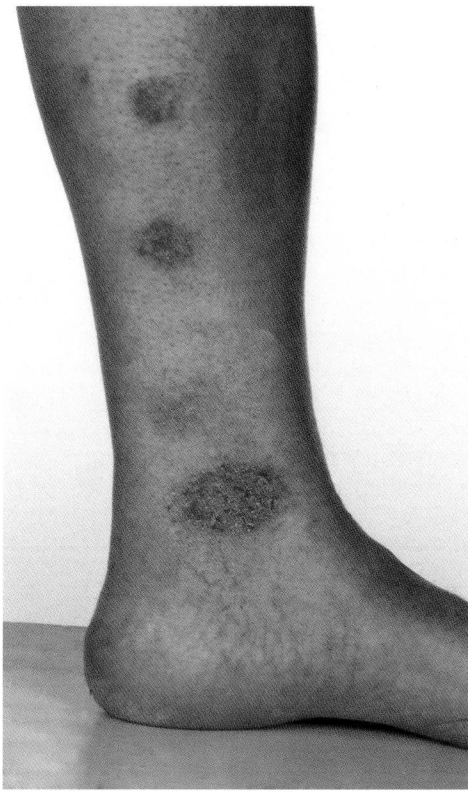

Figure 4.11 Discoid eczema.

Figure 4.12 Pompholyx eczema.

oedema, and ulceration may result. The mainstay of management is compression (see Chapter 11).

Investigations of eczema

Skin swabs should be taken from the skin if secondary bacterial (Figure 4.14) or viral infection is suspected. The swab should be moistened in the transport medium before being rolled thoroughly on the affected skin, coating all sides of the swab to ensure an adequate sample is sent to the laboratory. A significant growth of bacteria reported with its sensitivity and resistance pattern can be useful in guiding antibiotic usage. Nasal swabs should be performed in older children and adults with persistent facial eczema to check for nasal Staphylococcus carriage. If a secondary fungal infection is suspected then scrapings or brushings can be taken for mycological analysis.

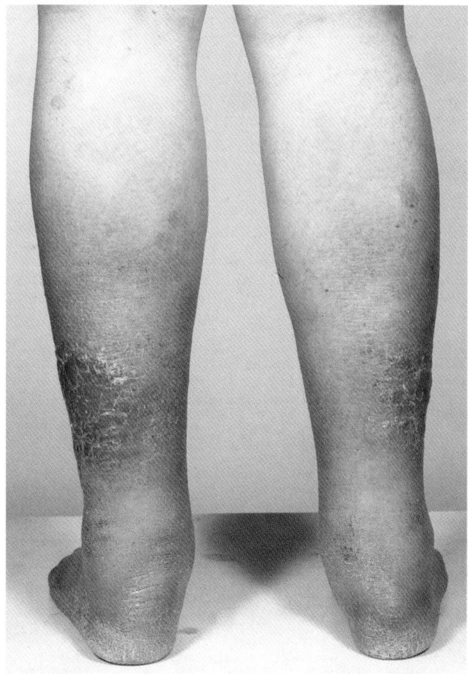

Figure 4.13 Varicose eczema.

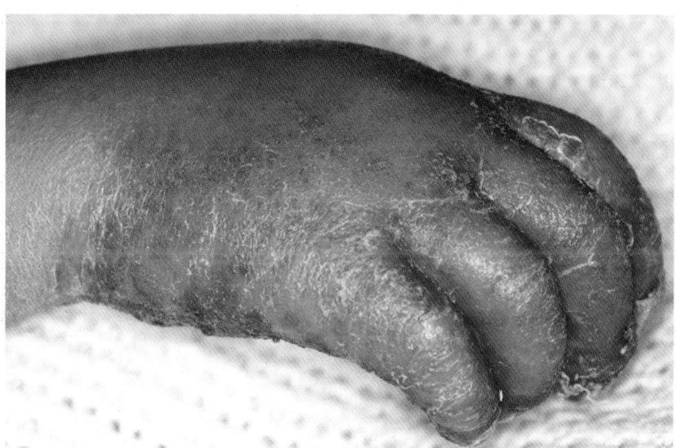

Figure 4.14 Infected eczema.

Routine blood tests are not necessary; however, an eosinophilia and raised immunoglobulin E (IgE) level may be seen. RAST (radioallergosorbent testing) looks for specific IgE levels against suspected allergens such as aeroallergens (pollens, house dust mite and animal dander) and foods (egg, cow's milk, wheat, fish, nuts and soya proteins). Skin prick testing may also be used to determine any specific allergies to aeroallergens or foods.

Skin biopsy (usually a punch biopsy) for histological analysis may be performed if the diagnosis is uncertain. Beware unilateral eczema of the areola, which could be Paget's disease of the nipple (Figure 4.15).

Varicose eczema (leg ulcer) patients should have their ABPI (ankle brachial pressure index) measured before compressing their legs with bandages. ABPI is the ratio of their arm:ankle systolic blood pressure.

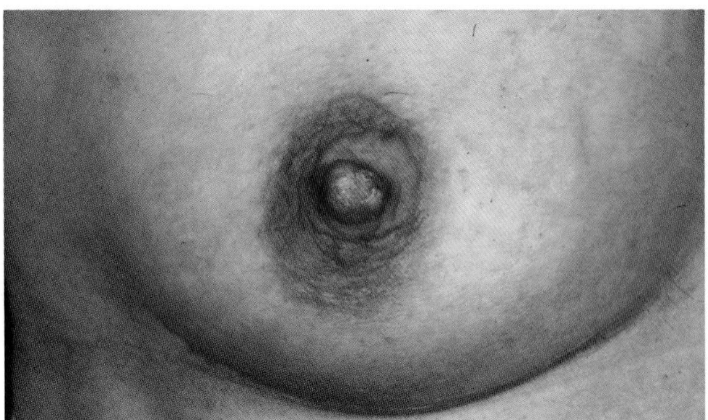

Figure 4.15 Paget's disease of the nipple – beware unilateral 'eczema'.

Classification of eczema

Endogenous (constitutional) eczema	Exogenous (contact) eczema	Secondary changes
Atopic	Irritant	Lichen simplex
Discoid	Allergic	Asteatotic
Pompholyx	Photodermatitis	Pompholyx
Varicose		Infection
Seborrhoeic (discussed later)		

Exogenous eczema

Contact dermatitis

Contact dermatitis can result from irritant or allergic reactions in the skin. Cutaneous contact allergy is not inherent but acquired because of exposure to environmental or occupational allergens (Box 4.1). In general, the more a person is exposed to a potential allergen (quantity and frequency) the more likely he or she is to develop an allergy. Patients with abnormal skin barrier function (e.g. those with eczema) are more likely to develop contact dermatitis and suffer from irritant reactions than those with normal skin. Patients develop an allergic skin reaction at the site of sensitisation to an allergen, and then on subsequent exposure at a distant skin site develop eczema simultaneously at previous sites of allergy.

Box 4.1 **Common contact allergens**

- Nickel/cobalt (jewellery, clothing, wristwatch, scissors and cooking utensils).
- Potassium dichromate (chemical used to tan leather; Figure 4.17).
- Perfumes, myroxylon pereirae (balsam of Peru, fragrances; Figure 4.20).
- Formaldehyde, parabens, quaternium, methylchloroisothiazolinone, methylisothiazolinone (MCI/MI) (preservatives).
- PPD (permanent hair dyes, temporary tattoos and textiles; Figure 4.22).
- Ethylenediamine (adhesives and medications).
- Chromates (cement and leather).
- Mercaptobenzothiazole, thiurams (rubber gloves and shoes).
- Neomycin, benzocaine (medicated ointments; Figure 4.21).
- Lanolin (wool alcohol, emollients and mediated ointments).

Clinical features

The clinical appearance of both allergic and irritant contact dermatitis may be similar, but there are specific changes that help in differentiating them. An acute allergic reaction tends to be intensely itchy and results in erythema, oedema and vesicles. The more chronic lesions are often lichenified. Irritant dermatitis may be itchy or sore and presents as slight scaling, erythema and fissuring.

The distribution of the skin changes is often helpful in identifying the underlying cause (Figure 4.16). For example, an itchy rash on the foot may indicate allergy to footwear (Figure 4.17) such as allergy to potassium dichromate, a chemical used to tan leather. An allergy to medications used for treating leg ulcers is a common cause of persistent dermatitis on the lower leg, or iodine used to clean the skin pre-operatively (Figure 4.18). Hand dermatitis can result from glove allergies (rubber and latex) or contact with an occupational exposure such as melamine formaldehyde resin (Figure 4.19) or irritation from sweat under gloves. Fragrance allergy is common

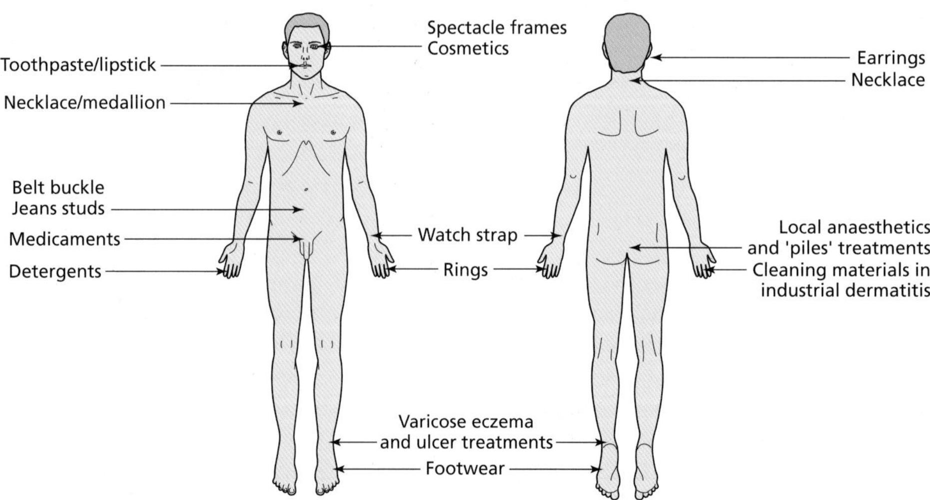

Figure 4.16 Common sources of contact dermatitis by body site.

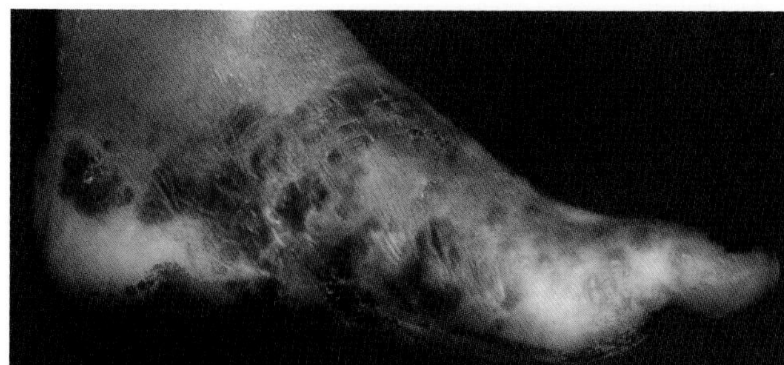

Figure 4.17 Severe contact dermatitis to potassium dichromate in leather shoes.

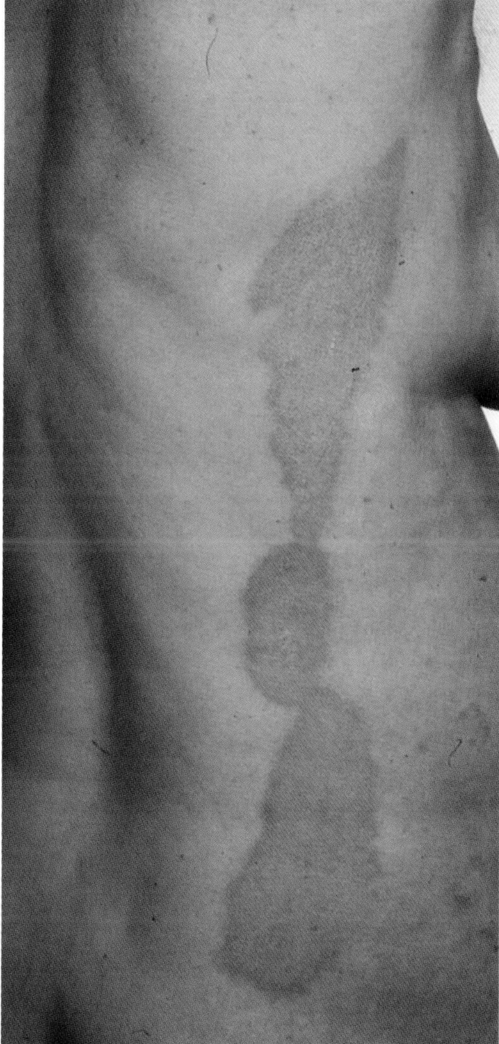

Figure 4.18 Contact dermatitis to iodine.

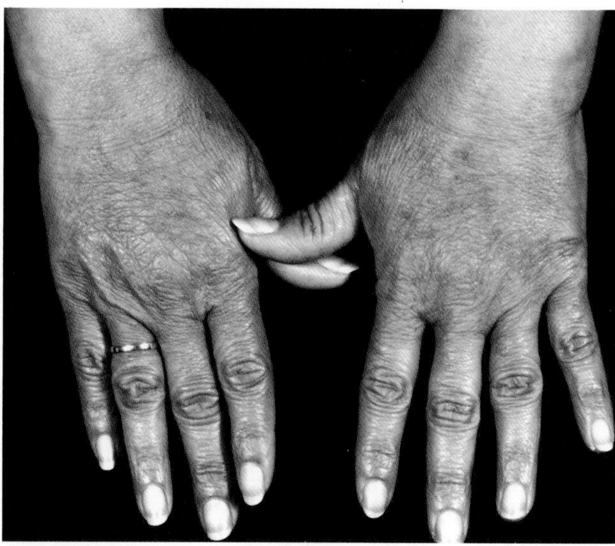

Figure 4.19 Allergic contact dermatitis to melamine formaldehyde resin.

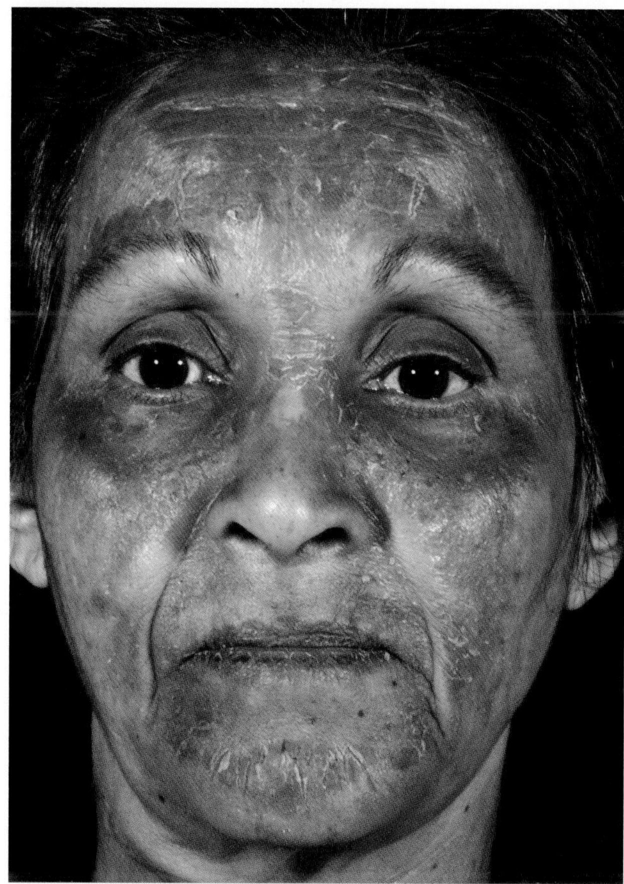

Figure 4.20 Contact dermatitis to fragrance in facial cream.

and can cause reactions to cosmetic products (Figure 4.20). Patients can develop allergies to medicaments such as those containing neomycin (Figure 4.21). Allergy to paraphenylenediamine (PPD) in a tattoo causes a very brisk vesicular reaction (Figure 4.22). Patients may also develop contact allergies to dressings/plasters applied to the skin (Figure 4.23). An irritant substance may produce a more diffuse eruption such as physical irritation to the skin caused by air conditioning.

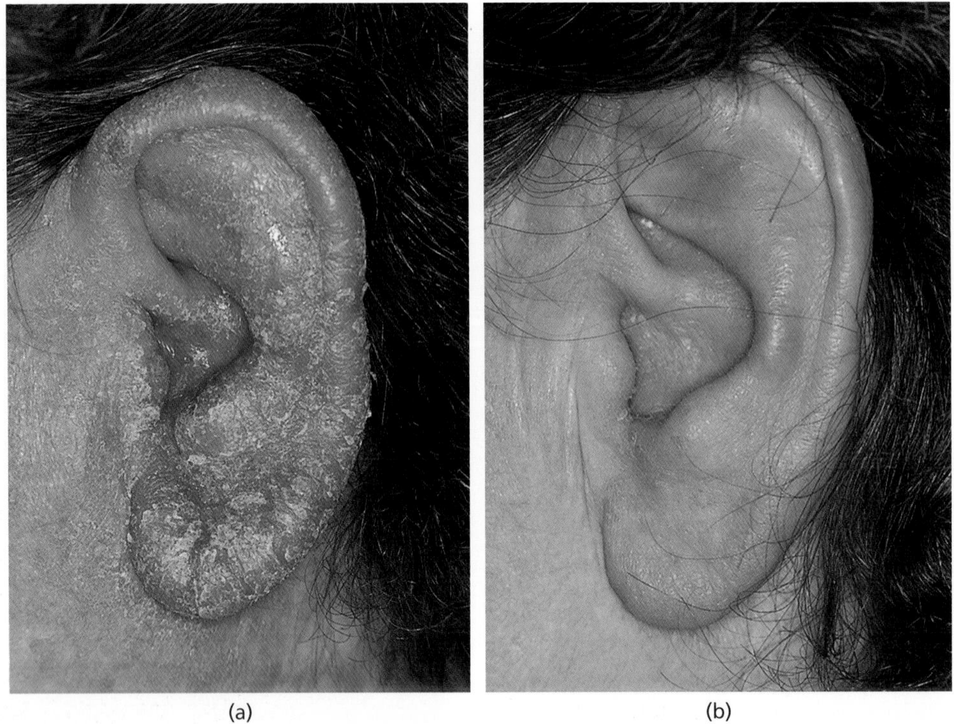

Figure 4.21 (a) Contact dermatitis to neomycin cream and (b) after stopping the treatment.

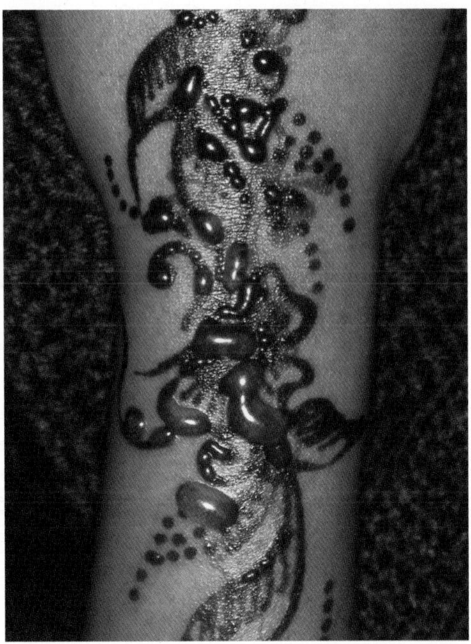

Figure 4.22 Acute PPD allergy in a 'henna' tattoo.

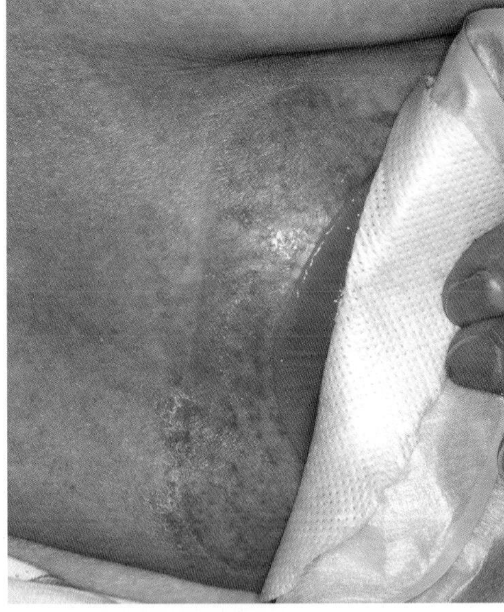

Figure 4.23 Contact allergy to stoma dressing.

Allergic contact dermatitis

The characteristics of allergic dermatitis are as follows:

- Previous exposure to the substance concerned.
- 48–96 h between contact and the development of changes in the skin.
- Activation of previously sensitised sites by contact with an allergen at a distant skin site.
- Persistence of the allergy for many years.

Immune mechanisms

Allergic dermatitis results from a type IV delayed hypersensitivity reaction in the skin. Specific antigens (usually proteins) penetrate the epidermis, combine with a protein mediator and are then picked

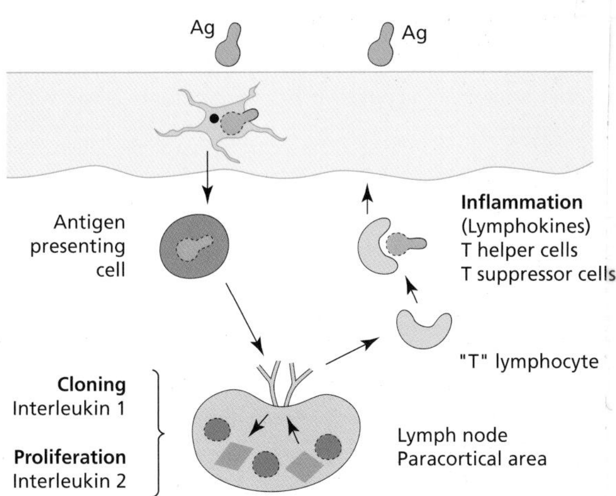

Figure 4.24 Immunological response leading to the development of contact dermatitis.

up by Langerhans cells. This causes T-lymphocytes in regional lymph nodes to become sensitised to the antigen. On subsequent exposure to the antigen, an allergic reaction occurs because of the accumulation of sensitised T-lymphocytes at the site of the antigen with a resultant inflammatory response. This takes 48 h and is amplified by interleukins that provide a positive feedback stimulus to the production of further sensitised T-lymphocytes (Figure 4.24).

Irritant contact dermatitis

This may be chemical or physical, has a less defined clinical course and is caused by a wide variety of substances with no predictable time interval between contact and the appearance of the rash. Physical irritants include air conditioning, prosthetic limbs, personnel protective clothing and repetitive mechanical trauma. Chemical irritants include detergents, solvents and acids. Dermatitis occurs soon after exposure and the severity varies with the quantity, concentration and length of exposure to the substance concerned. Previous contact is not required, unlike allergic dermatitis where previous sensitisation is necessary.

Photodermatitis

Photodermatitis is caused by the interaction of light and chemicals absorbed by the skin. It can result from (a) drugs taken internally, such as sulphonamides, phenothiazines, tetracycline and voriconazole or (b) substances in contact with the skin, such as topical antihistamines, local anaesthetics, cosmetics and antibacterials. Phytophotodermatitis is due to contact with plant material, often containing forms of psoralens (poison oak, common rue, lime juice and celery) and sunlight causing an allergic contact dermatitis. Patients with chronic actinic dermatitis (Figure 4.25) (chronic eczema on sun-exposed skin) are allergic to sunlight but in addition they may be allergic to compositae plants (daisy and sunflower family).

Occupational dermatitis

In the workplace, employees may have contact with allergens or irritants that can result in dermatitis. If an individual has an atopic

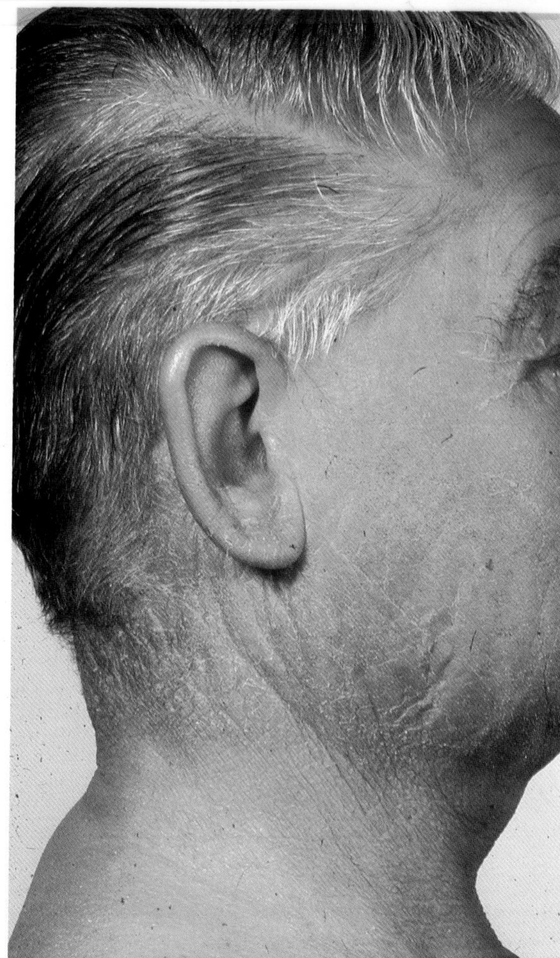

Figure 4.25 Chronic actinic dermatitis.

tendency to develop eczema he or she is at increased risk of developing occupational dermatitis. Secondary bacterial infection can play a role once dermatitis has occurred. Therefore, contact dermatitis, atopic eczema and infection may all be superimposed – for example, a nurse or hairdresser who is exposed to water, detergents and other factors that will exacerbate any pre-existing eczema. The skin then becomes broken because of scratching, and secondary infection occurs. The frequent use of alcohol-based hand gel in hospitals by health care professionals is leading to an increased frequency of irritant hand dermatitis which has implications for infection control.

An occupational dermatitis is likely if

- the dermatitis first occurred during a specific employment and had not been present before;
- the condition generally improves or clears when away from the workplace and
- there is exposure to known irritant/allergic substances and personnel protective measures are inadequate.

Persistence of dermatitis away from the workplace may occur in occupational dermatitis if the allergen is also present at home (e.g. rubber in gloves), if there is secondary infection and if there are

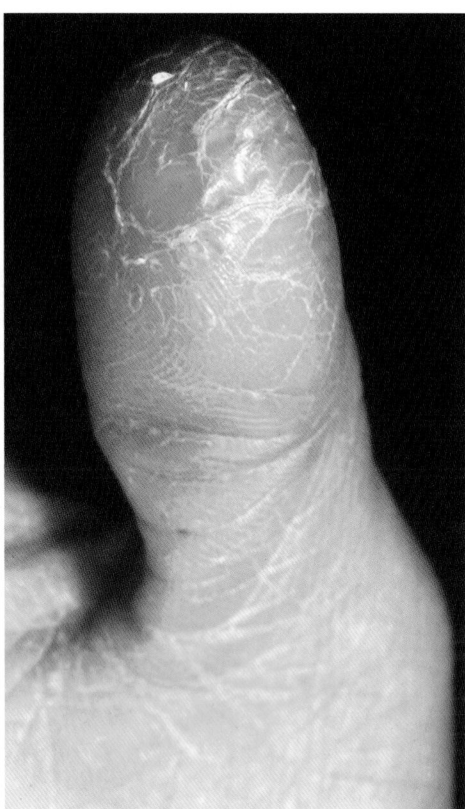

Figure 4.26 Irritant hand eczema in a chef.

chronic skin changes. The morphology of the skin eruption itself will be indistinguishable whatever the cause of the eczema.

Occupational irritant contact dermatitis can be acute or chronic. Acute reactions are usually associated with a clear history of exposure to a chemical or physical irritant. Chronic irritant dermatitis can be harder to assess as it develops insidiously in many cases. Individuals involved in frequent 'wet work' such as nurses, cleaners, chefs and those looking after small children can develop irritant hand dermatitis from repeated exposure to water (Figure 4.26). Initially, transient inflammation may clear; however, with each successive episode the damage becomes worse with an escalation of inflammatory changes that eventually become chronic and fixed. Once chronic damage has occurred the skin is vulnerable to any further irritation; therefore, the condition may flare up in the future even after removal of the causative factors. Individuals with atopic eczema are particularly liable to develop chronic irritant dermatitis, and secondary infection is an additional factor.

Occupational allergic contact dermatitis occurs as an allergic reaction to specific substances. There is no immediate reaction on first exposure; however, after repeated exposure a cell-mediated inflammatory response develops. Some substances are highly sensitising such as epoxy resin, whereas others such as cement need prolonged exposure over many years to trigger allergy. In addition to the capacity of the substance to produce an allergic reaction, individuals also vary considerably in the capacity to develop allergies.

Contact urticaria is an immediate-type sensitivity reaction that can occur to certain food proteins and latex glove allergy. Chefs may develop allergies to foods proteins (usually on their non-dominant hand as knives are usually held in the dominant hand) that can result in contact urticaria, or a more chronic irritant contact dermatitis.

Investigations of contact dermatitis

A full-detailed history is essential if the potential irritant or allergen is to be identified. Dermatology specialists should particularly assess those with a suspected occupational dermatitis as the investigations and subsequent results could affect the patients' future employment and possible compensation claims.

In relation to suspected occupational dermatitis, the exact details of the patient's job should be taken in careful detail. Occasionally, an 'on-site' visit to the work place may be required; for example, a worker in a plastics factory had severe hand dermatitis but the only positive result on patch testing was to nickel. On visiting the factory it became clear that the cause was a nickel-plated handle that he used several thousand times a day. It is also important to assess the working environment because exposure to dampness (on an oil rig) and irritants (dry air in aircraft cabins) can result in skin irritation.

Patch testing

Patch testing is used to determine the substances that cause contact dermatitis. The concentration used is critical to ensure a low false negative/positive rate. The optimum concentration and best vehicle have been ascertained for most common allergens. The standard series contains a 'battery' of tests that encompasses the most common allergens encountered. Additional specialist 'batteries' (dental, medicaments, metals, perfumes, etc.) may also be available in some specialist dermatology centres. It is important that patch testing is managed by experienced dermatologists to ensure that the most appropriate tests are performed, in the correct manner (timings and dilutions), interpreted correctly (irritant or allergic reactions) and then any relevance sought.

The test patches are usually placed on the upper back (sites marked) and left in place for 48 h, then removed and any positive reactions noted (Figures 4.27 and 4.28). A further examination

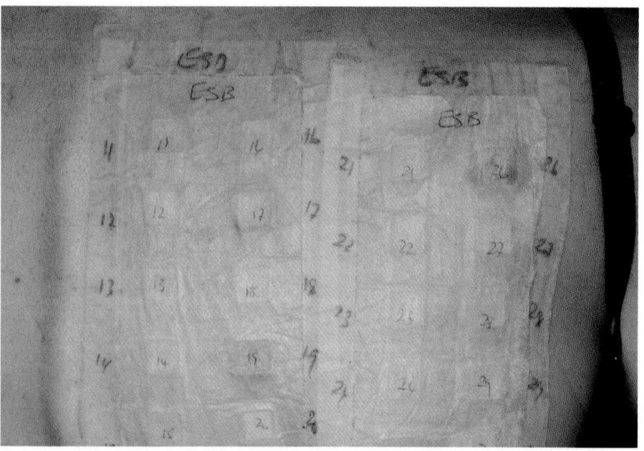

Figure 4.27 Test patches in place.

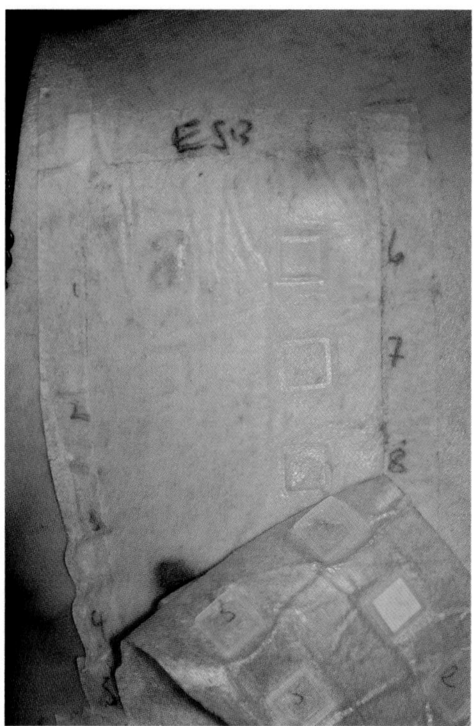

Figure 4.28 Patches being removed after 48 h.

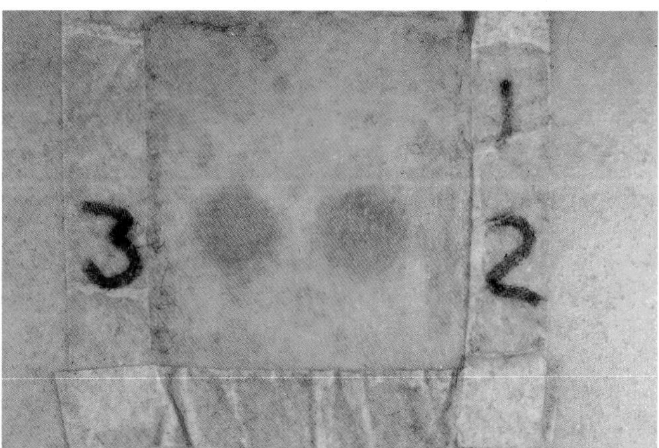

Figure 4.29 Positive patch test reactions.

is carried out at 96 h to detect any late reactions (Figure 4.29). Patients need to visit the unit three times in 1 week, be off systemic immunosuppressants and have an area of clear skin (usually the upper back) on which to perform the tests. Although rare, sensitisation may occur as a consequence of exposure to an allergen through patch testing.

General management of eczema

We must always remember to treat the patient and not just the rash. Many patients suffer considerably with their eczema whilst others seem less concerned. Many parents of children with AD are hoping for a quick 'cure' by the removal of triggers such as foods, but in the majority this is not the case. Management of atopic dermatitis patients should therefore include adequate time to discuss the aims of therapy and its limitations, namely, suppression rather than cure of the disease. Exogenous eczema may be transient and 'cured' after identification and avoidance of trigger factors.

Practitioners need to have realistic expectations about what patients can tolerate in terms of acceptability of topical formulations as some are greasy and smelly. Patients need to be physically capable and able to find the time to apply their own creams.

Many simple treatments can be purchased and applied by the individuals themselves without the need to consult a medical practitioner. Treatments usually start with simple emollients and mild topical steroids but with increasingly recalcitrant disease stronger therapies such as systemic immunosuppressants may be needed.

- Emollients. Patients with dry skin conditions have ready access to a wide range of emollients (moisturising creams) over the counter. In general, the oilier the cream the better its emollient properties; however, patients tend to prefer lighter creams. Moisturisers should be applied repeatedly throughout the day in generous amounts. Emollients help to restore barrier function and reduce itching.
- Cleansers. Normal soap contains surfactants which disrupt the lipid barrier and cause drying of the skin. Aqueous cream and emulsifying ointments are useful soap substitutes. Antibacterial moisturising washes have been shown to be very useful in those prone to infected eczema. There are numerous bath oils/shower washes available which help prevent drying of the skin caused by water alone. Soothing and de-scaling shampoos can be useful for dry, flaky and itchy scalps.
- Topical steroids – frequency and quantity. Topical steroids continue to be the mainstay of treatment for active eczema. Many patients are wary of using topical steroids as they are worried about skin thinning. We need to reassure patients that under careful medical supervision steroids should be safe and are highly effective. Ointments rather than creams should be used whenever possible (creams are more likely to cause irritation and have a higher risk of inducing contact allergies). Steroid should be applied once or twice daily to the affected skin only. One finger-tip-unit (a line of ointment from the tip of the finger to the first skin crease) is a sufficient amount to treat a hand-sized (palmar and dorsal surface) area of affected skin. Strength and frequency should be tailored to the severity and skin sites affected. Generally, they should be used twice daily on the affected skin.
- Topical steroids – potency. Very low potency steroids such as hydrocortisone may be purchased over the counter and used to treat mild eczema. For moderate to severe disease, the current approach is to prescribe potent topical steroids (mometasone, betamethasone and fluocinolone acetonide) for short periods followed by steroid 'holidays' rather than using daily low potency steroids, which rarely clear the eczema. For acute dermatitis start with a potent topical steroid for a few days or weeks and then reduce to a lower potency once the disease is controlled. Lower potency topical steroids should be used on the face and groin areas (hydrocortisone and clobetasone butyrate).
- Immunomodulators. These are useful topical preparations to control mild eczema and are usually prescribed and supervised

by an experienced dermatological practitioner. Tacrolimus (0.03% – children aged 2–15 years, 0.1% – adults) and pimecrolimus (1%) are applied twice daily to the affected skin. As yet, long-term safety data is unavailable for these topical calcineurin inhibitors and there is a theoretical risk of increased malignancies. Consequently, their use should be limited to those who have failed to respond adequately to first-line treatment (topical steroids). It is recommended that their use be for short periods rather than continuous use.

- Occlusion. Covering topical therapy with bandages, body suits, 'wet-wraps' and dressings can be very helpful in the management of chronic eczema (see Chapter 25). Prior to occlusion, the practitioner should ensure the eczema is not infected. Patients and their carers should be taught how to apply these occlusive aids which are generally worn overnight. Occlusive therapy helps relieve symptoms of itch, keep emollient creams on the skin and 'drive' topical therapy through the epidermis. The potency of topical steroids is enhanced 100-fold by occlusion; therefore, only very low potency steroids should be used under occlusion.
- Antibiotics. Occasionally, antibiotics are needed to treat infected eczema; they may be given topically or systemically. Topical antibiotics used include fusidic acid, silver sulfadiazine, polymyxins, neomycin and mupirocin. Formulations of antibiotics combined with topical steroids are available. It is recommended that topical antibiotics should be used for a maximum of 2 weeks continuously to try to reduce the risk of developing resistant bacteria. Systemic antibiotics used include flucloxacillin (amoxycillin and penicillin) erythromycin (clarithromycin and azithromycin) and ciprofloxacin (levofloxacin and ofloxacin). Antibacterial emollient washes can be useful in managing active cutaneous infections as well as preventing them by daily use.
- Phototherapy. Light treatment with narrow-band UVB (TL-01) or PUVA (psoralen with UVA) can be highly effective for generalised eczema. Each course of phototherapy lasts 6–8 weeks with patients attending 2–3 times per week. There is, however, a limit to the number of courses (cumulative dose) of phototherapy that any individual patient may receive before there is a significant increased risk of skin cancer.
- Systemic therapy. Severe widespread disease not controlled with topical therapy may require systemic immunosuppressants. Occasionally, dermatology specialists may prescribe a rapidly reducing course of oral prednisolone (30 mg for 5 days, then reducing by 5 mg every 5 days) to control very severe generalised acute eczema. However, long-term oral steroids should not be used to control eczema. Rather, azathioprine, ciclosporin, mycophenolate mofetil and methotrexate can be used for long-term management. If available, levels of thiopurine methyl transferase (TPMT) should be checked prior to initiation of azathioprine.

Pruritus

Pruritus is a term used to describe itching of the skin that is an unpleasant sensation that triggers rubbing or scratching. The sensation of pruritus can be extremely disturbing, leading to disrupted sleep and even depression. Pruritus may be localised/generalised and may be associated with skin changes or with normal skin.

Pruritus with skin changes

Pruritus may be localised or generalised.

Causes of localised pruritus with skin changes include eczema, psoriasis, lichen planus (flat-topped itchy papules of unknown cause), dermatitis herpetiformis (gluten allergy with rash, characteristically on elbows and buttocks), insect bites/stings, (nodular prurigo may develop after insect bites and is characterised by persistent itching, lichenified papules and nodules), head lice, contact dermatitis, polymorphic light eruption (an acute allergy to sunlight on sun-exposed skin), urticaria or angioedema ('hives' with swelling, especially of the face), fungal infections (particularly tinea pedis of the feet), pruritus ani (perianal itching, a common condition that may result from anal leakage, skin tags, haemorrhoids, thread worms, excessive washing, the use of medicated wipes or allergy to haemorrhoid creams containing Balsam of Peru) and pruritus vulvae (intense itching may result from lichen sclerosus et atrophicus, *Candida* infections or eczema).

Generalised pruritus with skin changes occurs in more widespread inflammatory skin diseases such as widespread eczema/psoriasis, scabies, allergic drug eruptions (antibiotics and anticonvulsants), graft versus host disease (following bone marrow transplantation), pre-bullous pemphigoid (dermatitic eruption before blisters appear), cutaneous lymphoma (may start over the buttocks as more localised disease), parasitophobia (belief that there are parasites under the skin, excoriations are seen), body lice or pubic lice (body lice live in the clothing), viral exanthems (rashes associated with systemic viral illness), urticaria (generalised 'hives') and xerosis (dry skin, especially in the elderly).

Investigation and management of pruritus with skin changes should be directed at the suspected underlying cause.

Pruritus with normal skin

Medical practitioners need to be alert to the patient with generalised pruritus and normal skin as itching may be the first symptom of a systemic disorder such as Hodgkin's disease, chronic renal failure and diabetes, or may be a side effect of mediation.

Systemic causes

- Endocrine – diabetes, myxoedema, hyperthyroidism, menopause and pregnancy.
- Metabolic – hepatic failure, biliary obstruction and chronic renal failure.
- Haematological – polycythaemia and iron deficiency anaemia.
- Malignancy – lymphoma, leukaemia, myeloma and carcinomatosis.
- Neurological/psychological – neuropathic pruritus, multiple sclerosis and anxiety.
- Infection – filariasis, hookworm and HIV.
- Drugs – opioids.

Investigations (pruritus with normal skin)

- Full blood count, erythrocyte sedimentation rate, liver and renal function.
- Serum iron, ferritin and total-iron binding capacity.
- Thyroid function and fasting glucose.

- Serum protein electrophoresis.
- HIV antibody.
- Urine analysis.
- Stools for blood and parasites/ova.
- Chest X-ray.
- Skin biopsy for direct immunofluorescence.

Management of pruritus

Identifying and treating the underlying cause of the pruritus is obviously desirable whenever possible. Patients themselves will find some short-term relief by scratching the skin, but this ultimately leads to further itching and scratching, the so-called 'itch-scratch cycle'. To break this cycle the sensation of itch needs to be suppressed, or the patient's behaviour changed by habit reversal techniques.

Individuals can purchase simple soothing emollients over the counter and apply these frequently to the pruritic areas. The soothing effect can be enhanced by storing the cream in the fridge and applying them cold. Menthol 1–2% in aqueous cream and calamine possess cooling and antipruritic properties. Camphor-containing preparations and crotamiton (Eurax) and topical doxepin hydrochloride applied thinly 3–4 times daily to localised areas may provide relief from itching.

Topical local anaesthetics (containing benzocaine, lidocaine or tetracaine) on sale to the public may give some temporary relief but intolerance may develop and allergic reactions can occur.

Topical and systemic antihistamines can provide relief from itching. Topical antihistamines (mepyramine and antazoline) are on sale to the public in various formulations which may give temporary relief to localised areas. Generally, non-sedating oral antihistamines are given during the day and sedating ones at night. Cutaneous itch responds readily to the histamine H1 blockers cetirizine, levocetirizine, desloratadine and fexofenadine during the day and hydroxyzine at night. H2 blockers (ranitidine and cimetidine) may be used in addition to H1 blockers in resistant cases.

Pruritus ani/vulvae. The affected area should be washed once daily; excessive washing should be avoided. Aqueous cream or emulsifying ointments can be used as a soap substitute. Patients should avoid perfumed/coloured/medicated toilet tissue or wipes. Simple paraffin or zinc cream can be used as a barrier ointment to prevent skin irritation from anal leakage/vaginal discharge. Weak topical steroids can help reduce inflammation and itching. If symptoms persist, patients should see a dermatology specialist who may do patch testing (contact dermatitis) or perform a skin biopsy (neoplasia, lichen sclerosus or lichen planus).

Further Reading

Bieber T, Leung DYM. *Atopic Dermatitis*, 2nd Edition, Informa Healthcare, New York, 2009.

Leung AKC, Hon KLE. *Atopic Dermatitis; A Review for Primary Healthcare Physicians*, Nova Science Publications, New York, 2012.

CHAPTER 5

Urticaria and Angio-oedema

Rachael Morris-Jones

Dermatology Department, Kings College Hospital, London, UK

> **OVERVIEW**
> - Definition and pathophysiology; the role of vasodilators.
> - Classification.
> - Clinical presentation of different types of urticaria.
> - Causes and investigation of non-physical urticarias.
> - Management and treatment.

Introduction

Urticaria describes transient pruritic swellings of the skin, often referred to as wheals, hives or nettle rash by the patient. Urticaria results from oedema in the superficial layers of the skin causing well-demarcated erythematous lesions. It may be associated with allergic reactions, infections or physical stimuli, but in most patients no cause can be found. Similar lesions may precede or be associated with vasculitis (urticarial vasculitis), pemphigoid or dermatitis herpetiformis.

Angio-oedema in contrast is usually painful rather than itchy and appears as a diffuse swelling that affects the deeper layers of the skin; it can occur rapidly and may involve the mucous membranes. Laryngeal oedema is the most serious complication and can be life threatening. Hereditary angio-oedema is a rare form with recurrent severe episodes of subcutaneous oedema, swelling of the mucous membranes and systemic symptoms.

Urticaria is a common skin disorder that affects 20% of the population at some point in their lives. Urticaria may occur as a single episode or be chronically recurrent. It is often self-limiting and is controlled with over-the-counter antihistamine. The prognosis is varied depending on the underlying cause, but in chronic idiopathic urticaria symptoms may persist for several years.

Pathophysiology

Urticaria results from histamine, bradykinin and proinflammatory mediators being released from basophils and mast cells in response to various trigger factors. The chemicals released by degranulation cause capillaries and venules to leak causing tissue oedema. Urticaria may be IgE mediated with cross-linking of two adjacent IgE receptors, or complement mediated (causing direct degranulation of mast cells), or mast cells may be directly stimulated by an exogenous or unknown substance. In patients with chronic urticaria, histamine can be released spontaneously or in response to non-specific stimuli and their vasculature is more sensitive to histamines.

Clinical history

Careful history-taking is of great importance in diagnosing patients with urticaria and/or angio-oedema because frequently there are no clinical signs for the medical practitioner to see. Ask about the onset, duration and course of lesions, rashes and swelling. Urticaria is very itchy and angio-oedema usually painful. Patients with urticaria complain of itchy spots or rashes lasting minutes or hours (usually less than 24 h) that resolve leaving no marks on the skin. Patients may complain of swelling (angio-oedema) of their face, particularly eyelids, lips and tongue, which may last hours or days.

If the skin eruption lasts for more than 24 h, is painful and resolves with bruising then urticarial vasculitis (Figure 5.1) is more likely than ordinary urticaria (Figure 5.2).

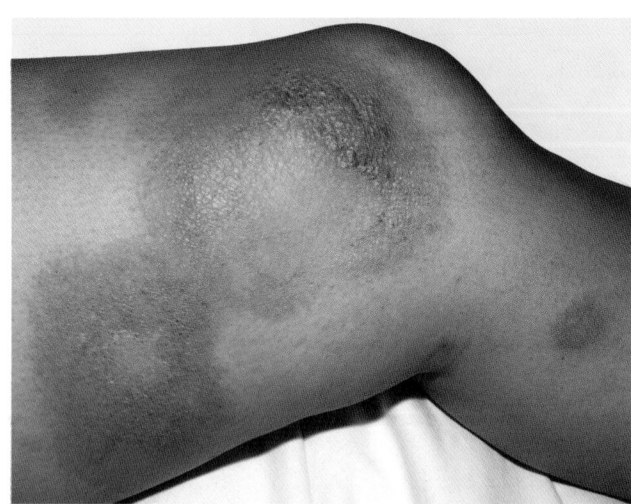

Figure 5.1 Urticarial vasculitis with bruising.

ABC of Dermatology, Sixth Edition. Edited by Rachael Morris-Jones.

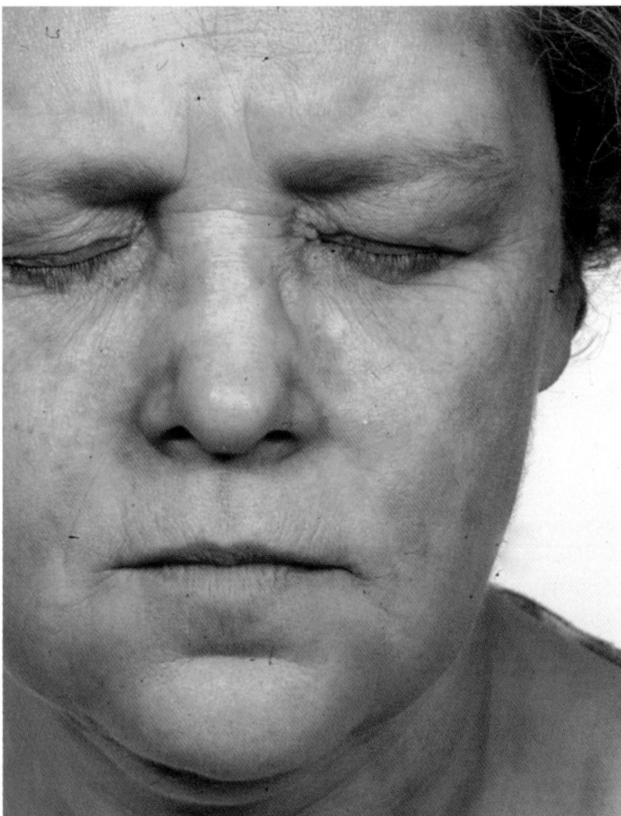

Figure 5.2 Ordinary urticaria.

Box 5.1 **Causes of non-physical urticaria**

- Food allergies: fish, eggs, dairy products, nuts and strawberries.
- Food additives: tartrazine dyes and sodium benzoates
- Salicylates: medication and foods.
- Infections: viral, bacterial and protozoal.
- Systemic disorders: autoimmune, connective tissue disease and carcinoma.
- Contact urticaria: meat, fish, vegetables and plants.
- Papular urticaria: persistent urticaria often secondary to insect bites.
- Aeroallergens: pollens, house dust mite and animal dander.

Box 5.2 **Causes of physical urticaria**

- Heat.
- Sunlight.
- Cold.
- Pressure.
- Water.

Patients may feel unwell before the onset of the rash or swelling and rarely in severe reactions anaphylaxis can occur. You should always ask about any associated respiratory distress. An attempt to identify possible triggers before the onset of symptoms is important. In particular, ask about any food eaten (nausea/vomiting), exercise, heat/cold, sun, medications/infusions, latex exposure, insect stings, animal contact, physical stimuli, infections, family history and any known medical conditions (Figures 5.3 and 5.4).

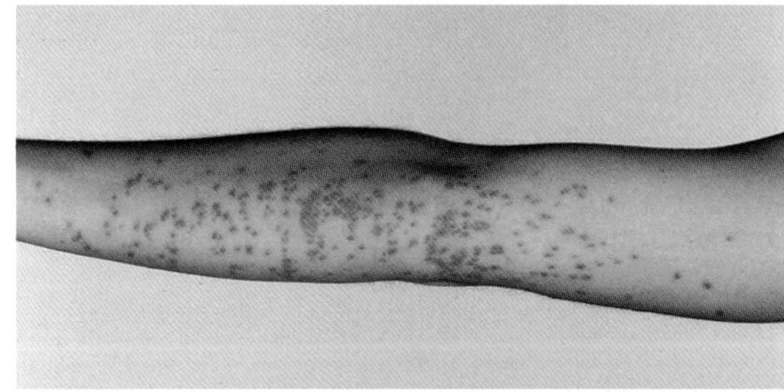

Figure 5.3 Urticaria from contact with brown caterpillar moths.

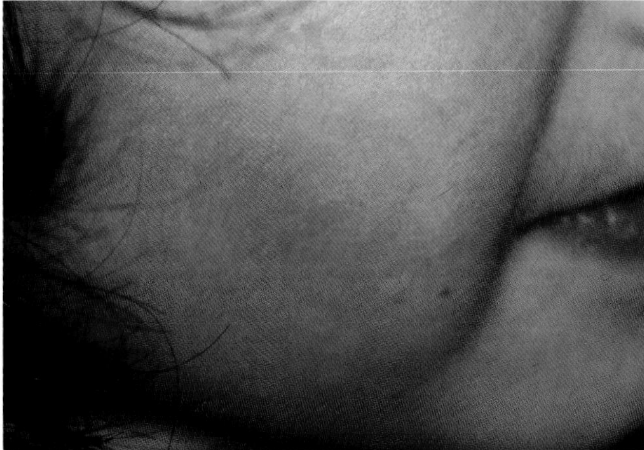

Figure 5.4 Cold-induced urticaria on the cheeks.

Classification of urticaria

Urticaria is traditionally classified as acute or chronic depending on whether symptoms last for less or more than 6 weeks. Another approach is to classify urticaria according to the underlying cause, but in 50% of cases no cause is identified (idiopathic). Urticaria can therefore broadly be divided into ordinary/idiopathic (acute/chronic), contact allergic, cholinergic, physical or urticarial vasculitis. See Boxes 5.1 and 5.2.

Ordinary urticaria

This is the most common form of urticaria characterised by intermittent fleeting wheals at any skin site, with or without angio-oedema (Figures 5.2 and 5.5). Lesions may be papular, annular (Figure 5.6) and even serpiginous. The urticarial lesions themselves last minutes to hours only and may recur over <6 weeks – acute urticaria, or attacks may become chronic (>6 weeks). In 50% of patients with ordinary urticaria no underlying cause is found. Possible triggers of acute urticaria include infections, vaccinations, medications and food. Generally, the more persistent the attacks of urticaria, the less likely that an underlying cause is identified; this is termed *chronic idiopathic urticaria*.

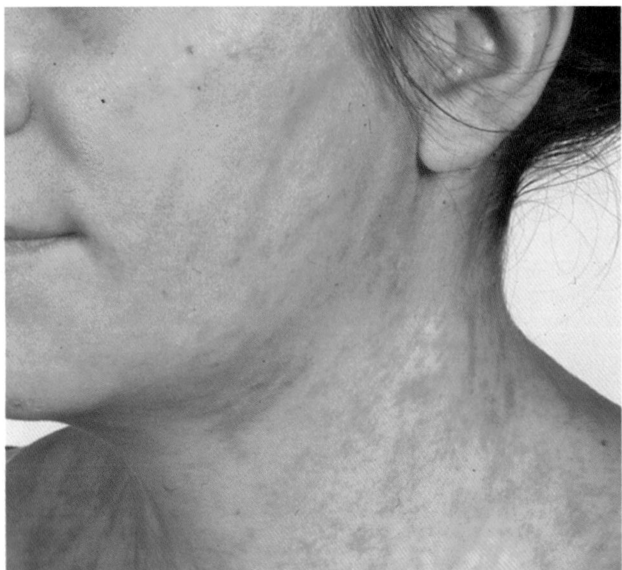

Figure 5.5 Ordinary urticaria with dermatographism.

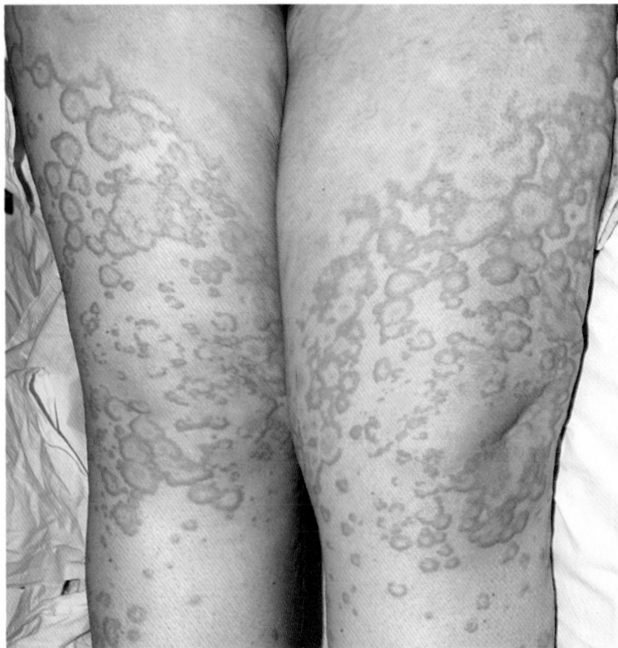

Figure 5.6 Annular urticaria.

Cholinergic urticaria

Patients are usually aged 10–30 years and typically report urticaria following a warm shower/bath, or after exercise. Patients report erythema and burning pruritus followed by extensive urticaria. The lesions consist of pinhead-sized wheals with a red flare around them. The underlying trigger is not fully understood, but deficiency in α_1-antitrypsin may predispose to urticaria in which sweat has been show to play a role and where serum histamine levels are raised following exertion. Avoidance of heat usually helps reduce the frequency and severity of symptoms.

A rarer form of cholinergic urticaria can result from exposure to the cold. Patients report urticaria on exposed skin during cold weather, lip/tongue/hand swelling following the holding and ingestion of cold beverages and a more generalised reaction following swimming in an outdoor pool. Affected individuals should avoid swimming in cold water and ingestion of ice-cold drinks as anaphylaxis and death have been reported.

Solar urticaria

Solar urticaria is a rare condition in which sunlight causes an acute urticarial eruption. Patients complain of stinging, burning and itching at exposed skin sites within 30 min of ultraviolet or artificial light source exposure. Lesions resolve rapidly (minutes to hours) when light exposure ceases. Photosensitive drug eruptions can present in a similar manner; so, a detailed drug history is important. Differential diagnosis may include porphyria (lesions resolve with scarring) and polymorphic light eruption (lesions take days to weeks to resolve). The pathophysiology is poorly understood but is thought to be mediated by antigen production as serum transfer can induce similar symptoms in asymptomatic controls. Light-testing confirms the diagnosis. Management can be difficult but avoidance of sunlight is helpful.

Pressure urticaria

Urticarial wheals occur at the site of pressure on the skin, characteristically around the waistband area (from clothing), shoulders (from carrying a backpack), soles of feet (from walking), hands (using tools or weight lifting), buttocks (from sitting) and genitals (sexual intercourse). The urticarial rash may occur immediately but a delay of up to 6 h can occur (delayed pressure urticaria), and lesions resolve over several days. Symptoms are usually recurrent over many years. The cause is unknown and although histamine is thought to play a role, patients are less likely to respond to antihistamines than in other forms of urticaria. Eosinophils and interleukin are thought to play a role. Investigation can include pressure challenge testing. Patients may respond to dapsone or montelukast.

Angio-oedema

Patients present with swelling plus or minus urticaria that develops over hours and resolves over days. Angio-oedema causes well-demarcated swelling of the subcutaneous tissues (Figure 5.7) and/or mucous membranes, from increased vascular permeability. A detailed drug history should be taken because allergy to medication (Angiotensin converting enzyme inhibitors, Non-steroidal anti-inflammatory drugs, bupropion, statins or proton pump inhibitors) may be the cause. Laryngeal swelling is the most serious complication and should ideally be managed by emergency medicine specialists.

A hereditary form of angio-oedema presents in young persons as recurrent severe attacks affecting the skin and mucous membranes. Tingling, tightness and pain are the main symptoms associated with the oedema. Patients may suffer associated gastrointestinal symptoms and life-threatening laryngeal oedema. Hereditary angio-oedema is caused by a deficiency in C1 (esterase) inhibitor. Serum complement C4 levels are low following attacks. Danazol can be used to reduce the frequency and severity of attacks and fresh frozen plasma can be used before elective surgery.

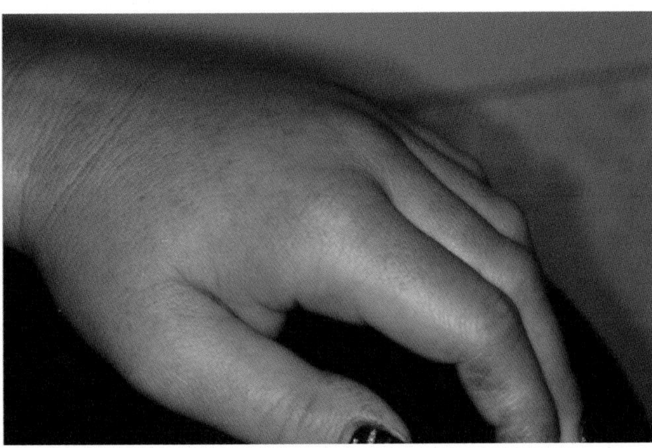

Figure 5.7 Angio-oedema of the hand.

General investigations

Apart from a detailed history and examination most patients need no further investigations. If food allergy is suspected patients can be asked to keep a food diary, particularly if their urticaria is recurrent and episodic. An attempt to elicit dermatographism (exaggerated release of histamine causing wheal and flare) should be made by firmly stroking the skin with a hard object such as the end of a pen; this is usually positive in physical urticaria (Figure 5.8).

A skin biopsy can be useful if urticarial vasculitis is suspected; plain lidocaine should be used for the local anaesthetic (as adrenaline causes release of histamine from mast cells). Histology from urticaria may show dermal oedema and vasodilatation. In urticarial vasculitis, there is a cellular infiltrate of lymphocytes, polymorphs and histiocytes.

In patients with more severe reactions a RAST (radioallergosorbent test) or skin prick testing (although not in patients with anaphylaxis) may help identify specific allergies. In addition, patch testing to identify contact urticaria can be undertaken in specialist centres.

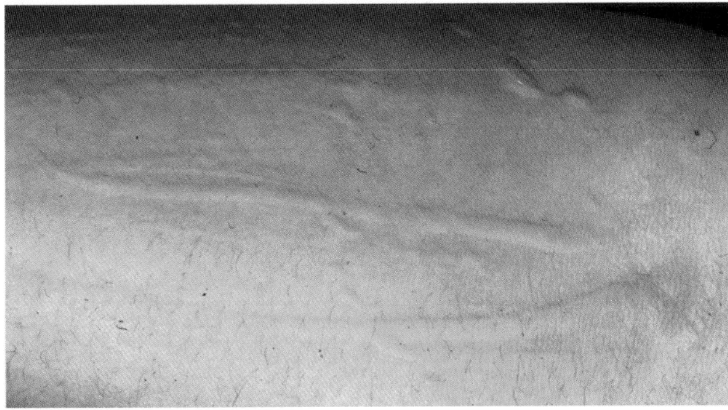

Figure 5.8 Dermatographism.

If you suspect hereditary angio-oedema check the complement C3 level and C1 esterase which are usually low.

If heat or cold are the possible precipitants then exercising for 5 min or placing an ice-cube on the skin for 20 min may be diagnostic. Physical urticaria can be elicited by firm pressure on the skin. Solar urticaria can be assessed in specialist centres using a solar simulator.

General management

Patients often make their own observations concerning trigger factors, especially food, medication and insect stings, and know what they should try to avoid. Treatment of any underlying medical condition identified should help settle the urticaria. Oral antihistamines are the mainstay of treatment/prevention of urticaria and angio-oedema. Patients can manage their own symptoms by purchasing antihistamines (cetirizine, loratadine or chlorphenamine) over the counter.

In severe recalcitrant cases, physicians may need to prescribe synergistic combinations of H1-receptor blockers (as above plus desloratadine, levocetirizine, terfenadine or hydroxyzine) plus H2 blockade (ranitidine or cimetidine) and leukotriene receptor antagonists (montelukast or zafirlukast) to control symptoms. Depending on the frequency of symptoms, antihistamines may be taken prophylactically daily or intermittently to treat symptoms.

Oral corticosteroids may be indicated in very severe eruptions, particularly those associated with urticarial vasculitis.

Patients known to be at risk of severe life-threatening urticaria/angio-oedema with respiratory distress may be asked to carry with them a pre-assembled syringe and needle (EpiPen®, or Anapen®) to inject adrenaline intramuscularly (300–500 μg). Management of the patient's airway is critical and once secured, oxygen and if necessary further intramuscular/intravenous adrenaline can then be administered by medical professionals.

Phase II clinical trials of single-dose subcutaneous omalizumab have shown encouraging results in patients whose urticaria is recalcitrant to the effects of H1-blockers.

Further reading

www.allergy-clinic.co.uk/urticaria

Kaplan AP, Greaves MW. *Urticaria and Angioedema.* Marcel Dekker Ltd., New York, 2004.

Zuberbier T, Grattan C, Maurer M. *Urticaria and Angioedema.* Springer, Heidelberg, 2010.

CHAPTER 6

Skin and Photosensitivity

Rachael Morris-Jones

Dermatology Department, Kings College Hospital, London, UK

OVERVIEW

- Ultraviolet radiation is a recognised carcinogen and the paler someone's skin the more susceptible they are to 'sun-damage'.
- Genetically inherited disorders such as albinism and xeroderma pigmentosum leave the skin and eyes vulnerable to UV light.
- Photosensitive eruptions have a typical appearance on sun exposed sites and can occur in any skin type.
- Photoprotection with clothing and sunscreen is important for vulnerable individuals.

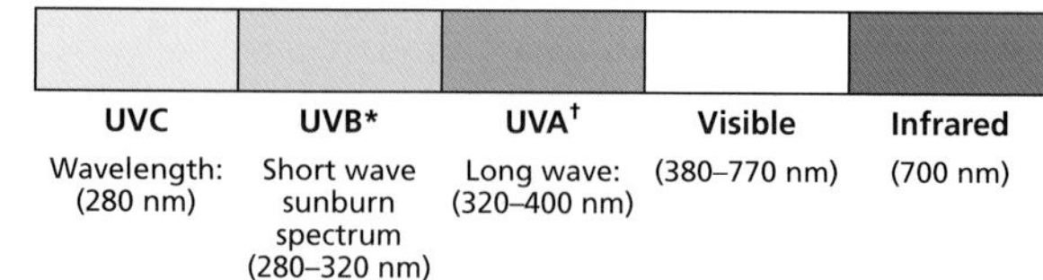

* The UVB band (280–320 nm) is responsible for erythema, sunburn, tanning and skin malignancy

† UVA light (320–400 nm) has the greatest penetration into the dermis and augments UVB erythema and skin malignancy

Figure 6.1 Light spectrum.

The term photosensitive is used to describe patients with cutaneous disorders that result from exposure to normal levels of ultraviolet (UV) light. Sun-exposed skin is predominately affected in acquired photosensitivity, particularly of the face, neck, dorsi of the arms/hands and lower legs. There is marked sparing of sun-protected sites, particularly the buttocks, behind the ears and under the chin, which can provide useful diagnostic clues.

Skin tolerance of UV light will depend on a number of factors including the intensity of UV light, skin type (Fitzpatrick skin types classified according to inherited levels of skin pigmentation), genetic disorders (sun-damage repair mechanisms may be defective), acquired allergic conditions and photosensitising medications.

Taking a thorough history of sun exposure and reactions to it is important in patients with suspected photosensitivity. Patients may not develop symptoms unless they are exposed to high intensity sunlight whereas others will be affected throughout the year with low intensity UV exposure. The time to onset of symptoms following UV exposure is an important part of the history as are the course of any skin eruption (frequency and duration) and whether any scarring or marks are left behind on the skin following the acute phase. Symptoms of itching, burning and even pain can be reported.

This chapter considers cutaneous disorders related to UV light; however, precancerous and cancerous skin lesions are discussed elsewhere (Chapters 21 and 22).

ABC of Dermatology, Sixth Edition. Edited by Rachael Morris-Jones.

Ultraviolet radiation

UV A and B radiation penetrate the earth's atmosphere and are known to play a role in sun-induced skin damage (Figure 6.1). UV intensity is greatest near the equator and at high altitudes. Environmental factors such as the season, time of day and reflective surfaces (water, snow and sand) can influence the intensity of UV light. There is evidence that holes in the ozone layer have led to pockets of high intensity UV.

UVB has a short wavelength and varies according to the season. UVB levels are at their highest in the summer months and during the middle of the day. UVB is important in both sunburn and the development of skin cancer. UVA has a longer wavelength and is present all year round and throughout the day at fairly constant levels. UVA can pass through glass and is known to induce immediate and persistent pigment darkening, delayed tanning and skin ageing. There is increasing evidence that UVA also plays a role in skin cancer development.

UV light can cause immediate effects on the skin in the form of photosensitivity and sunburn, and long-term effects such as skin ageing (wrinkling and solar keratoses) and skin cancer.

Fitzpatrick skin type classification

Natural skin pigmentation is formed by melanin which is synthesised by melanocytes. The quantity of melanin in the skin determines its ability to withstand UV radiation. In healthy skin, the number of melanocytes remains constant; however, the amount of melanin they synthesise is genetically determined, leading to different levels of skin pigmentation. Fitzpatrick devised a classification based on skin type according to inherited pigmentation and the skin's response to UV light. Patients with type I skin are likely to burn even if the UV intensity is low, whereas patients with type VI skin will not usually suffer sun-damage. An assessment of a patient's skin type will help the physician determine the patient's susceptibility to UV as well as in guiding certain therapies, such as phototherapy and laser treatments. Fitzpatrick skin type can be used to determine the starting doses and increments of UVA/TL-01 during phototherapy.

- Type I (very fair skin/freckled/red hair) – always burns, never tans.
- Type II (fair skin) – usually burns, tans eventually.
- Type III (fair to olive skin) – occasionally burns, tans easily.
- Type IV (brown skin) – rarely burns, tans easily.
- Type V (dark brown skin) – very rarely burns, tans easily.
- Type VI (black skin) – never burns, tans easily.

Genetic disorders causing photosensitivity

Oculocutaneous albinism

Genetic mutations that control melanin synthesis, distribution and degradation result in a group of inherited disorders that lead to loss of skin/hair/eye pigment. Oculocutaneous albinism is an autosomal recessive condition characterised by little or absent melanin pigment at birth (Figure 6.2). Oculocutaneous albinism affects skin, hair and ocular pigmentation, resulting in sun-induced skin changes, photophobia, nystagmus and reduced visual acuity.

Oculocutaneous albinism is traditionally classified into two groups – tyrosinase positive or negative – depending on whether the enzyme is absent or dysfunctional; however, there are numerous subtypes depending on the specific genetic mutation.

Affected individuals should be assessed in the neonatal period by a dermatologist and an ophthalmologist. The family may wish to consult a geneticist. A sunscreen blocking UVA and UVB light (broad-spectrum) should be applied to the skin on a daily basis and reapplied as necessary. Protective clothing and sun avoidance behaviour should be encouraged. Skin checks for any evidence of sun-damage or skin cancer should be undertaken regularly. Corrective spectacles may improve visual acuity.

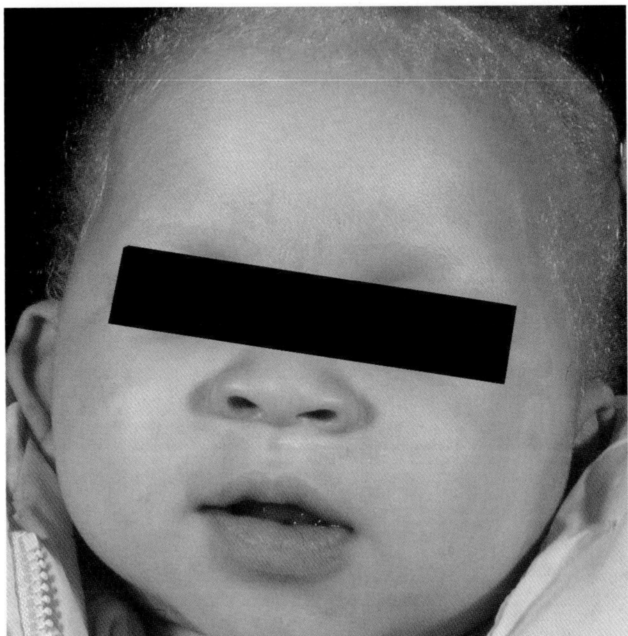

Figure 6.2 Oculocutaneous albinism.

Other genetic conditions associated with loss of skin pigment include piebaldism, phenylketonuria, tuberous sclerosis and Waardenburg and Apert syndromes.

Xeroderma pigmentosum

A group of autosomal recessive conditions result from deficient cutaneous nucleotide excision repair mechanisms which lead to defective DNA repair. Patients have accelerated UV-associated changes in the skin characterised by photosensitivity, pigmentary changes, premature skin ageing and tumour formation during the first decade of life. Ocular damage also results from photosensitivity. The diagnosis is usually apparent between the ages of 1 and 2 years. Early signs of the disorder include excessive persistent sunburn, freckling, mottled pigmentation (poikiloderma), telangiectasia and skin thinning. Later, patients develop multiple skin cancers including melanoma and squamous and basal cell carcinomas. Early ocular signs include photosensitivity and conjunctivitis and later fibrosis and malignancies. Patients may also suffer from neurological problems including deafness and mental retardation. Strict sun avoidance (skin and eyes) is paramount for these patients. Photoprotective clothing, broad-rimmed hats, sunglasses and physical sunscreen should be regularly used. Oral retinoids can help reduce the rate and number of skin cancers. The use of imiquimod and 5-fluorouricil to treat the sun-damaged skin has been shown to help reduce skin tumour development. In the future, it may be possible to correct DNA damage by delivering topical liposomal DNA repair enzymes. Ultimately, gene therapy may be utilised to manage this disease.

Metabolic disorders of photosensitivity

Porphyrias are a group of disorders associated with the accumulation of intermediate metabolites in the metabolic pathway of haem biosynthesis. Most porphyrias are inherited but some may be triggered by alcohol, oestrogens or hepatitis on a background of hereditary predisposition.

The most common form is porphyria cutanea tarda, which results in photosensitivity (Figure 6.3). Patients develop cutaneous fragility and blisters that heal with scarring, pigment changes and milia on sun-exposed skin, particularly on the face and dorsi of the hands. Patients may have scarring alopecia, facial hypertrichosis and onycholysis. Men with excessive alcohol intake are most frequently affected.

Hepatic porphyrias lead to skin fragility and blistering from exposure to sunlight or minor trauma. Patients with erythropoietic and erythrohepatic photoporphyrias are highly photosensitive (Figures 6.4 and 6.5) to UVB and UVA (the latter can pass through the glass of windows of a house/car). Patients with acute intermittent porphyria do not have cutaneous involvement.

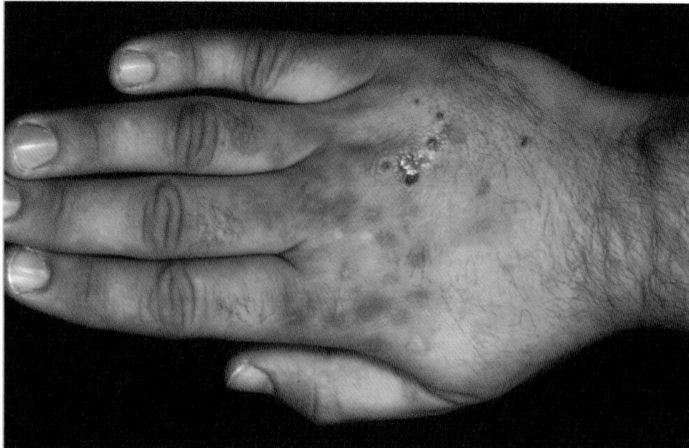

Figure 6.3 Porphyia cutanea tarda hand.

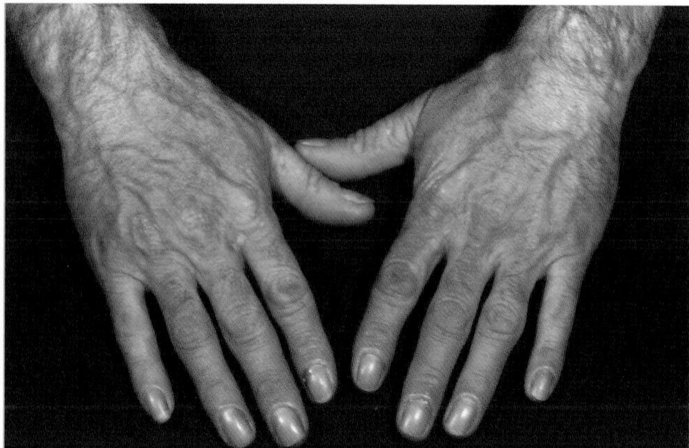

Figure 6.4 Erythropoietic porphyria.

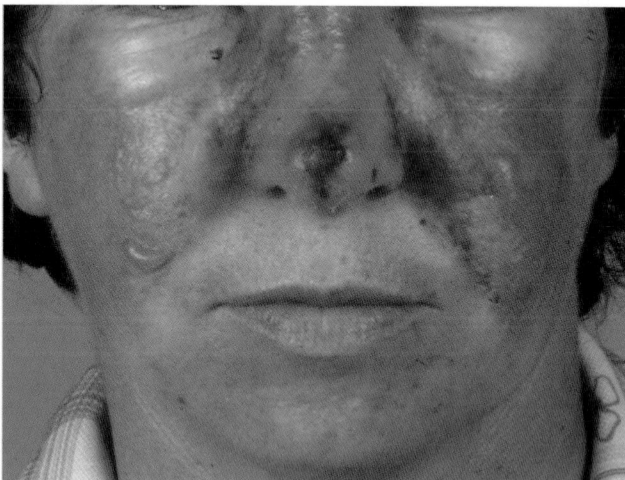

Figure 6.5 Varigate porphyria.

Patients need to be given sun avoidance advice including keeping out of midday sun, protective tight-weave clothing (long sleeves, gloves and hat), high factor broad-spectrum sunscreen (Dundee cream), application of tinted films to windows, β-carotene and avoidance of precipitants.

Exogenous substances causing photosensitivity

Medications causing photosensitivity

Topical and systemic medications can lead to localised and generalised photosensitive eruptions (see Chapter 7) (Figure 6.6). The combination of UV light and the chemicals result in a skin reaction. Reactions may be rapid onset phototoxic (occur in most individuals if they are exposed to sufficient drug doses and UV – resembles sunburn) or delayed photoallergic (can occur even at low drug doses, reaction is eczematous, resembles allergic type IV hypersensitivity contact dermatitis) reactions. Phototoxic reactions are confined to the sun-exposed skin only whereas photoallergic reactions can spread from the sun-exposed to sun-protected areas in severe reactions. Some drug-induced skin reactions appear lichenoid in nature with multiple purplish papules occurring on sun-exposed sites. Skin biopsy from affected skin shows lichenoid changes consistent with a lichenoid drug eruption.

Pseudoporphyria can be induced by medications and haemodialysis. Clinically, pseudoporphyria resembles porphyria cutanea tarda, which is characterised by fragile skin with blisters on sun-exposed sites, in the absence of raised porphyrins. Medications can induce or reactivate subacute cutaneous lupus (SCLE) which presents with erythematous annular scaly lesions usually on the upper trunk. More than 100 medications have been reported to cause SCLE, but most commonly hydrochlorothiazide, calcium channel blockers, angiotensin-converting enzyme inhibitors,

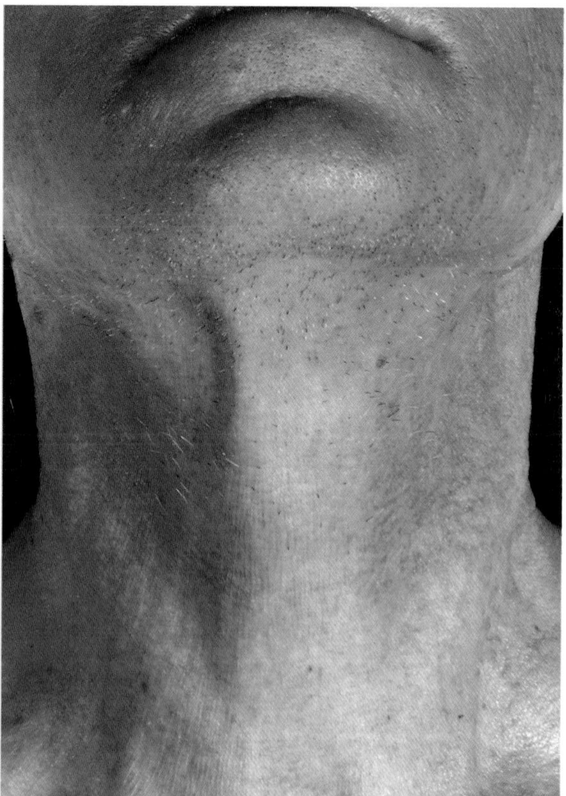

Figure 6.6 Photosensitive drug eruption (sparing under the chin).

terbinafine and tumour necrosis factor antagonists. In all cases of severe photosensitive drug reactions, the medication should be stopped if possible. Once the skin condition has settled with topical/oral steroids then the culprit drug may only be cautiously reintroduced in the context of vigorous photoprotection using clothing, sunscreen and sun avoidance.

Medication	Phototoxic reaction	Photoallergic reaction	Other reactions
Amiodarone	Yes	No	Pseudoporphyria
Ciprofloxacin	Yes	No	
Diltiazem	Yes	No	Subacute lupus
Enalapril	No	No	Subacute lupus
Furosemide	Yes	No	Pseudoporphyria
Imatinib	No	No	Pseudoporphyria and skin lightening
Isotretinoin	Yes	No	
Itraconazole	Yes	Yes	
Naproxen	Yes	No	Lichenoid eruption
Oral contraceptive	No	Yes	Pseudoporphyria
Phenothiazines	Yes	Yes	Lichenoid eruption
Salicylates	No	Yes	
Statins	Yes	Yes	Lichenoid eruption
Sulphonylureas	No	Yes	Pseudoporphyria
Tetracyclines	Yes	No	Lichenoid eruption Photo-onycholysis
Voriconazole	Yes	No	Pseudoporphyria

Phytophotodermatitis

Phytophotodermatitis is an acute onset blistering skin rash resulting from photosensitizing plant material in contact with the skin plus UVA light (Figure 6.7). This is a phototoxic skin reaction not requiring any previous exposure to the plant. Children and agricultural works are particularly affected because of outdoor activities. Implicated plant materials include meadow grass, common rue, poison ivy/oak, celery, parsley, lemons and limes. The cutaneous rashes usually appear within hours of exposure and present with blisters on an erythematous background, which looks exogenous with bizarre linear streaks on the legs and 'drip marks' down the arms. Phytophotodermatitis should be treated with a potent topical steroid and the causative plant material subsequently avoided on the skin if possible.

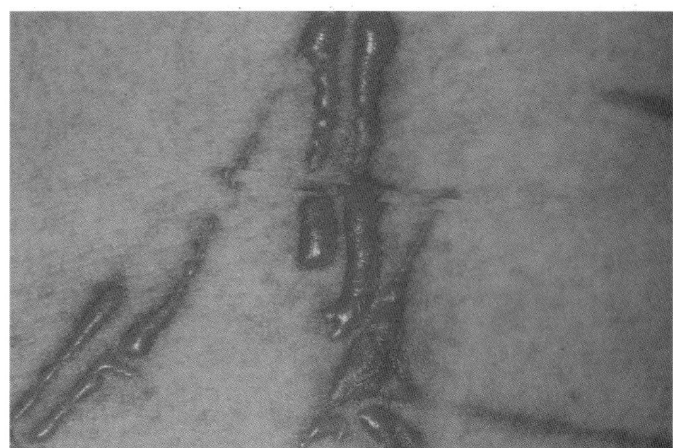

Figure 6.7 Phytophotodermatitis to lime juice.

Idiopathic disorders causing photosensitivity

Polymorphous light eruption (PMLE)

Polymorphous light eruption (PMLE) manifests as a pruritic papulovesicular reaction on exposed skin after sunlight exposure in the early spring/summer. The underling cause of PMLE is not fully understood but there is evidence that it is an allergic type IV hypersensitivity reaction to sunlight. UVA is the most common trigger; however, there are reports of UVB and UVC (from welding devices) causing PMLE. The disease is most common in women in the first three decades. Any skin type can be affected. PMLE is triggered after 30 min to a few hours of exposure to sunlight or occasionally an artificial UV source. The rash is itchy and most commonly affects the forearms and anterior neck. The rash is usually papular – but as its name suggests this disorder can have a varied morphology, including blisters and widespread inflamed oedematous lesions (Figure 6.8a and b). The eruption of PMLE

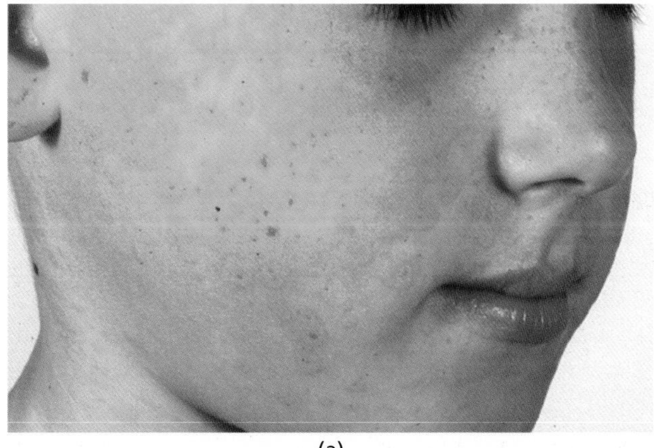

(a)

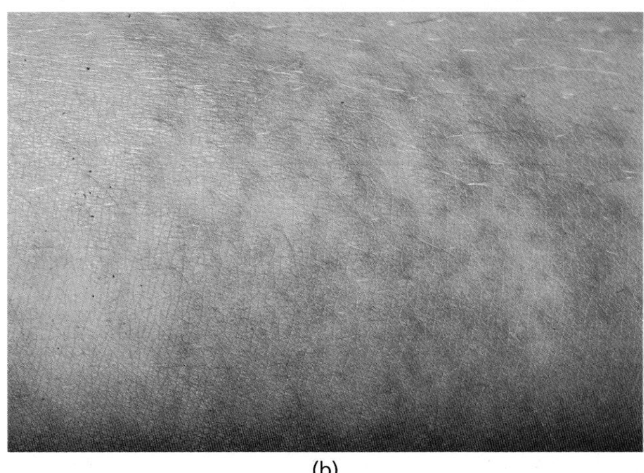

(b)

Figure 6.8 (a) Polymorphous light eruption (PMLE). (b). PMLE papular and erythematous eruption.

usually takes several weeks to resolve and heals without scarring, although post-inflammatory pigment changes can result.

Management includes sun avoidance, seeking shade, protective clothing and sunscreens; topical or even oral corticosteroids may be needed in severe cases. A course of desensitizing TL-01 (narrow-band UVB) or PUVA (oral psoralen plus UVA) prior to sun exposure the following year can be effective. Recent studies have shown that a combination of topical antioxidant plus sunscreen was more effective than either component alone. Topical vitamin D and E have also been applied to sun-exposed skin for secondary prophylaxis effects with some success.

Solar urticaria

This relatively rare photoallergic skin condition presents with rapid onset of an itchy, stinging erythema and urticaria following less than 30 min of sun exposure (or an artificial light source). Careful history-taking is the key to making the diagnosis as the rash is transient, resolving within minutes or hours after retreating from the light. A wide range of UV wavelengths can reportedly trigger the reaction, which is thought to be antigen mediated. Studies have shown that injection of serum from those affected into the dermis of healthy individuals can passively transfer the condition. The diagnosis can be confirmed by a solar simulator or TL-01 light tests. Solar urticaria can be very debilitating and difficult to manage. Patients quickly learn to avoid sunlight and often become reclusive. Oral antihistamines, high factor broad-spectrum sunscreen and, paradoxically, phototherapy may prevent or control symptoms.

Chronic actinic dermatitis (CAD)

Middle-aged or elderly men are most commonly affected by this itchy photosensitive eruption that affects the face, posterior and 'V' of the neck, and dorsi of the hands (Figure 6.9). Sunlight all year round can trigger chronic actinic dermatitis (CAD), and consequently the rash usually resembles chronic lichenified eczema. UVB, UVA, visible and artificial light sources have all been implicated; therefore, sunscreen should be used daily all year round and even if patients remain indoors. Patch and photopatch testing can be very useful in identifying compounding contact allergies, especially to compositae plants (daisy family), perfumes, sunscreen and colophony (pine trees and elastoplast). Apart from sun-protective measures, patients should be managed in a similar way to those with eczema, with topical steroids and emollients. Patients may, however, require short courses of systemic corticosteroids and in recalcitrant cases, azathioprine may be needed.

Photoprotective behaviour

The benefits versus dangers of UV exposure are hotly debated within the field of medicine. Some experts suggest that the only safe tan is an artificial one whist others argue vitamin D levels may be inadequate and the frequency of some systemic cancers increased if the sun is avoided.

Although not universal, current fashions in many societies view a tanned skin as desirable and 'healthy'. Fifty years ago, a tanned skin was mainly a consequence of outdoor work. Nowadays, a tanned skin is associated with increased leisure time, relative ease of travel to sunny climates and deliberate tanning through sun-bed use. There is, however, some evidence that the link between skin ageing and UV exposure is increasingly recognised by women who photo-protect to stay looking younger for longer.

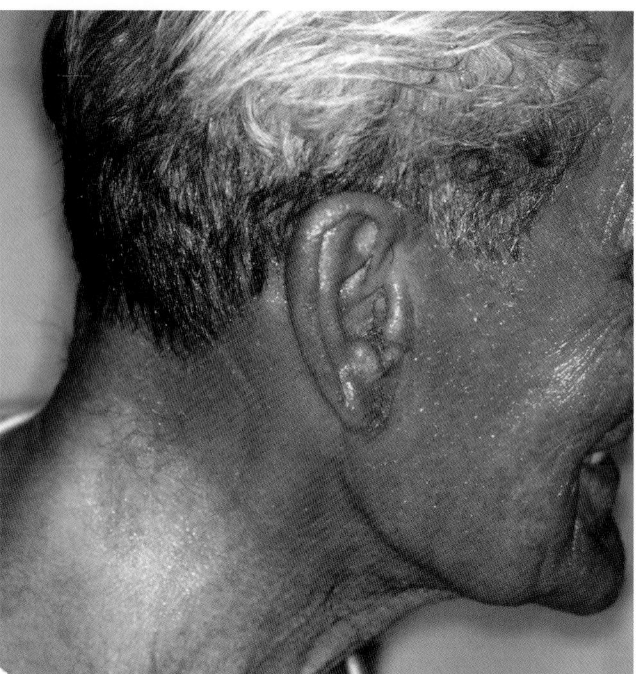

Figure 6.9 Chronic actinic dermatitis.

A sensible approach to sun protection is advisable according to each individual's susceptibility to burning and ability to tan. Fitzpatrick skin type shows that those with type I skin are more at risk than those with type VI skin. Simple measures to avoid excessive UV exposure in susceptible individuals include avoidance of midday sun (between 11 AM and 3 PM), sitting in the shade (equivalent to SPF 9, i.e. not 'out of the sun'), protective clothing (tighter weaves give greater protection), regular application of sunscreen and sun-protective eyewear.

Vitamin D levels and systemic disease

Over the past decade, there has been growing concern amongst physicians that Vitamin D deficiency may be linked to underlying diseases such as multiple sclerosis, allergic asthma, type I diabetes and numerous systemic cancers. Consequently, advising individuals to avoid sunlight exposure to limit the incidence of skin cancer has come into question. The majority of human vitamin D is attained through sunlight (UVB, resulting in metabolism of vitamin D within the exposed skin) rather than diet. The amount of Vitamin D metabolised in the skin depends on multiple factors including the intensity of the UVB, exposure time, Fitzpatrick skin type, surface area of skin exposed and current level of serum Vitamin D. 25(OH) vitamin D_3 is the storage form of the enzyme and reflects an individual's vitamin status. Measurement of serum vitamin D levels is technically difficult and varies from one laboratory to another. This has hampered global attempts to define the normal range for serum vitamin D in a population. The current consensus is that normal adult 25(OH) vitamin D should be above 50 nmol/l (20 ng/ml) for healthy bones; however, levels required for a healthy immune, cardiovascular system and anti-tumour activity is less well defined. It has been suggested that levels greater than 75 nmol/l should be sufficient.

To date, studies where vitamin D supplementation has been given to patients with multiple sclerosis, asthma and type I diabetes have been disappointing in their results. Some researchers have therefore concluded that the cause of these systemic diseases may not be vitamin D deficiency itself but some other immunoregulatory effect from UV. Advice to patients on safe/desirable levels of sun exposure must be made on an individual basis with the general consensus favouring prolonged exposure to small areas of skin rather than repeated short exposure to large areas of skin. A sensible approach would be moderate sunlight exposure (avoiding sunburn) and supplementation of vitamin D through dietary supplementation and/or fortification of common foods (such as bread, butter or milk).

Sunscreen

Sunscreens are formulated to protect the skin from UV radiation. However, some experts believe that when people apply sunscreen they stay out in higher intensity UV light for longer than they would without the sunscreen, and therefore its use may in fact increase their sun-seeking behaviour.

There are two main types of sunscreen – physical and chemical. As a general rule, physical sunscreens look opaque when applied to the skin and are therefore viewed as less cosmetically acceptable; however, they are highly effective and generally hypoallogenic. Chemical sunscreens are more likely to cause skin irritation or allergy.

Physical sunscreens contain minute particles of titanium dioxide or zinc/ferric oxide that reflect and scatter UV radiation. Chemical sunscreens contain combinations of *p*-amino benzoic acid (PABA), cinnamates and benzophenones that absorb UV radiation.

The degree of protection provided by each sunscreen is formally measured in terms of its UVB (SPF number) and UVA (number or star rating) blocking activity. SPF is the ratio of the minimum UV radiation required to cause minimal skin erythema, with and without sunscreen. The level of protections is calculated by using a specific number of grams of cream applied to a specific surface area of skin and irradiated with a known dose of UV. Unfortunately, there is evidence that in reality individuals do not apply their sunscreen in similar quantities and therefore tend to achieve 1/3 to $^1/_2$ of the predicted SPF/star rating specified on the bottle.

The apparent failure of sunscreens to protect the skin from sun-damage usually results from not using high protection sunscreen, inadequate application (not put on before going outside, insufficient amounts, infrequently reapplied), washed off by water/sweat and breakdown of photoprotective chemicals by UV light itself.

Further reading

Collignon LN and Normand CB. *Photobiology: Principles, Applications and Effects*. Nova Science Publishers, New York, 2010.

Lim HW, Honigsmann H and Hawk JLM. *Photodermatology (Basic and Clinical Dermatology)*, Informa Healthcare, New York, 2007.

CHAPTER 7

Drug Rashes

Sarah Walsh

Dermatology Consultant, Kings College Hospital, London, UK

OVERVIEW

- Drug reactions in the skin are common. Cutaneous adverse reactions account for a third of all adverse reactions to drugs.
- Drugs can cause adverse reactions in several ways: by changing normal skin function, by exacerbating an existing dermatosis, by causing an idiopathic dermatosis such as urticaria, by causing a specific drug eruption (lichenoid drug rashes) or by precipitating a severe drug reaction (toxic epidermal necrolysis).
- Identifying the culprit drug requires careful history-taking and knowledge of the notoriety of certain drugs in the causation of certain reactions.
- Careful skin examination is required to identify the morphology of the rash and the correct classification of the drug reaction.
- The most important step in management of drug rashes is identification and withdrawal of the culprit medication.
- Some drug reactions are mild and resolve quickly (maculopapular exanthems); others are more severe and carry considerable morbidity and mortality (Stevens–Johnson syndrome and toxic epidermal necrolysis).

Introduction

Adverse reactions in the skin to medications are very common and are an important cause of iatrogenic illness. Drug rashes are usually self-limiting and resolve completely upon withdrawal of the culprit medication, but a small number (<2%) can cause serious morbidity and mortality. This may not only have medicolegal and economic implications but may undermine the patient's confidence in the prescriber and affect future adherence. Diagnosis of drug-induced skin disease may be difficult for a number of reasons:

- Almost any drug can cause any rash.
- Unrelated drugs can cause similar reactions.
- The same medication can cause a different rash in different individuals.
- Patients may not volunteer information about medicines that they have taken, which they deem not to be relevant (over-the-counter (OTC) preparations and complementary medicines).

ABC of Dermatology, Sixth Edition. Edited by Rachael Morris-Jones.

History

It is imperative to take a thorough history from patients in whom a drug reaction is suspected. Eliciting the temporal association of the ingestion of the drug and the onset of the eruption is key (Table 7.2). Apart from noting any medications taken for the first time in the 3 months prior to the appearance of the rash, patients should be specifically asked about any recent changes to brand, dosing or preparation of long-term medications. Patients may not volunteer information about drugs they have taken that they assume are not relevant, such as paracetamol taken for a headache, or an antihistamine taken for hay fever. Direct questioning about OTC preparations should always form part of a thorough drug history. Medications recommended by alternative/complementary health practitioners may not be revealed spontaneously and should be asked about directly. Both generic and brand names of all drugs should be recorded, and the patient should be asked about any history of sensitivity to medications. Knowledge of whether the patient has been previously exposed to suspected culprit drugs is also relevant.

Examination

The patient should be exposed fully to allow complete examination of the skin. The morphology of the rash should be described – for example, lichenoid, urticated, vasculitic, maculopapular or bullous. The distribution of the rash should be noted: Is it widespread? Limited? Acral (hands and feet)? Photo-distributed? These features will help to classify the eruption and may give a pointer as to the causative drug. Special attention should be paid to the mucosal sites – eyes, mouth, genitalia – as involvement at these sites can indicate one of the severe cutaneous adverse reaction (SCAR) syndromes. Early diagnosis of these syndromes is crucial as patients may become unwell and deteriorate quickly. Careful examination of the appendageal structures such as hair, nails and teeth should also be carried out as these can be affected by certain medications.

Investigations

In most cases, careful history and examination will provide all the necessary clues to make a confident diagnosis of a drug rash. A skin biopsy can be helpful to confirm the diagnosis, but the result of this is likely to be delayed following an acute presentation, and so action based on clinical assessment will usually precede this. Exclusion of differential diagnoses such as infection may require other investigations such as blood tests (white cell counts and CRP levels). There are no consistently reproducible diagnostic tests which confirm specific drug allergy in the convalescent period; however, certain investigations such as measurement of specific IgE, patch testing, intradermal testing and in vitro tests such as lymphocyte transformation tests and cytokine release assays may be helpful. However, these investigations should be carried out by experts as their interpretation is highly specialised.

Classification of drug reactions in the skin

Cutaneous reactions to medications are extremely varied. They may be classified in a number of ways. Pathogenetically, drug reactions in the skin may be classified as *immune-mediated* or *non-immune mediated*. *Immune-mediated* rashes are the most common and include hypersensitivity reactions from types I to IV. Type I reactions (immediate reactions, usually mediated by IgE or drug-specific receptors bound to mast cells and other immune cell membranes) tend to manifest in the skin as urticaria or angio-oedema. Type II reactions (cytotoxic reactions) result in cutaneous purpura. Type III (immune complex-mediated) reactions lead to cutaneous vasculitis. Type IV delayed hypersensitivity reactions are by far the most common group of drug rashes resulting in generalized exanthems, phototoxic rashes and severe drug reactions such as toxic epidermal necrolysis (TEN).

Non-immune-mediated rashes include accumulation of medications in the skin (causing pigment changes), instability of mast cells (causing histamine release), slow acetylators (metabolism of drugs affected) and photosensitivity reactions (increased susceptibility to UV light).

However, drug reactions in the skin may also be classified clinically, and this is the approach adopted here. Drug reactions in the skin are discussed under the following headings:

1 Drugs which alter normal skin function.
2 Drugs which exacerbate an existing dermatosis.
3 Common drug-induced rashes – maculopapular exanthem, urticaria, vasculitis, lichenoid drug reaction and fixed drug eruption.
4 Severe drug-induced rashes – Stevens–Johnson syndrome (SJS) and TEN, acute generalised exanthematous pustulosis (AGEP) and drug reaction with eosinophilia and systemic symptoms (DRESS).

Drugs which alter normal skin function

Photosensitivity

Drugs may cause excessive sensitivity to light in two ways: phototoxic reactions and photoallergic reactions. Phototoxic reactions (Figure 7.1a and b) are the more common, and resemble sunburn and may blister. The reaction is confined to light-exposed sites and may be characterised by a sharp demarcation between covered and uncovered skin. The onset will typically be fast (within 5–15 h of taking the drug and exposure to light) and recovery is quick on withdrawal of the medication. Photoallergic reactions are usually eczematous, but may be lichenoid, uriticarial, purpuric or bullous. The onset may be delayed by weeks or months following introduction of the medication, and similarly, recovery may be slow on withdrawal. Patients taking medication known to cause light sensitivity (amiodarone, tetracycline antibiotics and retinoids) should be advised to avoid excess sun exposure, and to wear a broad-spectrum sun screen year-round. Drugs causing photosensitivity are detailed in Table 7.1.

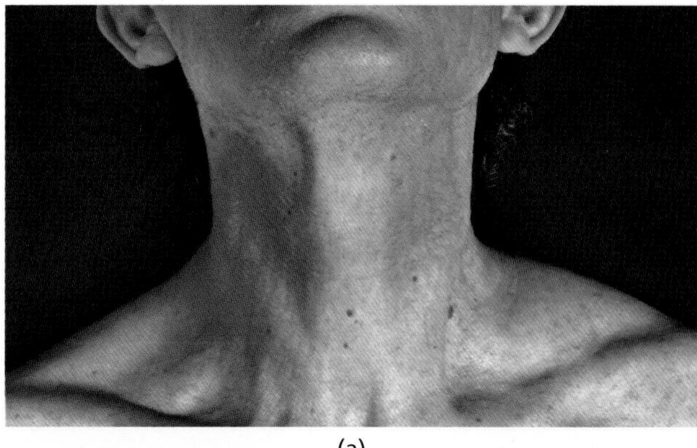

(a)

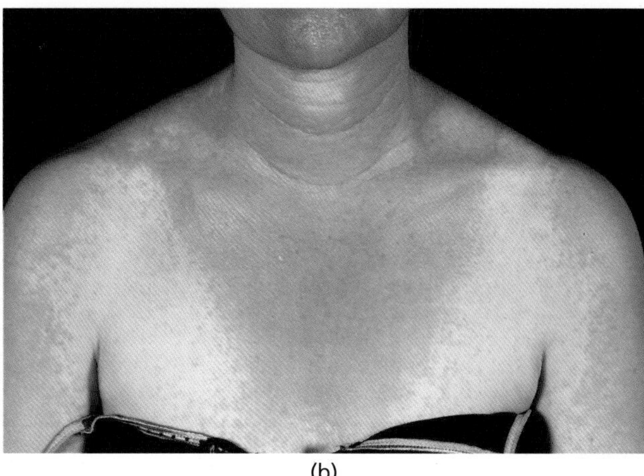

(b)

Figure 7.1 (a) Photosensitive eruption. (b) Phototoxic eruption.

Pigmentation

Hyperpigmentation, hypopigmentation and discolouration are all associated with certain drugs (Figure 7.2). The pigmentary change may require light exposure to manifest. Common examples would include the development of melasma in female patients taking the oral contraceptive pill, or the facial blue-black pigmentation which may be caused by amiodarone. Tetracycline antibiotics may also cause a slate-grey pigmentation. Mechanisms for drug-induced pigmentation are unclear, but may involve deposition of the drug or its metabolite in the dermis, or enhanced melanin production.

Hair and nails

Excessive hair: Hypertrichosis is the growth of hair at sites which are not normally hair-bearing; hirsutism is excessive growth of hair in the male pattern of hair growth, especially in women. Both hormonal and non-hormonal treatments may bring about this

Table 7.1 Cutaneous reactions and the most commonly implicated drugs

Skin reaction	Drugs
Phototoxic reactions	Amiodarone, NSAIDs, tetracyclines, chlorpromazine
Photosensitive reactions	Amiodarone, tetracyclines, calcium channel blockers, diuretics, voriconazole, itraconazole, terbinafine, ritonavir, saquinavir
Photoallergic reactions	NSAIDs, antibiotics, thiazides, anticonvulsants, allopurinol, quinolones, nelfinavir
Pigmentation changes	Chlorpromazine, phenytoin, hydroxychloroquine, cyclofosphamide, bleomycin, amiodarone, clofazimine, minocycline, mepacrine
Urticaria/angio-oedema	NSAIDs, opioid analgesics, ACE inhibitors, antibiotics, anti-retrovirals (didanosine/nelfinavir/zidovudine), infliximab, proton-pump inhibitors, IV contrast media
Drug-induced lupus	Terbinafine, hydralazine, procainamide, quinidine, isoniazid, diltiazem, and minocycline
Drug-induced vasculitis	Antibiotics, NSAIDs, phenytoin, ramipril, proton-pump inhibitors, allopurinol, thiazides, adalimumab, indinavir
Lichenoid drug eruption	Gold, mepacrine, tetracyclines, diuretics, amlodipine, carbamazepine, propranolol, NSAIDs, ACE inhibitors, proton-pump inhibitors, statins
Erythema nodosum	Oral contraceptives, antibiotics, gold, sulphonylurea
Fixed drug eruption	Antibiotics, NSAIDs, oral contraceptive, barbiturates
SJS/TEN	Antibiotics, anticonvulsants, NSAIDs, anti-retrovirals, allopurinol (didanosine/indinavir/saquinavir), barbiturates, ramipril, diltiazem
DRESS	Allopurinol, anticonvulsants, antibiotics, anti-retrovirals, imatinib (Gleevec), NSAIDs, ACE inhibitors, calcium channel blockers, terbinafine
AGEP	Antibiotics, anticonvulsants, anti-tubercular medications

Antibiotics: most commonly sulphonamides, penicillins, ampicillin, tetracyclines and vancomycin.
Anticonvulsants: most commonly phenytoin, carbamazepine, sodium valproate and lamotrigine.
Calcium channel blockers: most commonly diltiazem, nifedipine and amlodipine.
NSAIDs: most commonly aspirin and ibuprofen.

effect; the most commonly implicated would include ciclosporin and phenytoin.

Hair loss: Loss of hair may be dramatic or insidious in onset, and if the latter, may not be immediately noticed by the patient. The temporal relationship between the onset of the hair loss and the introduction of the medication depends on the part of the hair cycle which the drug is interfering with. Cytotoxic agents interrupt the anagen ('growth') phase of the hair cycle, and so loss is rapid and complete; delayed, insidious hair loss generally results from interference with the telogen ('shedding') phase of the hair cycle. Drugs such as acitretin, statins and anti-thyroid drugs may have this effect. Androgenic drugs promote shrinkage of the hair follicles and shortening of anagen, and so can cause hair loss. An example would be exogenously administered testosterone used to treat hypogonadism in male patients.

Table 7.2 Time from drug commencement to drug rash.

Time to onset of rash after starting the drug	Cutaneous drug reaction
Hours/days	Urticaria/angio-oedema, contact urticaria, fixed drug eruption, vasculitis/urticarial vasculitis
Weeks	Toxic erythema, Stevens–Johnson syndrome, toxic epidermal necrolysis, erythema multiforme, acute generalized exanthematous pustulosis, contact dermatitis, erythroderma, photosensitive eruptions
Months	DRESS, Stevens–Johnson syndrome, pigmentation changes, contact dermatitis

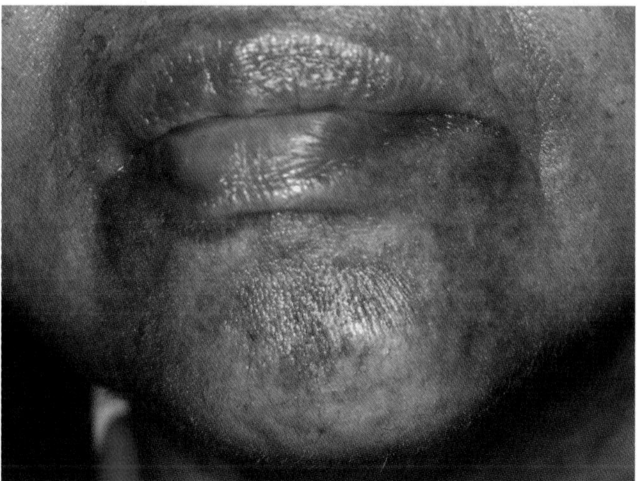

Figure 7.2 Diltiazem pigmentation on the face.

Nails

Nails may become discoloured with use of mepacrine or hydroxyurea. Onycholysis, which is separation of the nail plate from the nail bed, may be caused by cytotoxic agents.

Drugs which exacerbate pre-existing dermatoses

Medications may exacerbate skin conditions which the patient already has. The following summarises the most common associations:

Psoriasis – this is a common condition affecting approximately 2% of the population; however, some medications are known to worsen psoriasis. These are classically described as beta blockers, lithium and antimalarial medications, though newer drugs such as ACE (angiotensin converting enzyme) inhibitors can also worsen psoriasis. Non-prescribed drug such as alcohol have a detrimental effect on psoriasis.

Eczema – statins and diuretics such as hydrochlorothiazide may worsen eczema.

Acne – some forms of the oral contraceptive pill, particularly progesterone-only pills, may worse acne. Corticosteroids, ciclosporin and anti-epileptics such as phenytoin may also have the same effect.

Figure 7.3 Maculopapular exanthem.

Urticaria – non-steroidal anti-inflammatory drugs (NSAIDs) and opiate analgesics may worsen urticaria in a susceptible individual, by lowering the threshold for mast cell degranulation. ACE inhibitors and angiotensin receptor blockers may exacerbate angio-oedema. This is non-allergic urticaria/angio-oedema; allergic uritcaria/angio-oedema is described in the next section.

Common drug-induced rashes

Drug-induced exanthems

The most common cutaneous reaction to a drug is an exanthem, meaning a widespread rash. Such rashes may be morbilliform (resembling measles) or maculopapular (consisting of a mixture of raised and flat areas) (Figure 7.3). The patient may be symptomatic with burning, itch or discomfort arising from the skin. Onset is typically within 7–10 days of starting the drug, representing a delayed-type hypersensitivity. However, subsequent reactions on inadvertent re-exposure to a culprit drug may provoke a reaction in the skin more quickly, because of the presence of memory T cells in the lymph nodes. The proportion of the body surface area (BSA) involved may vary, and in cases where it exceeds 90%, the patient may be described as erythrodermic. Following withdrawal of the culprit drug, application of a potent topical corticosteroid and emollient will help alleviate discomfort and itch, and hasten resolution of the eruption. Any drug may cause a drug-induced exanthem but antibiotics of any class, anti-hypertensive agents and cholesterol-lowering drugs are amongst the most common precipitants.

Urticaria/angio-oedema

The appearance of raised, red itchy weals in the skin (Figure 7.4) may occur alone or in combination with angio-oedema, which is head and neck soft-tissue swelling. The latter may be serious, and when it involves the soft tissue of the airway, may cause respiratory embarrassment. It may be non-allergic (described above) or allergic; in the latter, a reaction occurs between a drug or its metabolite and a specific mast cell-bound IgE. A drug may cause anaphylaxis, occurring rapidly after drug ingestion (type I drug hypersensitivity) or may be delayed by a number of days following exposure to the drug (type IV hypersensitivity).

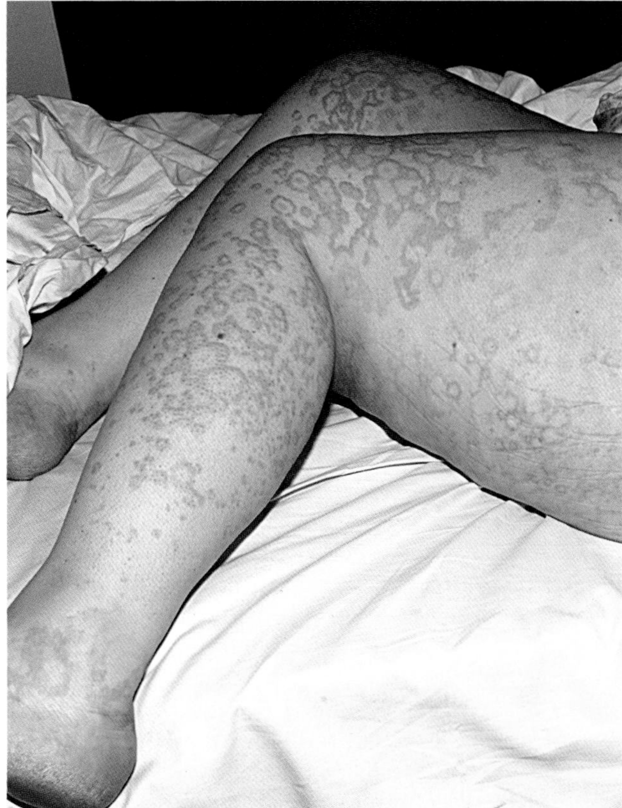

Figure 7.4 Urticaria secondary to penicillin.

Drug-induced lupus

Medication may produce an eruption indistinguishable from cutaneous lupus – in particular, the rash of sub-acute cutaneous lupus (SCLE) (Figure 7.5). The patient does not have any pre-existing autoimmune disease, and the condition remits on withdrawal of the culprit drug. The most common drugs to cause drug-induced lupus are listed in Table 7.1, but a recent study named terbinafine

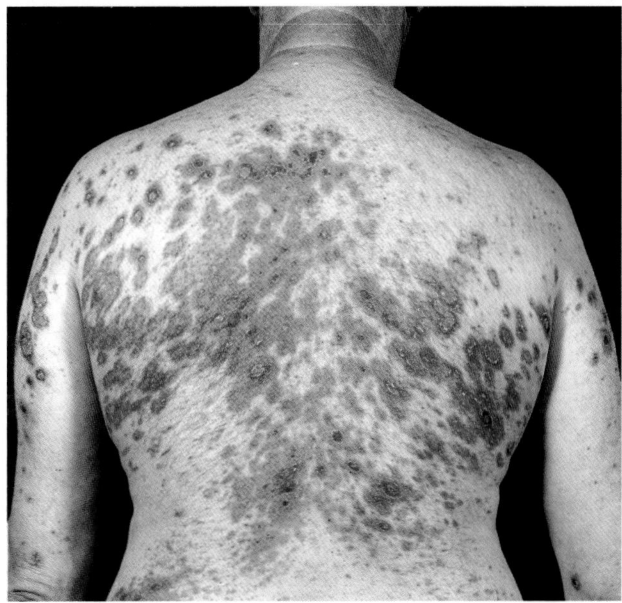

Figure 7.5 Drug-induced lupus.

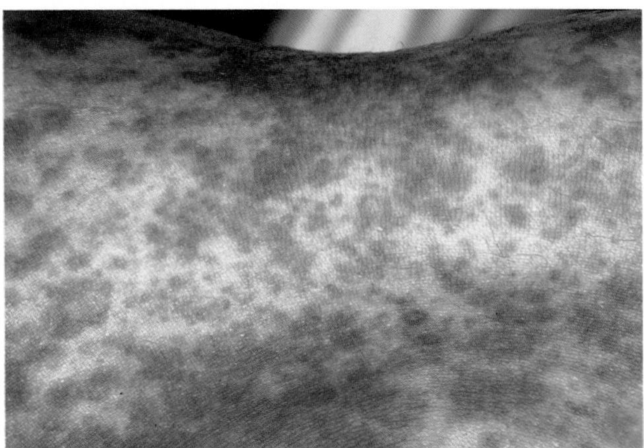

Figure 7.6 Drug-induced vasculitis.

as the most common culprit. Antihistone antibodies are present in >95% of cases, but dsDNA is usually negative and complement levels are normal.

Drug-induced vasculitis

Medication may cause a purpuric eruption that is indistinguishable from vasculitis (Figure 7.6). The distribution is usually predominantly in the lower limbs. As viral and bacterial infections may also cause vasculitis, it is often difficult to ascribe causality to a drug, as in cases where an antibiotic is suspected, the patient may also have had a recent infectious episode. In practice, in the absence of overt clinical signs of infection, causality is best determined by withdrawing the suspected culprit drug; if this brings about resolution of the vasculitis, then this adds weight to the diagnosis of a drug-induced phenomenon. Drugs associated with vasculitic eruptions include antibiotics, anticonvulsants and NSAIDs.

Lichenoid drug eruptions

Lichenoid drug eruptions resemble idiopathic lichen planus, but may not be confined to the classic sites of predilection of the latter. They consist of purplish papules which may have a lace-like white change on their surface (Figure 7.7a and b). The sites of predilection are the forearms, the neck and inner thighs, but the eruptions can appear anywhere. Onset may be delayed by a number of months following introduction of the culprit medication, leading to difficulties in diagnosing the eruption as drug induced. Resolution following drug withdrawal can be slow and take up to 2 months, and the post-inflammatory hyperpigmentation left behind may be dramatic. Table 7.1 illustrates the drugs which most commonly cause lichenoid eruptions.

Erythema nodosum

This is a tender, nodular eruption which classically appears on the anterior aspect of the legs. It is characterised histologically by septal panniculitis (inflammation in the subcutaneous fat). Although infective and inflammatory triggers are recognised (such as tuberculosis, *Yersinia* infections, rheumatoid arthritis, lupus and inflammatory bowel disease), EN may also be a drug-induced phenomenon. Drugs which commonly cause this include the oral contraceptive pill, penicillin and sulphonamide antibiotics and salicylates.

On page 52, Figures 7.7a and 7.7b are incorrect and should appear as follows:

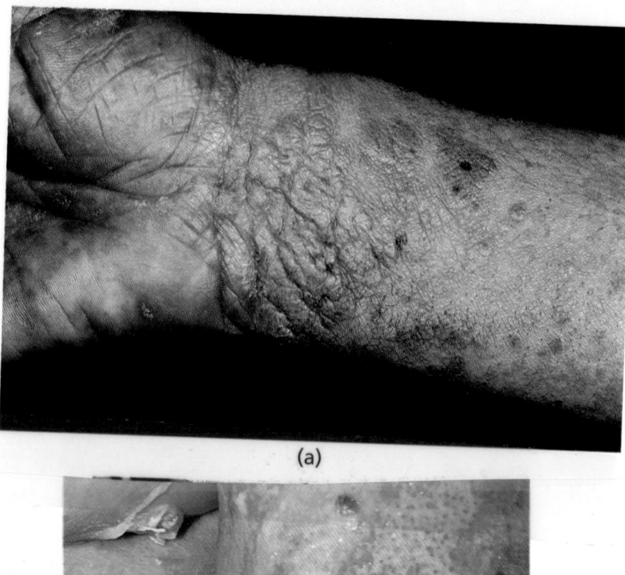

(a)

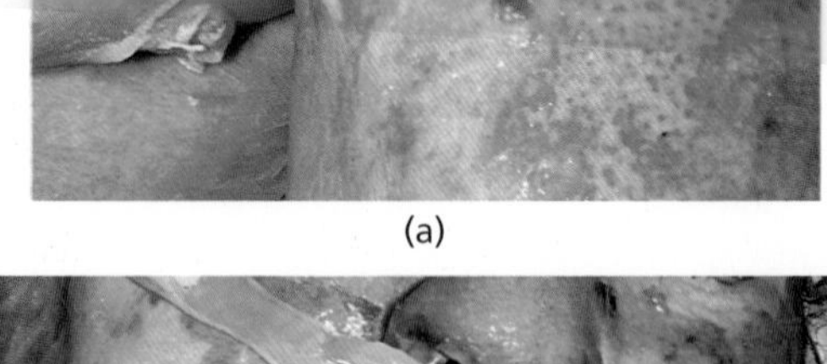

(a)

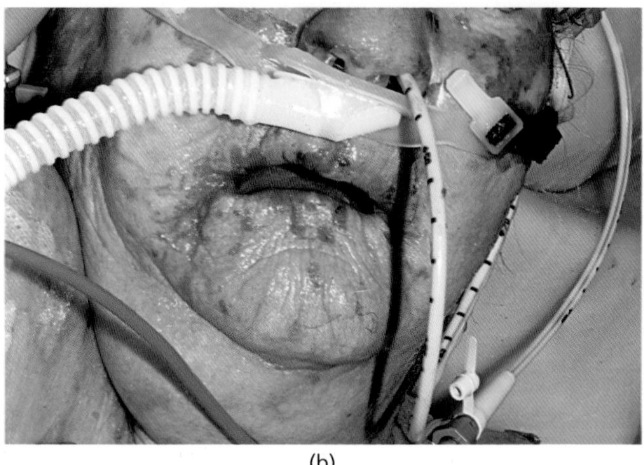

(b)

Figure 7.7 (a) Lichenoid drug reaction to nifedipine. (b) Lichenoid drug reaction to nifedipine; note swollen ankles which is a side effect of calcium channel blockers.

Fixed drug eruption

This is peculiar phenomenon whereby one or more inflammatory patches appear at the same cutaneous or mucosal site on each occasion that the patient ingests a culprit drug (Figure 7.8). The time frame for developing the lesion at the characteristic site can vary from 2 to 24 h. Common sites include the torso, hands, feet, face and genitalia. The patches resolve sometimes leaving post-inflammatory hyperpigmentation in the skin. Any drug can potentially cause a fixed drug eruption, but those more commonly associated are listed in Table 7.1.

Severe drug reactions in the skin

Stevens–Johnson syndrome (SJS) and toxic epidermal necrolysis (TEN)

SJS and TEN are rare, life-threatening drug-induced hypersensitivity reactions in the skin and mucous membranes. This mucocutaneous disorder is characterised by widespread, painful areas of epidermal detachment, and erosions of the mucous membranes,

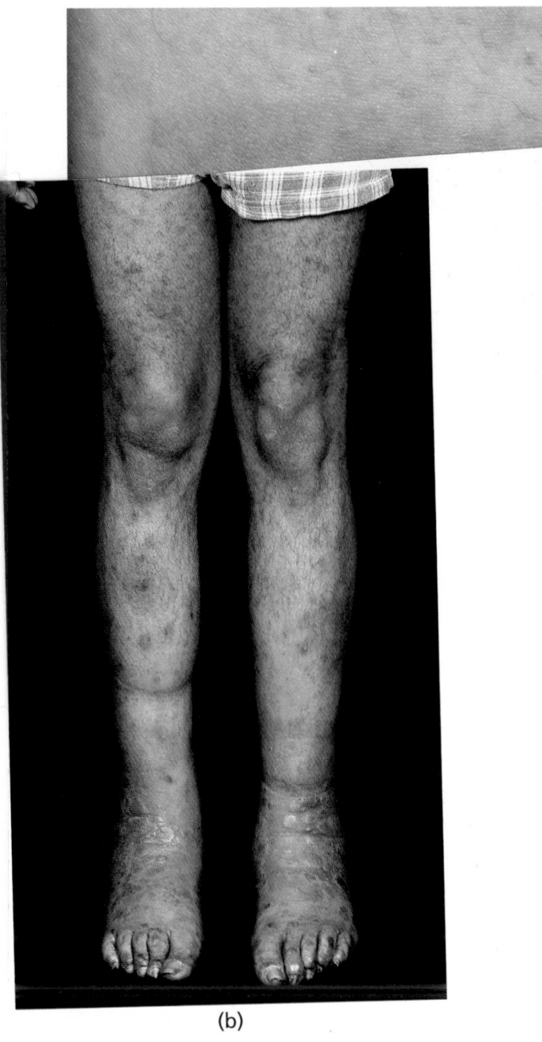

(b)

ure 7.7 (a) Lichenoid drug reaction to nifedipine. (b) Lichenoid drug ction to nifedipine; note swollen ankles which is a side effect of calcium nnel blockers.

ct (Figure 7.9a
preceded by a
nd skin *pain* is
appearance of
ng a spectrum
A detachment,
erm 'SJS–TEN
10% and 30%
id is estimated
neters.
the priority is
de anticonvul-
sulphonamide
upportive care.
intensive care
inical state. In
ive care physi-
licine, urology
involvement.
... and fragility demand specialist dermatology nursing care, with anti-shear handling, non-adherent dressings, and careful attention to antisepsis to prevent systemic infection. Expectant management of mucosal involvement will help prevent serious sequelae of the illness, described below.

Table 7.3 SCORTEN Parameters

SCORTEN parameters (1 point for each)	
Age (≥40 years)	
Heart rate (≥120 bpm)	
Cancer/haematological malignancy	
Body surface area (BSA) involvement (>10%)	
Serum urea (>10 mmol/L)	
Serum bicarbonate (<20 mmol/L)	
Serum glucose (>14 mmol/L)	
SCORTEN SCORE	Mortality
0–1	3%
2	12%
3	35%
4	58%
≥5	90%

The use of a number of active agents in the treatment of SJS/TEN has been described, including intravenous immunoglobulin, ciclosporin, corticosteroids, thalidomide, and infliximab, but there is insufficient evidence to conclusively support the use of any of these.

If the patient survives the acute phase of illness, a number of sequelae may be experienced. Corneal involvement in the acute phase may lead to blindness, involvement of the genital tract may lead to stenoses and the patient may experience dry mouth as a consequence of oral cavity involvement.

Drug reaction with eosinophilia and systemic symptoms (DRESS)

DRESS is a drug-induced phenomenon comprising a constellation of clinical features: a characteristic rash (usually a maculopapular exanthema, associated with head and neck oedema; Figures 7.10a and b), fever, lymphadenopathy, eosinophilia and involvement of one or more solid organs (usually the liver). Mortality is estimated at 5%, this being largely attributable to the small number of cases who develop fulminant liver failure in the context of DRESS. Other solid organs may also be involved, including the pancreas, the kidneys, the lungs, the heart and thyroid gland. The latency period following drug exposure is generally more protracted that in other

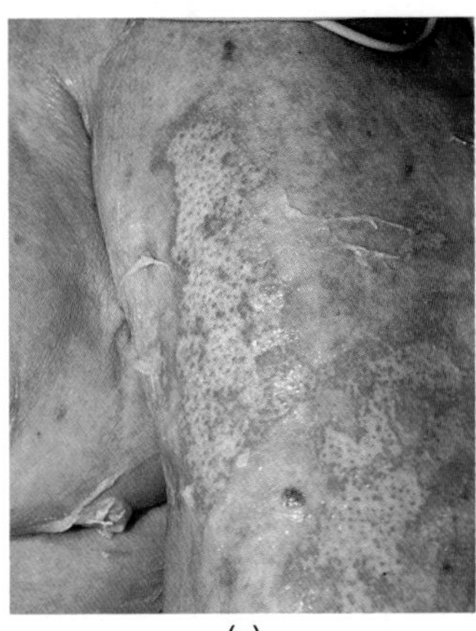

(a)

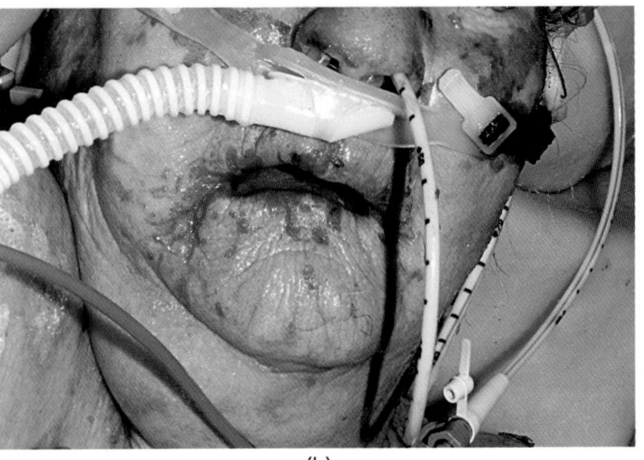

(b)

Figure 7.9 (a) Toxic epidermal necrolysis on the trunk. (b) Toxic epidermal necrolysis mucosal involvement.

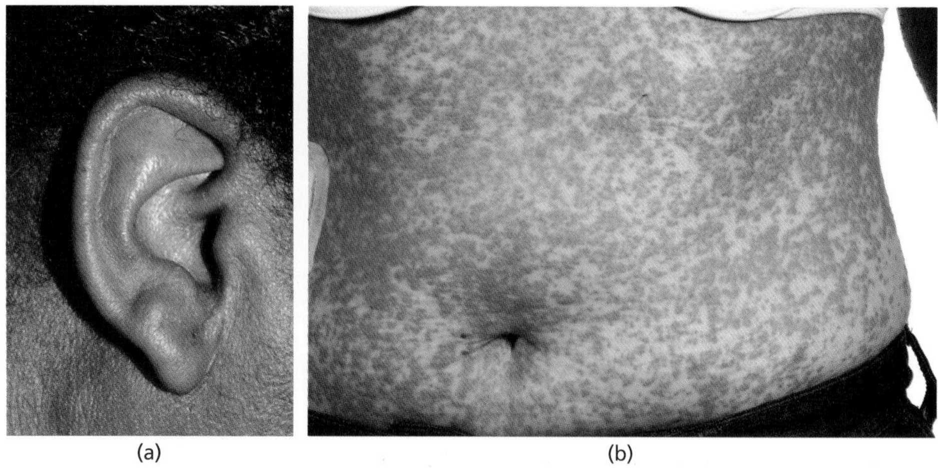

Figure 7.10 (a) DRESS swollen ears. (b) DRESS cutaneous eruption.

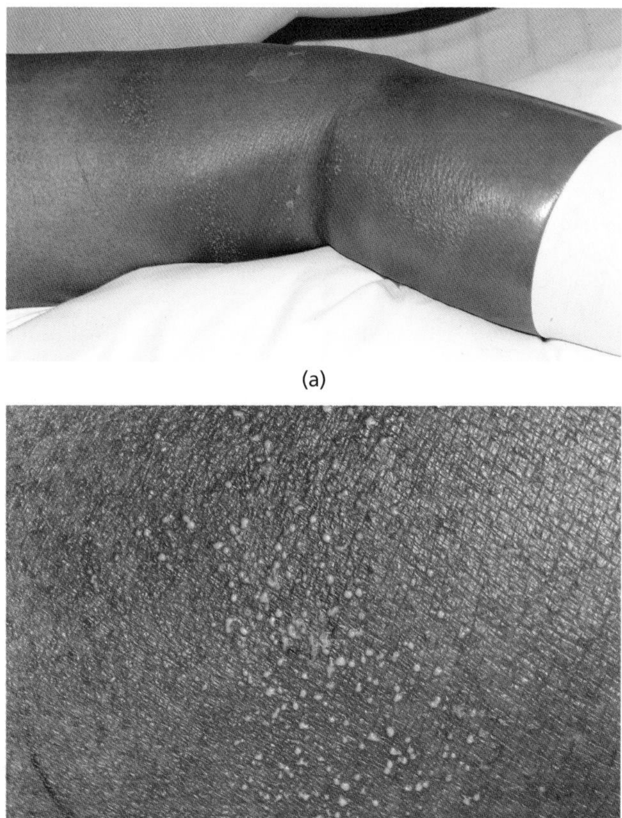

Figure 7.11 (a) Acute generalised exanthematous pustulosis multiple pustules on an erythematous base. (b) Acute generalised exanthematous pustulosis – inflammatory pustules which are non-follicular.

drug-induced syndromes, being 15–60 days. For this reason, the diagnosis is often overlooked, and symptoms of rash, fever and lymphadenopathy attributed incorrectly to infection. Management consists of withdrawal of the offending drug plus administration of corticosteroids. The latter may be given topically in the mildest cases, but generally either oral corticosteroids in the form of prednisolone or intravenously in the form of methylprednisolone will be required. Drugs with high notoriety for causing this condition are listed in Table 7.1, with the anticonvulsants and allopurinol accounting for a large proportion of cases.

Acute generalized exanthematous pustulosis (AGEP)

This is a rare pustular drug reaction recognisable by the appearance of sheets of non-follicular pustules which have a predilection for the major flexures (axillae, groin and neck) appearing 3–7 days after ingestion of a culprit medication (Figure 7.11a and b). The pustules resolve over 3–7 days, in a phase characterised by post-pustular desquamation. The rash may be accompanied by fever and oedema, and in a small number of cases by systemic upset with involvement of the lungs or the liver. Recovery may be accelerated by the use of topical or oral corticosteroids. Antibiotics are the most common culprit drugs.

Further reading

Bastuji-Garin S, Fouchard N, Bertocci M, et al. SCORTEN: a severity-of-illness score for Toxic Epidermal Necrolysis. *J Inv Dermatol* **115**:149–153, 2000.

Kardaun SH. *Severe Cutaneous Adverse Drug Reactions: Challenges in Diagnosis and Treatment*. Uitgeverij Boxpress, Groningen, 2012.

Revuz J *et al. Life Threatening Dermatoses and Emergencies in Dermatology*, Springer, Berlin, 2009.

CHAPTER 8

Immunobullous and Other Blistering Disorders

Rachael Morris-Jones

Dermatology Department, Kings College Hospital, London, UK

OVERVIEW

- Blisters arise from destruction or separation of epidermal cells by trauma, viral infection, immune reactions, oedema as in eczema or inflammatory causes such as vasculitis.
- Immune reactions at the dermoepidermal junction and intraepidermally cause blisters.
- Susceptibility is inherited; trigger factors include drugs, foods, viral infections, hormones and ultraviolet radiation.
- Differential diagnosis depends on specific features, in particular the duration, durability and distribution of lesions.
- The most important immunobullous conditions are bullous pemphigoid, pemphigus, dermatitis herpetiformis (DH) and linear IgA.
- Investigations should identify underlying causes and the site and nature of any immune reaction in the skin.
- Management includes topical treatment, immunosuppressive drugs and a gluten-free diet.

Introduction

Blisters, whether large bullae or small vesicles, can arise in a variety of conditions. Blisters may result from *destruction* of epidermal cells (a burn or a herpes virus infection). *Loss of adhesion* between the cells may occur within the epidermis (pemphigus) or at the basement membrane (pemphigoid). In eczema there is *oedema* between the epidermal cells, resulting in spongiosis. Sometimes, there are associated *inflammatory* changes in the dermis (erythema multiforme/vasculitis) or a metabolic defect (as in porphyria).

The integrity of normal skin depends on intricate connecting structures between cells (Figure 8.1). In autoimmune blistering conditions autoantibodies attack these adhesion structures. The level of the separation of epidermal cells within the epidermis is determined by the specific structure that is the target antigen. Clinically, these splits are visualised as superficial blisters which may be fragile and flaccid (intraepidermal split) or deep mainly intact blisters (subepidermal split). Therefore, the clinical features can be used to predict the level of the underlying target antigen in the skin.

ABC of Dermatology, Sixth Edition. Edited by Rachael Morris-Jones.

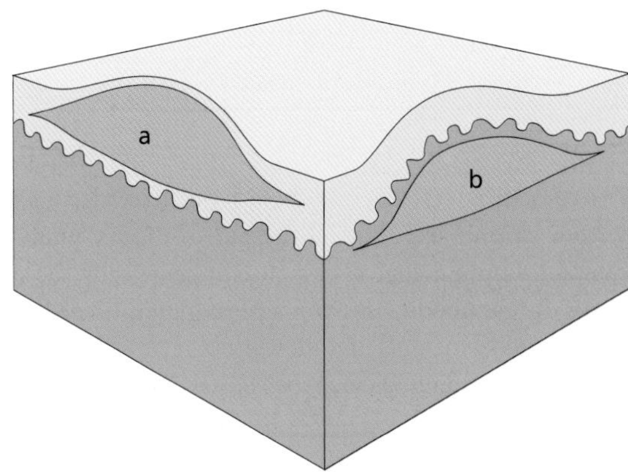

Figure 8.1 Section through the skin with (a) intraepidermal blister and (b) subepidermal blister.

Pathophysiology

Susceptibility to develop autoimmune disorders may be inherited, but the triggers for the production of these skin-damaging autoantibodies remains unknown. In some patients possible triggers have been identified including drugs (rifampicin, captopril and D-penicillamine), certain foods (garlic, onions and leeks), viral infections, hormones, UV radiation and X-rays.

Bullous pemphigoid results from IgG autoantibodies that target the basement membrane cells (hemidesmosome proteins BP180 and BP230). Studies have demonstrated a reduction in circulating regulatory T cells (Treg) and reduced levels of interleukin-10 (IL-10) in patients with bullous pemphigoid, which partially correct following treatment. Complement activates an inflammatory cascade, leading to disruption of skin cell adhesion and blister formation. The subepidermal split leads to tense bullae formation.

Pemphigus vulgaris results from autoantibodies directed against desmosomal cadherin desmoglein 3 (Dsg3) found between epidermal cells in mucous membranes and skin. This causes the epidermal cells to separate, resulting in intraepidermal blister formation. This relatively superficial split leads to flaccid blisters and erosions (where the blister roof has sloughed off). Pemphigus foliaceus (PF) is a rare autoimmune skin disease characterised by subcorneal blistering and IgG antibodies directed against desmoglein 1 (Dsg1) usually manifested at UV-irradiated skin sites.

Table 8.1 Differential diagnosis of immunobullous disorders – other causes of cutaneous blistering.

Other causes of cutaneous blistering	Key clinical features	Diagnostic tests	Further reading
Erythema multiforme	Target lesions with a central blister, acral sites	Skin biopsy for histology	Chapter 7
Stevens–Johnson syndrome/toxic epidermal necrolysis	Mucous membrane involvement, Nikolsky-positive, eroded areas of skin	Skin biopsy for histology	Chapter 7
Chicken pox	Scattered blisters in crops appear over days	Viral swab to detect VZV; serology	Chapter 14
Herpes simplex/varicella zoster virus	Localised blistering of mucous membranes or dermatomal	Vesicle fluid for viral analysis	Chapter 14
Staphylococcus impetigo	Golden crusting associated with blisters	Bacterial swab for culture	Chapter 13
Insect bite reactions	Linear or clusters of blisters, very itchy	Clinical diagnosis	Chapter 17
Contact dermatitis	Exogenous pattern of blisters	Patch testing	Chapter 4
Phytophotodermatitis	Blisters where plants/extracts touched the skin plus sunlight exposure	Clinical diagnosis	Chapter 6
Porphyria	Fragile skin with scarring at sun-exposed sites	Urine, blood, faecal analysis for porphyrins	Chapter 6
Fixed drug eruption	Blistering purplish lesion/s at a fixed site each time drug taken	Skin biopsy for histology	Chapter 7

DH is caused by IgA deposits in the papillary dermis which results from chronic exposure of the gut to dietary gluten triggering an auto-immunological response in genetically susceptible individuals. IgA antibodies develop against gluten-tissue transglutaminase (found in the gut) and these cross react with epidermal-transglutaminase leading to cutaneous blistering.

Differential diagnosis

Many cutaneous disorders present with blister formation. Presentations include large single bullae through to multiple small vesicles, and differentiating the underlying cause can be a clinical challenge (Table 8.1). The history of the blister formation can give important clues to the diagnosis, in particular the development, duration, durability and distribution of the lesions – the 'four Ds'.

Development

If erosions or blisters are present at birth then genodermatoses must be considered in addition to cutaneous infections. Preceding systemic symptoms may suggest an infectious cause such as chicken pox or hand, foot and mouth disease. A tingling sensation may herald herpes simplex, and pain, herpes zoster. If the lesions are pruritic, then consider DH or pompholyx eczema. Eczema may precede bullous pemphigoid.

Duration

Some types of blistering arise rapidly (allergic reactions, impetigo, erythema multiforme and pemphigus), while others have a more gradual onset and follow a chronic course (DH, pityriasis lichenoides, porphyria cutanea tarda and bullous pemphigoid). The rare genetic disorder epidermolysis bullosa is present from, or soon after, birth and has a chronic course.

Durability

The blisters themselves may remain intact or rupture easily and this sign can help elude the underlying diagnosis. Superficial blisters in the epidermis have a fragile roof that sloughs off easily leaving eroded areas typically seen in pemphigus vulgaris, porphyria, Stevens–Johnson syndrome, toxic epidermal necrolysis, staphylococcal scalded skin and herpes viruses. Subepidermal blisters have a stronger roof and usually remain intact and are classically seen in bullous pemphigoid, linear IgA and erythema multiforme. Scratching can result in traumatic removal of blister roofs, which may confuse the clinical picture.

Distribution

The distribution of blistering rashes helps considerably in making a clinical diagnosis (Boxes 8.1 and 8.2). In general, immunobullous diseases present with widespread eruptions with frequent mucous membrane involvement. Herpes infections usually remain localised to lips, genitals or dermatomes. Photosensitive blistering disorders involve sun-exposed skin.

Box 8.1 **Widespread blistering eruptions**

- Bullous pemphigoid.
- Pemphigus vulgaris.
- DH (or localised).
- Erythema multiforme.
- Drug rashes: Stevens–Johnson syndrome, toxic epidermal necrolysis.
- Chicken pox.

Box 8.2 **Localised blistering eruptions**

- DH (knees, elbows and buttocks).
- Pemphigus gestationis (abdomen).
- PF (upper trunk, face and scalp).
- Porphyria (sun-exposed sites).
- Pompholyx eczema (hands and feet).
- Contact dermatitis.
- Fixed drug eruption.
- Insect bite reactions (often in clusters or linear patterns).
- Infections: herpes simplex, herpes zoster and staphylococcus (impetigo).

Table 8.2 Clinical features of immunobullous disorders.

Immunobullous disorder	Typical patient	Distribution of rash	Morphology of lesions	Mucous membrane involvement	Associated conditions
Bullous pemphigoid	Elderly	Generalised	Intact blisters	Common	None
Mucous membrane pemphigoid	Middle aged or older	Varied	Erosions, flaccid blisters, scarring	Severe and extensive	Autoimmune disease
Pemphigoid gestationis	Pregnant	Periumbilical	Intact blisters, urticated lesions	Rare	Thyroid disease
Pemphigus vulgaris	Middle aged	Flexures, head	Flaccid blisters, erosions	Common	Autoimmune disease
Dermatitis herpetiformis	Young adults	Elbows, knees, buttocks	Vesicles, papules, excoriations	Rare	Small bowel enteropathy (gluten-sensitive), lymphoma
Linear IgA	Children and adults	Face and perineum (children) Trunk and limbs (adults)	Annular urticated plaques with peripheral vesicles	Common	Lymphoproliferative disorders

Clinical features of immunobullous disorders

Clinical features of the different immunobullous disorders (Table 8.2) are discussed in the following subsections.

Bullous pemphigoid

This usually presents over the age of 65 years with tense blisters and erosions on a background of dermatitis or normal skin (Figure 8.2). The condition may present acutely or be insidious in onset, but usually enters a chronic intermittent phase before remitting after approximately 5 years. Some patients have a prolonged prebullous period in which persistent pruritic urticated plaques (Figure 8.3), or eczema, precedes the blisters. Characteristically, blisters have a predilection for flexural sites on the limbs and trunk. Mucous membrane involvement occurs in about 20% of cases (Figure 8.4). Blisters heal without scarring. Potential triggers include vaccinations, drugs (NSAIDs, furosemide, ACE (angiotensin converting enzyme) inhibitors and antibiotics), UV radiation and X-rays. In children bullous pemphigoid usually follows vaccination, where the condition characteristically affects the face, palms and soles.

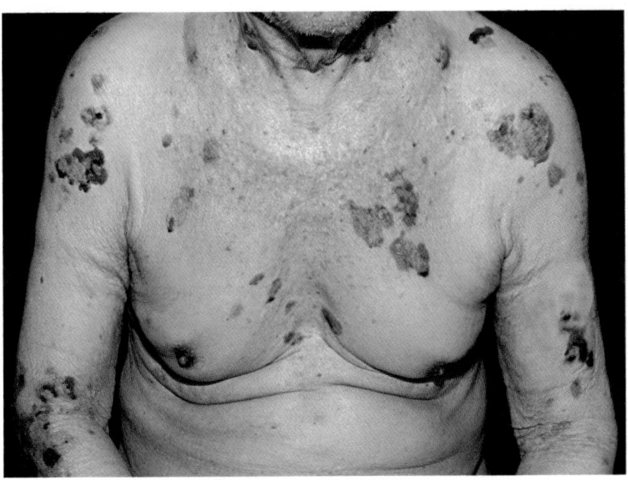

Figure 8.2 Bullous pemphigoid.

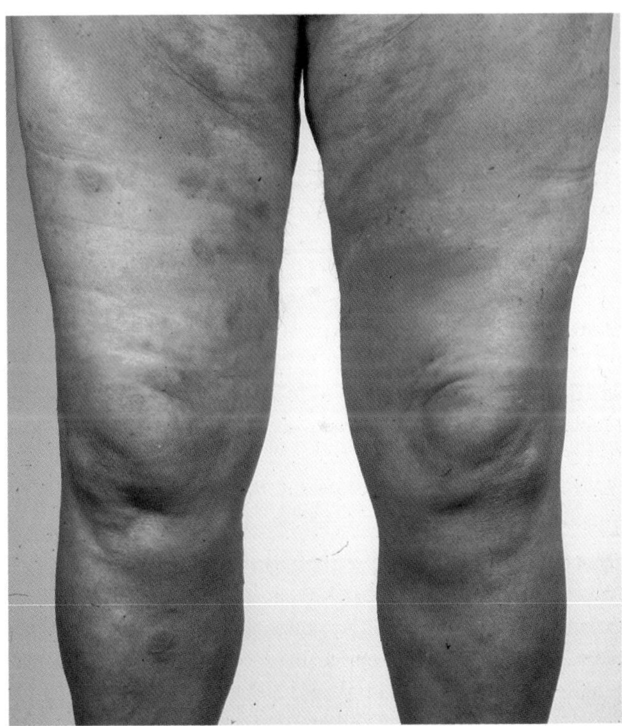

Figure 8.3 Urticated plaques in pre-bullous pemphigoid.

Pemphigoid gestationis

This rare autoimmune disorder usually occurs in the second/third trimester of pregnancy. Mothers may have other associated autoimmune conditions. Acute-onset intensely pruritic papules, plaques and blisters spread from the periumbilical area outwards (Figure 8.5). Mucous membrane involvement can occur. Babies may be born prematurely or small for dates and can have a transient blistering eruption that rapidly resolves. The maternal cutaneous

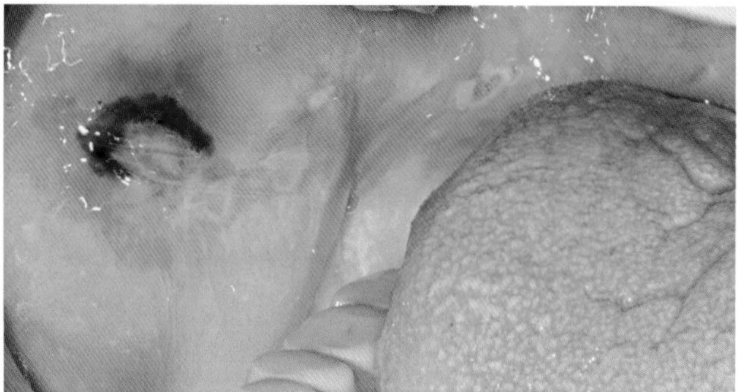

Figure 8.4 Bullous pemphigoid: showing mouth erosions.

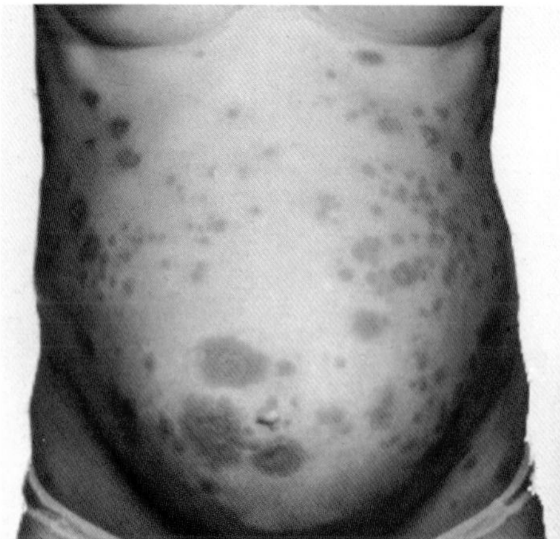

Figure 8.5 Pemphigoid gestationis on the abdomen.

eruption usually resolves within weeks after birth, but may flare immediately postpartum.

Mucous membrane pemphigoid (cicatricial pemphigoid)

Patients usually present with painful sores in their mouth, nasal and genital mucosae, and may complain of a gritty feeling in their eyes. Cutaneous lesions occur in around 30% of patients; tense blisters may be haemorrhagic and heal with scarring (Figure 8.6). Scalp involvement can lead to scarring alopecia (Figure 8.7). Symptoms from mucous membrane sites can be very severe with chronic painful erosions and ulceration that heals with scarring.

Ocular damage (Figure 8.8) can include symblepharon (tethering of conjunctival epithelium), synechiae (adhesion of iris to cornea) and fibrosis of the lacrimal duct (dry eyes) resulting in opacification, fixed globe and eventually blindness.

Pemphigus vulgaris

Seventy percent of patients develop oral lesions in chronic progressive pemphigus vulgaris. Mucous membrane involvement may precede cutaneous signs by several months. Skin lesions do, however, occur in most patients and are characterised by painful flaccid blisters and erosions arising on normal skin (Figure 8.9). The bullae are easily broken, and even rubbing apparently normal skin causes the superficial epidermis to slough off (Nikolsky sign positive).

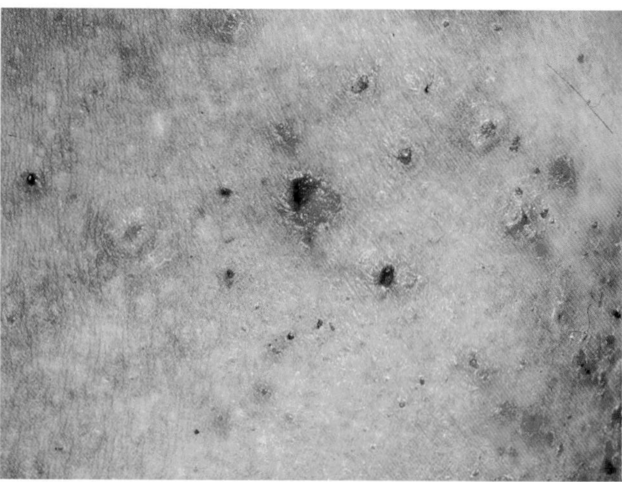

Figure 8.6 Mucous membrane pemphigoid: scarring skin eruption.

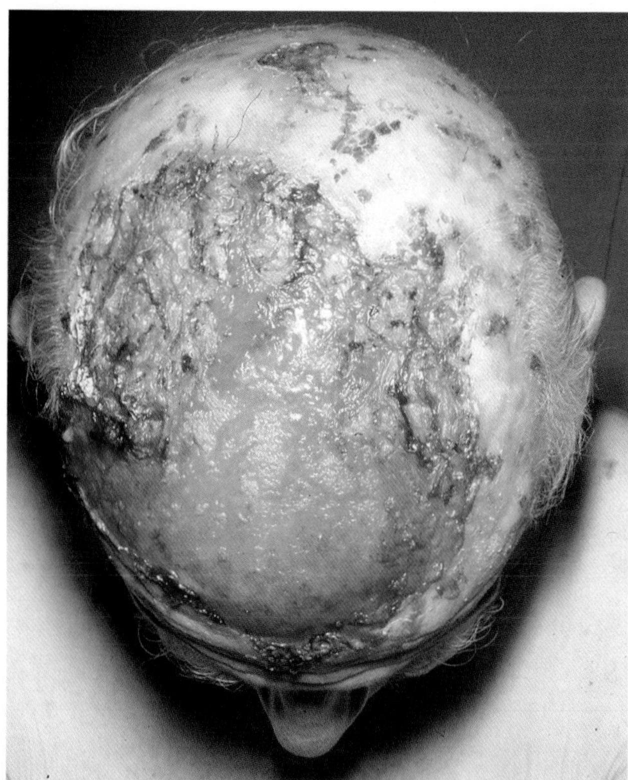

Figure 8.7 Mucous membrane pemphigoid on the scalp.

Slow-healing painful erosions occur in the mouth, particularly on the soft/hard palate and buccal mucosae, but the larynx may also be affected. The oral cavity lesions may be so severe that patients have difficulty eating, drinking and brushing their teeth (Figure 8.10). Recognised drug triggers of pemphigus vulgaris include rifampicin, ACE inhibitors and penicillamine. Paraneoplastic pemphigus is clinically similar to pemphigus vulgaris but with an associated underlying malignancy such as non-Hodgkin's lymphoma or chronic lymphocytic leukaemia.

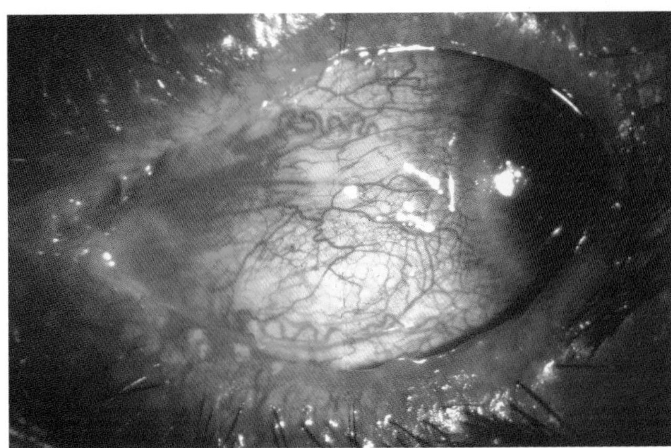

Figure 8.8 Mucous membrane pemphigoid: eyes.

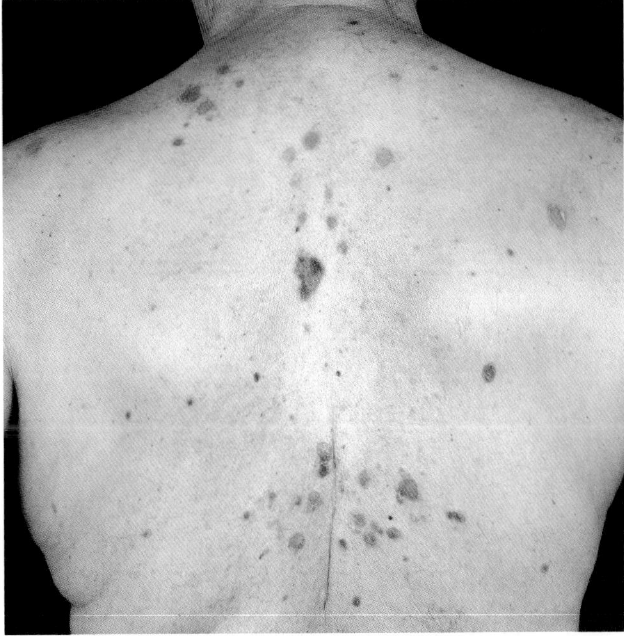

Figure 8.9 Pemphigus vulgaris on the trunk.

Pemphigus foliaceus (PF) tends to affect patients in middle age and is characterised by flaccid small bullae on the trunk, face and scalp that rapidly erode and crust. Dugs may induce PF; the most commonly reported are penicillamine, nifedipine, captopril and NSAIDs.

Dermatitis herpetiformis (DH)

This is an intensely pruritic autoimmune blistering disorder that affects young/middle-aged adults and is associated with an underlying gluten-sensitive enteropathy. Several HLA types have been identified in patients with DH (HLA-DR3, B8, DQ2 and A1) and 10% of patients report an affected relative. Cutaneous lesions are characteristically intermittent and mainly affect the buttocks, knees (Figure 8.11) and elbows. The intense pruritus leads to excoriation of the small vesicles which are consequently rarely seen intact by clinicians. Most patients do not report any bowel symptoms unless prompted, but may experience bloating and diarrhoea. Low ferritin and folate can result from malabsorption. Interestingly, small bowel investigation reveals abnormalities (villous atrophy, raised lymphocyte count) in 90% of patients. There is an increased frequency of small bowel lymphoma in patients with enteropathy.

DH patients should be encouraged to follow a strict gluten-free diet, as this should control the cutaneous and gastrointestinal

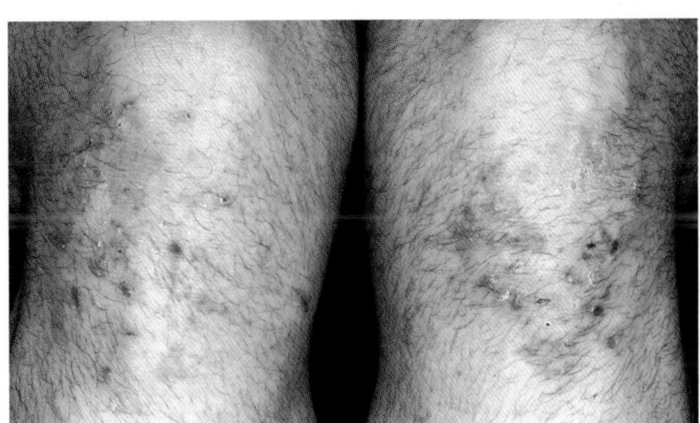

Figure 8.11 Dermatitis herpetiformis on the knees.

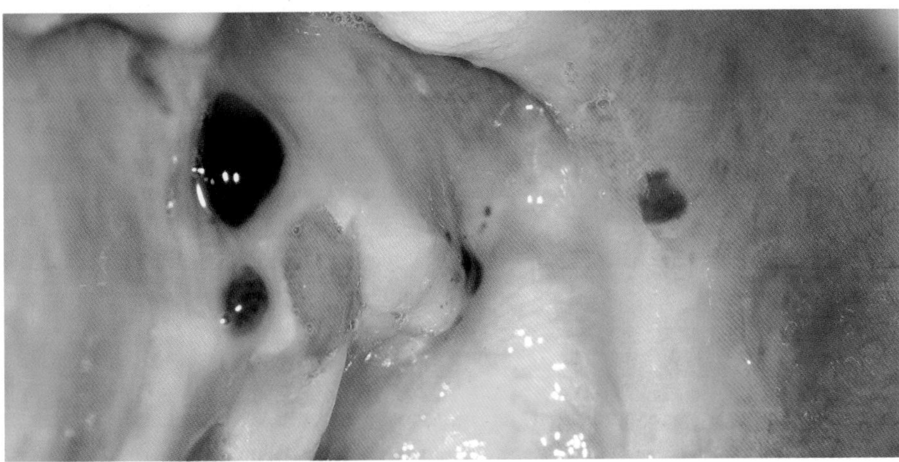

Figure 8.10 Pemphigus vulgaris in the mouth.

symptoms and is thought to reduce the risk of small bowel lymphoma. Patients should avoid wheat, rye and barley. Dapsone and sulphapyridine can be used to control symptoms if dietary manipulation is unsuccessful. DH is a chronic condition and therefore lifelong management is needed.

Linear IgA

Children and adults can be affected by this autoimmune subepidermal blistering disorder. The clinical picture is heterogeneous, ranging from acute onset of blistering to insidious pruritus before chronic tense bullae. In children, the blisters tend to affect the lower abdomen and perineum, whereas in adults the limbs and trunk are most commonly affected (Figure 8.12). Blisters are usually intact and are classically seen around the periphery of annular lesions ('string of beads sign') or in clusters ('jewel sign'). Mucous membrane involvement is common. Reported drug triggers include vancomycin, ampicillin and amiodarone. Management is similar to that for DH, with patients responding to dapsone and sulphapyridine.

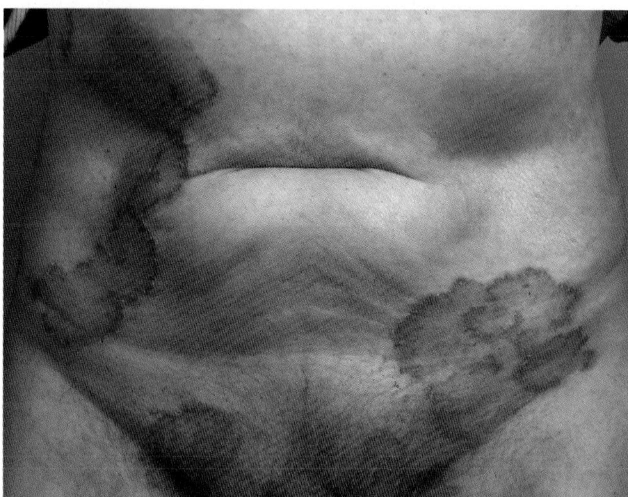

Figure 8.12 Linear IgA on the trunk.

Investigation of immunobullous disease

The gold standard for diagnosing immunobullous disease is direct immunofluorescent analysis of perilesional skin. Skin biopsies are taken across a blister/erosion; the lesional part is sent for histopathology and the adjacent skin sent for direct immunofluorescence (Table 8.3). The histological features can be diagnostic or supportive of the diagnosis. The level and pattern of immunoglobulin staining on direct immunofluorescence is usually diagnostic. Indirect tests involve taking the patients serum and applying this to a substrate such as monkey oesophagus or salt-split human skin substrate (Figures 8.13–8.16). Circulating intercellular

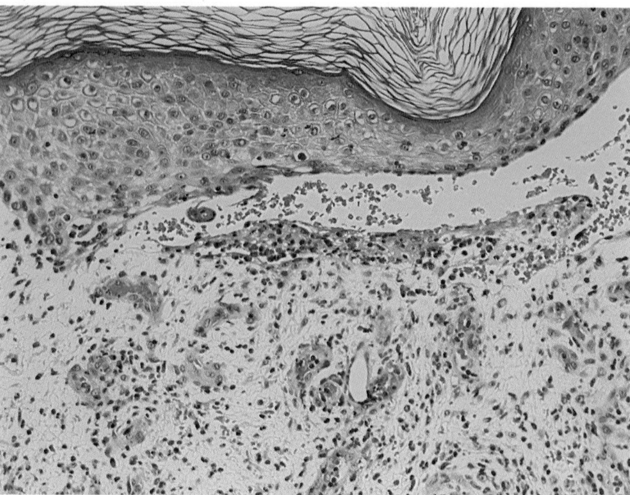

Figure 8.13 Histopathology of bullous pemphigoid.

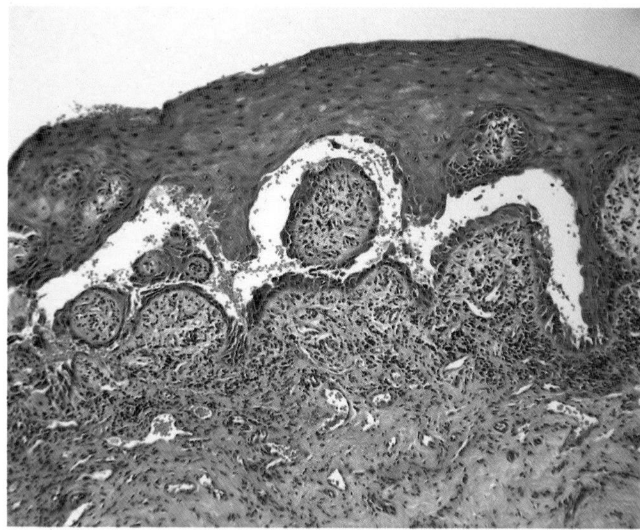

Figure 8.14 Histopathology of pemphigus vulgaris.

Table 8.3 Skin biopsy findings in immunobullous disorders.

Immunobullous disorder	Histology features	Immunofluorescence features
Bullous pemphigoid	Subepidermal blister containing mainly eosinophils	Linear band of IgG at the basement membrane zone
Pemphigoid gestationis	Subepidermal blister containing mainly eosinophils	Linear band of C3 at the basement membrane zone
Mucous membrane pemphigoid	Subepidermal blister with variable cellular infiltrate	Linear band of IgG/C3 at the basement membrane zone
Pemphigus vulgaris	Suprabasal split (basal cells remain attached to basement membrane, looking like 'tombstones')	IgG deposited on surface of keratinocytes in a 'chicken-wire' pattern
Dermatitis herpetiformis	Small vesicles containing neutrophils and eosinophils in the upper dermis	Granular deposits of IgA in the upper dermis (dermal papillae)
Linear IgA	Subepidermal blisters with neutrophils or eosinophils	Linear deposition of IgA at the basement membrane zone

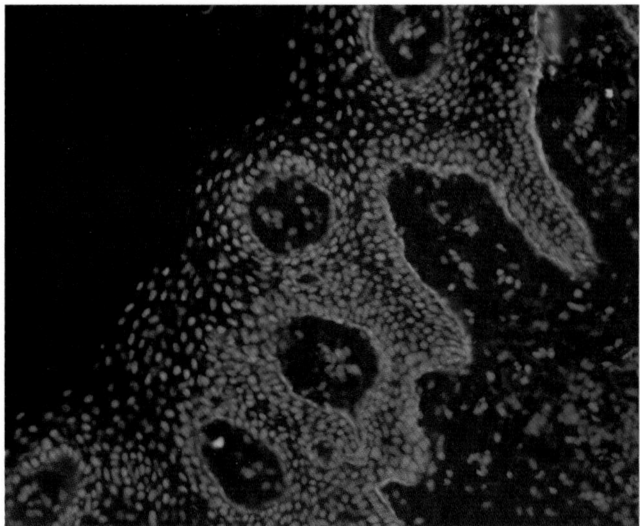

Figure 8.15 Immunofluorescence of bullous pemphigoid.

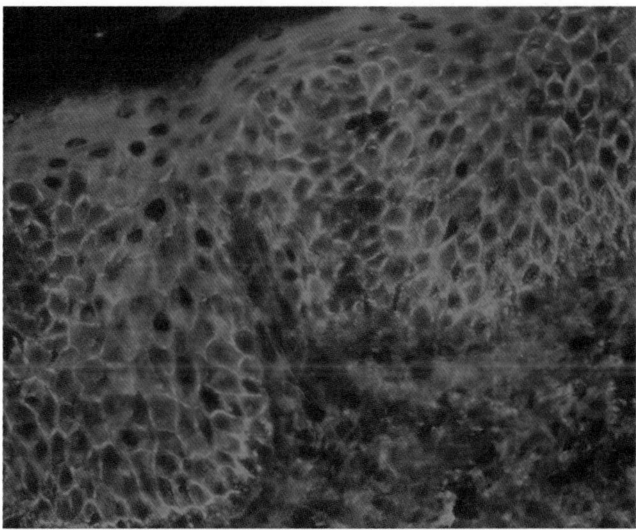

Figure 8.16 Immunofluorescence of pemphigus vulgaris.

antibodies may be detected in patients with pemphigus, leading to titre measurement which may help guide management.

Management of immunobullous disease

Tense intact blisters can be deflated using a sterile needle (the roof of the blister should be preserved as this provides a 'natural wound covering'). Use of non-adherent dressings or a bodysuit can be used to cover painful cutaneous erosions. Liquid paraffin should be applied regularly to eroded areas to help retain fluid and prevent secondary infection.

In most cases of immunobullous disease immunosuppressive treatments are required. Bullous pemphigoid presenting in an elderly patient may respond to intensive potent topical steroids to affected skin. Reducing courses of systemic corticosteroids can be helpful in the short term, but most patients are maintained on azathioprine or minocycline (anti-inflammatory properties). Other treatments used include methotrexate, cyclophosphamide, mycophenolate mofetil and the anti CD-20 biological agent rituximab.

Severe forms of pemphigoid gestationis may require high doses of systemic corticosteroids which can usually be rapidly reduced during the postpartum period. Care should be taken if mothers are breastfeeding as most drugs pass into breast milk.

Mucous membrane pemphigoid is chronic and resistant to many treatments, making management difficult. Oral disease may respond to topical steroids and tetracycline mouthwashes. Ophthalmic disease should be managed carefully as scarring can result in blindness. Topical steroid drops and mitomycin may be useful, but usually systemic immunosuppression such as mycophenolate mofetil is required.

The management of pemphigus vulgaris has been transformed by the use of rituximab which is a biological agent with anti-CD20 activity that depletes antibody-producing B-cells. A dose of 1 g of rituximab given at day 1 and 15 induces remission in 70% of patients by 70 days and 86% of patients at 6 months. About 40% of patients will subsequently relapse after two infusions of rituximab usually after many months and studies show that when they receive further infusions of rituximab at 500 mg, further disease remission can be achieved. In most cases, all other immunosuppressive medications can be stopped, leading to a reduction in long-term morbidity and mortality induced by medications.

A gluten-free diet is an effective way of controlling the cutaneous eruption of DH as well as relieving gastrointestinal symptoms and reducing the risk of developing small bowel lymphoma. Dapsone or sulphapyridine are both helpful in controlling the disease.

Further reading

Boehncke W-H and Radeke HH. *Biologics in General Medicine*, Springer, Berlin, 2007.

Burge S and Wallis D. *Oxford Handbook of Medical Dermatology*, Oxford University Press, 2011.

Hertl M. *Autoimmune Diseases of the Skin: Pathogenesis, Diagnosis, Management*, Springer-Verlag/Wein, New York, 2011.

CHAPTER 9

Connective Tissue Disease, Vasculitis and Related Disorders

Rachael Morris-Jones

Dermatology Department, Kings College Hospital, London, UK

OVERVIEW

- Many connective tissues disorders affect the skin.
- Fibrosis in connective tissue is a feature of systemic sclerosis, morphoea, CREST syndrome and lichen sclerosus.
- Lupus erythematosus may be solely cutaneous or cause severe systemic disease.
- Dermatomyositis results in characteristic skin involvement and muscle weakness, it may be a marker of internal malignancy.
- Lichen planus is a common chronic inflammatory condition of the skin of unknown cause that can affect mouth, eyes and ears.
- Vasculitis results from changes in capillaries and arterioles and may involve internal organs in addition to the skin.
- Causes of cutaneous vasculitis include inflammatory, viral and haematological conditions. A wide range of investigations may be indicated.

Introduction

The skin is a dynamic interface of trafficking immune cells that may remain localised and respond to nearby stimuli, or migrate through the skin in response to more distant triggers. The skin has been called 'the immunological battleground of the body' and immune cells involved in inflammatory reactions may be part of a local immune reaction or migrate to the skin as a result of antigenic stimuli at distant sites. Malfunction of the sophisticated human immune system may result in the body attacking its own tissues, that is, failure to distinguish 'self' from 'non-self'. These autoimmune responses may develop against a tissue in a specific organ such as the thyroid gland, or to tissues within and between organs resulting in connective tissue diseases.

Connective tissue disease

Connective tissue disease can be difficult to define but encompasses disorders that involve tissues connecting and surrounding organs.

Connective tissues include the extracellular matrix and support proteins such as collagen and elastin. Acquired disorders of connective tissue are thought to have an autoimmune basis, many of which have distinctive clinical features and patterns in laboratory investigations. However, at times classification may not be easy. What triggers dysregulation of the immune system is usually unknown; however, some recognised factors include sunlight, infections and medication. Patients may have an underlying hereditary susceptibility to develop autoimmune diseases, marked by specific HLA (human lymphocyte antigen) types in some cases.

In autoimmune disorders immune cells may be attracted to particular targets within the skin locally (pemphigus and pemphigoid – Chapter 8) or accumulate at sites of connective tissues in multiple organs (systemic lupus erythematosus (SLE) and dermatomyositis). Once at their destination these immune cells trigger a cascade of chemical messages leading to inflammation.

The possibility of an underlying connective tissue disorder should be considered if a patient complains of any combination of symptoms including cutaneous lesions (especially face and fingers), joint pains, muscle aches, malaise, weakness, photosensitivity, Raynaud's phenomenon and alopecia. Linking the clinical symptoms and signs with the most appropriate investigations in order to arrive at a unifying diagnosis is a challenge to even the most experienced medical practitioner (Box 9.1).

Box 9.1 **Investigations might include the following**

- Full blood count (FBC)
- Antinuclear antibodies (ANAs)
- Extractable nuclear antibodies (ENA), (Ro, La)
- Erythrocyte sedimentation rate (ESR)
- Renal and liver function
- ANCA (antineutrophil cytoplasmic antibodies)
- Hepatitis serology
- Streptococcal serology (ASOT)
- Rheumatoid factor
- Angiotensin-converting enzyme (ACE)
- Antiphospholipid antibodies
- Coagulation screen, lupus anticoagulant
- Anticardiolipin antibodies
- Factor V Leiden, antithrombin III, proteins S and C
- Urine dipstick and microscopy
- Blood pressure
- Chest X ray

ABC of Dermatology, Sixth Edition. Edited by Rachael Morris-Jones.

Vasculitis

Complex reactions occurring specifically in the capillaries and arterioles of the skin may lead to cutaneous erythema (redness). The erythema may be macular or papular and may be transient or last for weeks. Blood vessels can become leaky, leading to pouring out (extravasation) of red blood cells into the tissue with or without inflammation of the blood vessel walls. Inflammation of blood vessel walls is called vasculitis and may involve arteries and/or veins. Vasculitis can also lead to stenosis, occlusion and ischaemia.

Symptoms can include pain in the skin, general malaise, fever, abdominal pain and arthropathy. Clinically, patients have a non-blanching skin eruption that is most commonly seen on the lower limbs (Figure 9.1). Individual skin lesions may be macular or palpable purpura, blistering, ulcerated and necrotic (Figure 9.2). Vasculitis confined to the skin can be painful and unpleasant, but systemic vasculitis may be life threatening.

There are numerous possible underlying causes of vasculitis including infections, medications, connective tissue disease, underlying malignancy, vascular/coagulopathy disorders, inflammatory bowel disease and sarcoidosis (Box 9.1. indicates appropriate investigations in patients with a vasculitis of unknown cause).

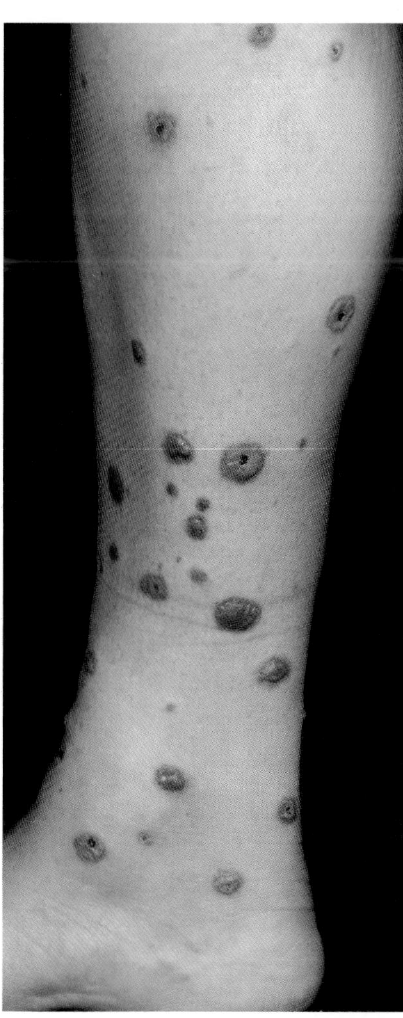

Figure 9.1 Vasculitis.

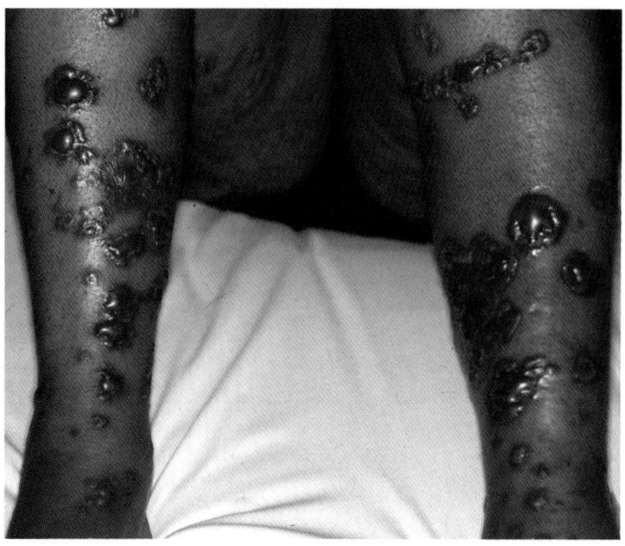

Figure 9.2 Bullous vasculitis with necrosis.

The pathophysiology of vasculitis is complex and poorly characterised but is thought to be antibody or immune complex mediated. Blood vessel endothelial lining cells become damaged as a result of immune complex deposition, antibody targeting and consequent inflammatory cascades. Inflammation involves activation of complement and the release of inflammatory mediators resulting in vasodilatation and polymorph accumulation. The resultant leakage and occlusion of blood vessels leads to ischemia.

Confirmation of cutaneous vasculitis from a skin biopsy for histology and immunofluorescence (IMF) can be helpful but is not usually diagnostic of the underlying cause (Box 9.2). However, in Henoch–Schönlein purpura the IMF from the skin biopsy usually shows IgA deposition.

Box 9.2 **Possible causes of cutaneous vasculitis**

- Drug hypersensitivity
- Hepatitis
- Endocarditis
- Inflammatory bowel disease
- Connective tissue disease
- Coagulopathies
- Behçet's syndrome
- Kawasaki disease
- Sarcoidosis

Polyarteritis nodosa (PAN)

PAN is a systemic vasculitis of small- to medium-sized arterioles that most commonly affects the skin and joints. Immune complexes mediate the disease, activating the complement cascade leading to inflammatory damage to vessels. The sites of blood vessel bifurcation are commonly affected and this leads to micro-aneurysm formation with resultant occlusion and haemorrhage. ANCA may be positive. Patients present with general malaise, fever, weight loss, weakness, arthralgia, neuropathies and skin lesions. Of the patients,

60% develop renal involvement, which may lead to renal failure. Cutaneous manifestations may include a subtle lacy/mottled pattern (livedo reticularis), purpura, tender subcutaneous nodules, ulceration and necrosis, particularly on the lower limbs. Investigations may include angiography and tissue biopsy (skin, sural nerve or muscle). Management relies on oral steroids with the addition of cyclophosphamide in severe cases.

Henoch–Schönlein purpura

This usually occurs in children (75% of cases) or young adults (M > F); the aetiology is unknown, but up to 50% of patients have preceding upper respiratory tract symptoms and a positive antistreptolysin O titre (ASOT). The skin, kidneys (IgA nephropathy), GI tract and joints are mainly affected. IgA, complement and immune complexes are deposited in small vessels (arterioles, capillaries, venules), leading to systemic vasculitis. HSP is characterised by a vasculitic rash on the buttocks and lower legs (which may associated with oedema of scrotum/hands/ears), abdominal pain and vomiting, joint pains in the knees/ankles and haematuria. Skin/renal biopsy may demonstrate deposition of IgA on immunofluorescence, which can support the diagnosis. Treatment is mainly supportive and most patients recover within weeks. Occasionally, the condition can persist and systemic corticosteroids have been used to treat skin, gastrointestinal and arthritis symptoms but steroids have not been shown to prevent or treat renal disease.

Management of cutaneous vasculitis

Treat any underlying cause. For mild to moderate cutaneous involvement a potent topical steroid can be applied to the affected skin. If the lower legs are affected then support hosiery should be used and the legs elevated on sitting.

In more severe cases, systemic corticosteroids (30–60 mg) are usually required. Anticoagulation with heparin or warfarin may be needed. If the vasculitis persists then an alternative immunosuppressant may be needed in the long term such as azathioprine or methotrexate.

Raynaud's phenomenon

Recurrent reversible vasospasm of peripheral arterioles secondary to cold exposure leads to transient ischaemia of the digits associated with an underlying autoimmune disease (Raynaud's disease is the same phenomenon without any underlying systemic disease). Raynaud's phenomenon is most commonly associated with systemic sclerosis, mixed connective tissue disease (MCTD), SLE and cryoglobulinemia. In the cold, the affected digits characteristically turn white (vasospasm), then blue (cyanosis) and finally red (hyperemia); these colour changes may be associated with pain or numbness. The condition most frequently affects the fingers in a bilateral and symmetrical pattern but may also affect the toes, nose and ears. Consider investigating patients with full blood count, renal and liver function, coagulation profile, thyroid function, serum glucose, creatinine kinase, hepatitis serology and antinuclear antibodies. Management involves keeping peripheries warm, nifedipine and iloprost (prostacycline analogue).

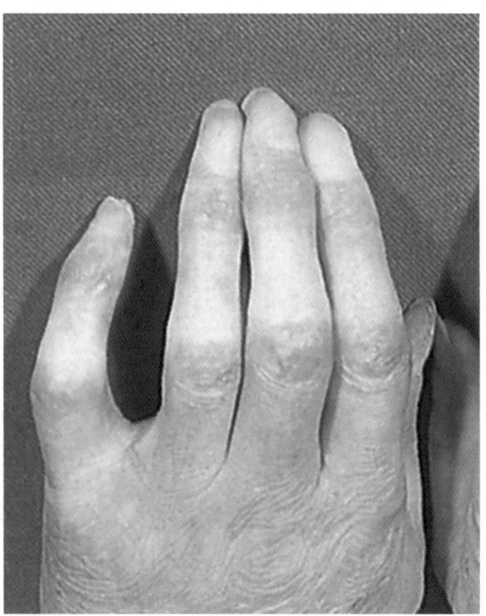

Figure 9.3 Systemic sclerosis.

Systemic sclerosis (SSc)

This is a condition in which there is extensive sclerosis (excessive collagen deposition and fibrosis) of the subcutaneous tissues in the fingers and toes as well as around the mouth (scleroderma), with similar changes affecting the internal organs, particularly the lung and kidneys. Blood vessels can be affected, leading to Raynaud's phenomenon (fingers) and telangiectasia (mouth and fingers) (Figure 9.3). The main types of SSc are limited (lSSc) and disseminated (dSSc), the former mainly affecting females. About 90% of patients with SSc will have at least one positive ANA. Antibodies against topoisomerase I DNA (Scl 70) are found in about 30% of patients (70% of those with dSSc and interstitial lung disease). About 38% of patients with SSc and skin involvement have a positive anticentromere antibody (most commonly in lSSc). Other positive ANAs include anti-SSA/Ro/RNA polymerase III. Additional investigations that may be helpful include CRP/ESR (raised), high resolution CT scan of the lungs (thickening of the alveolar walls), lung function tests (impaired ventilation–perfusion) and skin biopsy (fibrotic changes seen on histology). Clinically, there is considerable tethering of the skin on the fingers/toes, which becomes very tight with a waxy appearance and considerable limitation of movement. There are many other forms of scleroderma including undifferentiated connective tissue disease and the so-called 'CREST syndrome' (Box 9.3).

Box 9.3 **CREST syndrome**

C Calcinosis cutis
R Raynaud's phenomenon
E Oesophageal dysmotility
S Sclerodactyly
T Telangiectasia

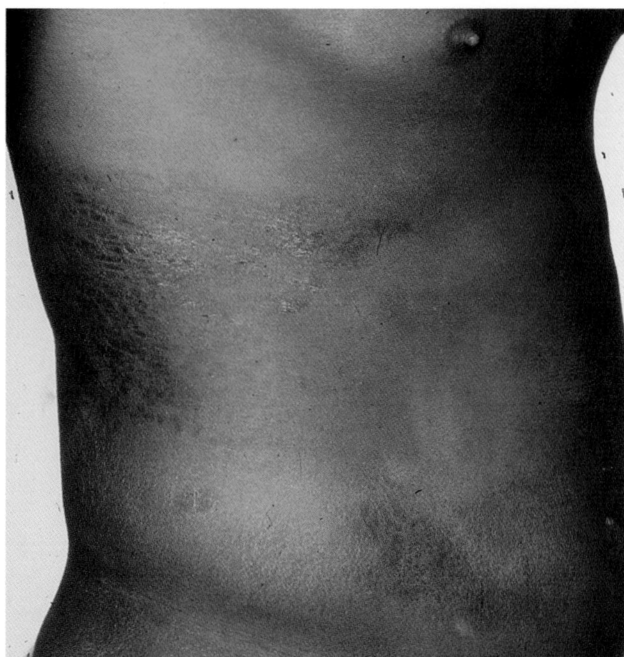

Figure 9.4 Morphoea.

Morphoea is a benign form of localised systemic sclerosis in which there is localised sclerosis with very slight inflammation. There is atrophy of the overlying epidermis. In the early stages the skin may have a dusky appearance, but as the disease progresses the skin becomes discoloured and feels very firm (Figure 9.4). Localised morphoea in the frontoparietal area ('en coup de sabre') is associated with alopecia and a sunken groove of firm sclerotic skin.

Patients who develop CREST usually first complain of Raynaud's phenomenon, followed by thickening of the skin of the digits due to scleroderma (progressive fibrosis) leading to sclerodactyly. Calcium deposits in the skin are seen as chalky-white material which can be painful (Figure 9.5). Patients then develop multiple telangiectasia, usually first seen on the face (Figure 9.6) but mucous membranes and the gastrointestinal tract may also be affected. Dysmotility of the oesophagus is usually a late development.

Investigations should include an FBC, ANA, anticentromere antibody and anti-Scl-70.

A multidisciplinary team approach to management is usually needed, including psychological support. Patients should keep themselves warm, especially their hands. Calcium-channel blockers

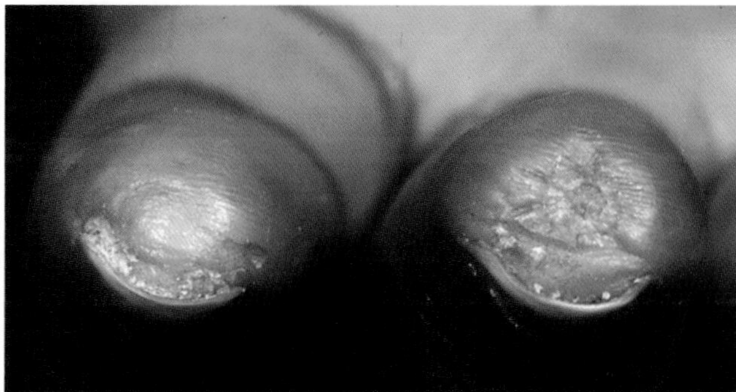

Figure 9.5 Calcinosis cutis.

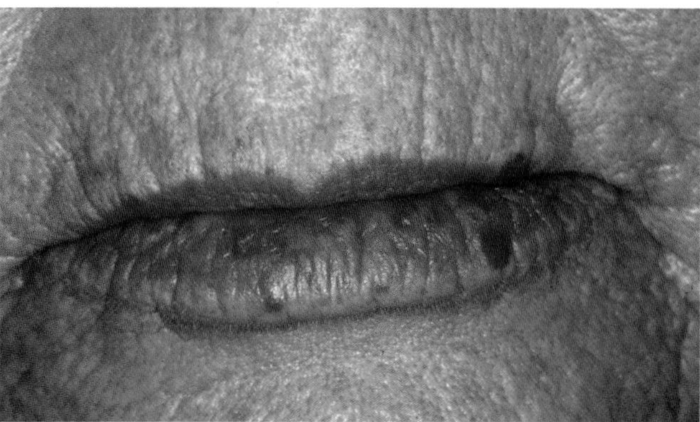

Figure 9.6 CREST syndrome.

and prostaglandins/protacycline may help prevent and treat Raynaud's phenomenon. Calcitriol may soften the sclerodactyly, and pulsed dye laser may treat facial telangiectasia.

Lichen sclerosus (LS)

This is an itchy eruption which mainly affects the genital and perineal regions in women. The disorder is characterised by well-demarcated atrophic patches and plaques with a distinctive ivory white colour. There is fibrosis of the underlying tissues with associated loss of normal genital architecture. It frequently affects the vulva (Figure 9.7) and perineum, but may also affect the penis

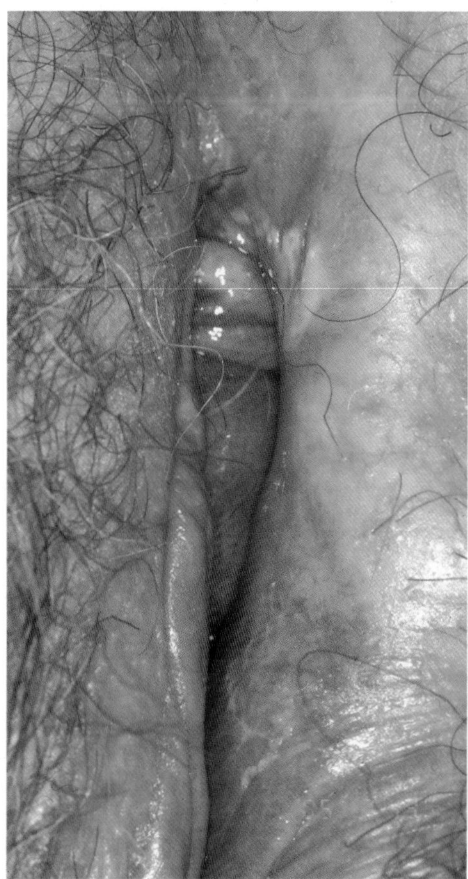

Figure 9.7 Lichen sclerosus.

and extragenital skin. A more acute form can affect children, which tends to resolve but in adults it is a chronic condition. LS can rarely be associated with the development of squamous cell carcinoma (SCC). The cause of the hyalinised collagen and epidermal atrophy is unknown, but in early lesions there is an infiltrate of lymphocytes with CD3, CD4, CD8 and CD68 markers. An immunological basis for the disease has been suggested because patients have an increased incidence of autoimmune disease. Histologically, there are some similarities between LS and lichen planus; however, they usually present with different clinical features. Treatment is with intermittent potent topical steroids, which usually controls the itching. If pruritus is not controlled by potent topical steroids or soreness develops, then review by an experienced dermatologist is indicated to rule out the development of SCC.

Lichen planus (LP)

Clinically, patients have an itchy eruption consisting of shiny purple-coloured flat-topped papules that characteristically appear on the wrists (Figure 9.8) and ankles. White lines called Wickham's striae may appear on the surface of the lesions at any site. Lesions may appear in clusters or in linear scratches/surgical scars (Koebner phenomenon).The underlying cause is unknown, but the condition is thought to have an immunological aetiology. The histological features are characterised by a band of lymphocytes attacking the basal keratinocytes which results in oedema, subepidermal clefts and death of some keratinocytes. In patients with black skin, LP may be very hypertrophic and heal with marked post-inflammatory hyperpigmentation. The mouth (especially, buccal mucosa; Figure 9.9) and genitals (erosions on labia minora) may also be involved and distinctive linear ridges may affect the nails. Scalp lesions are often scaly with marked follicular plugging that may result in scarring alopecia. Severe acute lichen planus can manifest as bullous lesions (Figure 9.10). Most cases resolve over 1–2 years. Hypertrophic LP may, however, persist for decades. Potent topical steroid applied to the itchy active lesions is usually effective. Occlusion of the steroid for treatment of hypertrophic lesions is usually more effective than steroid alone. Severe lichen planus can be treated with systemic corticosteroids, mycophenolate mofetil, methotrexate or azathioprine.

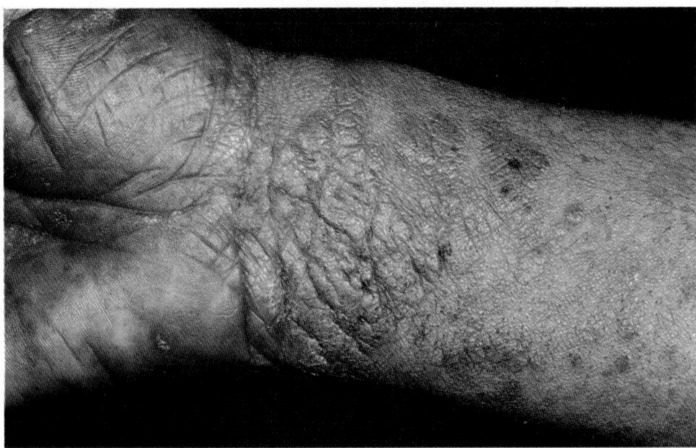

Figure 9.8 Lichen planus on the wrist.

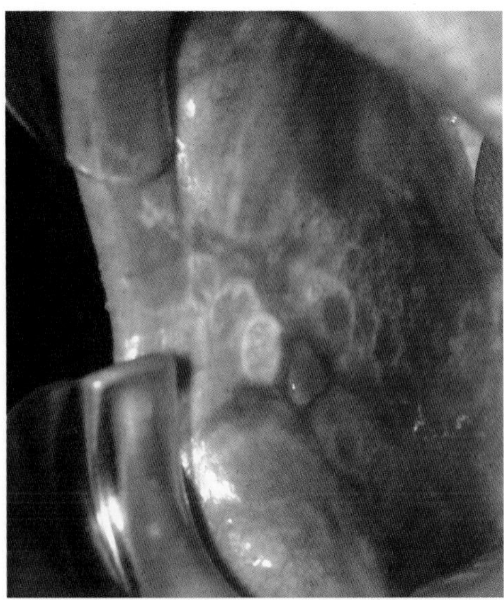

Figure 9.9 Lichen planus in the mouth.

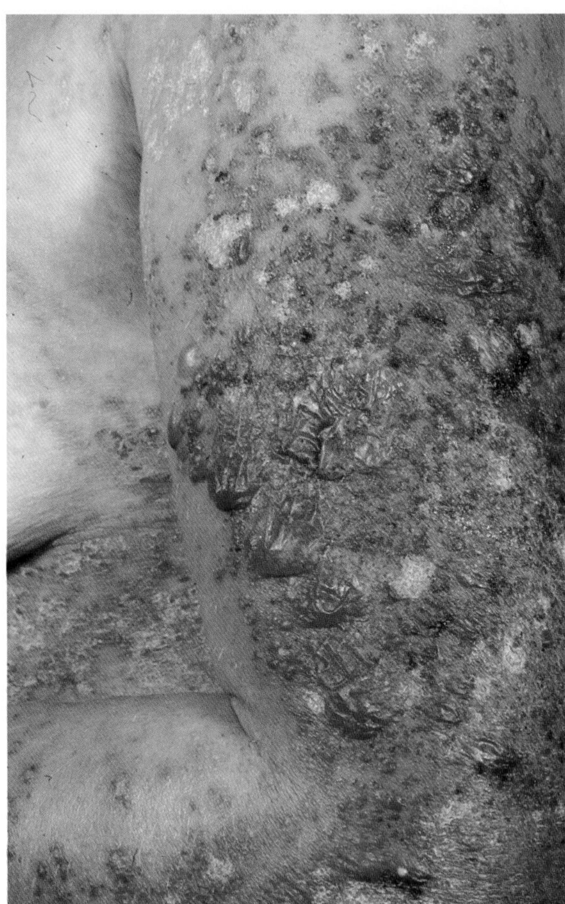

Figure 9.10 Bullous lichen planus

Lichenoid drug eruptions are clinically similar to LP but lesions are usually more extensive and oral involvement is rare (see Chapter 7). Lesions only resolve very slowly after the drug is stopped, generally taking 1–4 months to settle and usually leaving hyperpigmentation on the skin.

Lupus erythematosus (LE)

There are four main clinical variants of lupus erythematosus: systemic, subacute, discoid and neonatal (Box 9.4).

Box 9.4 **Clinical variants of lupus erythematosus**

- Systemic
- Subacute cutaneous
- Discoid
- Neonatal

SLE is an autoimmune disorder characterised by the presence of antibodies against various components of the cell nucleus. SLE has been triggered by drugs including chlorpromazine, quinine and isoniazid. SLE is a multisystem disease; 75% of patients have skin involvement, most commonly an erythematous 'butterfly' distribution rash on the face (Figure 9.11). Photosensitivity, hair loss and areas of cutaneous vasculitis may occur. As the disease progresses the cutaneous manifestations can become extensive (Figure 9.12). Systemic changes include fever, arthritis and renal involvement, but there may be involvement of a wide range of organs.

Diagnostic criteria for SLE include four of the following at any given time:

- malar rash
- serositis
- discoid plaques
- neurological disorders
- photosensitivity
- haematological changes
- arthritis
- immunological changes
- mouth ulcers
- antinuclear antibodies
- renal changes.

Subacute lupus erythematosus (SLE) is a variant that presents with an erythematous annular and serpiginous eruption on the skin (Figure 9.13). Systemic involvement is less common/severe than in SLE. It is associated with a high incidence of neonatal lupus erythematosus in children born to mothers with the condition. The ENA test is positive in 60% and anticytoplasmic antibodies are present in 80% of patients.

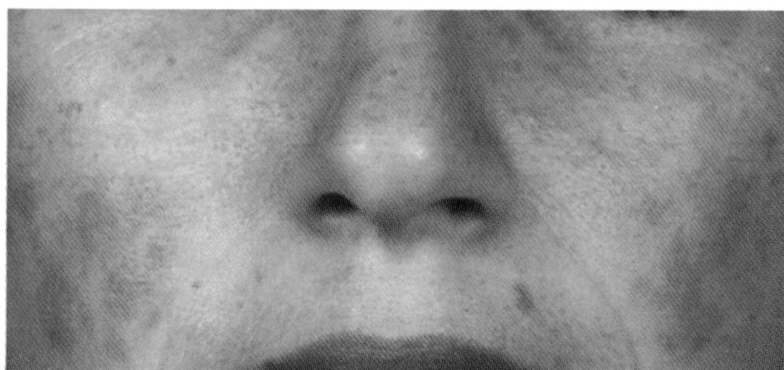

Figure 9.11 Systemic lupus erythematosus: butterfly rash.

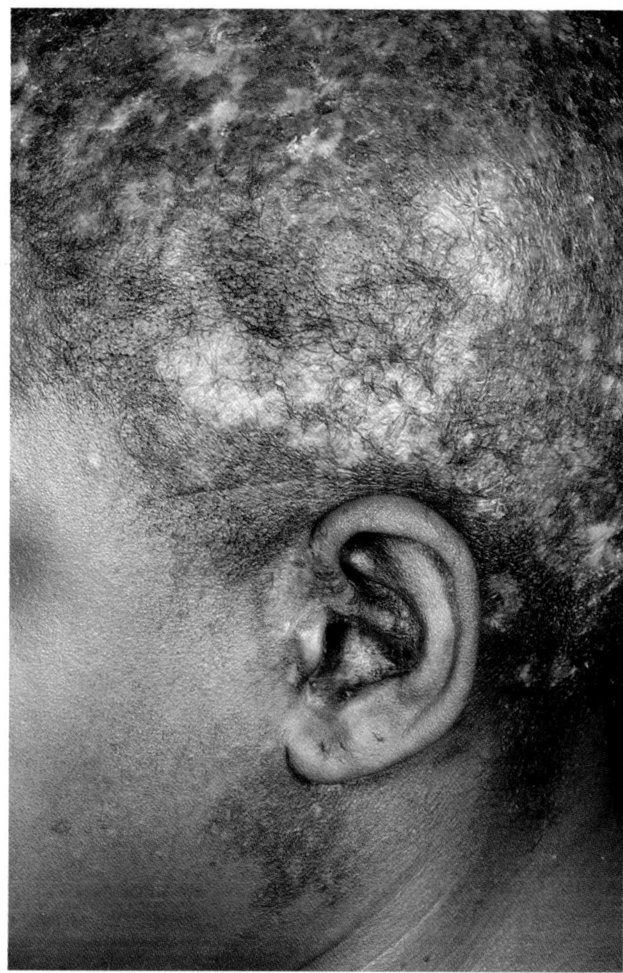

Figure 9.12 Extensive severe systemic lupus erythematosus.

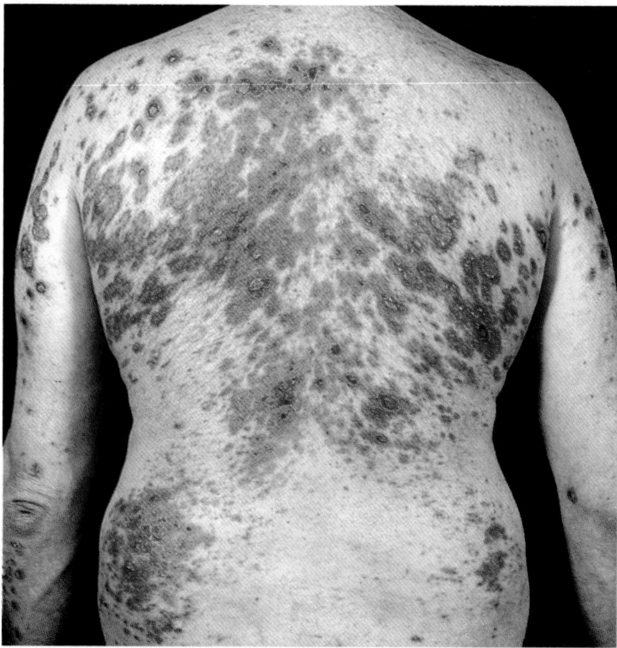

Figure 9.13 Subacute lupus erythematosus.

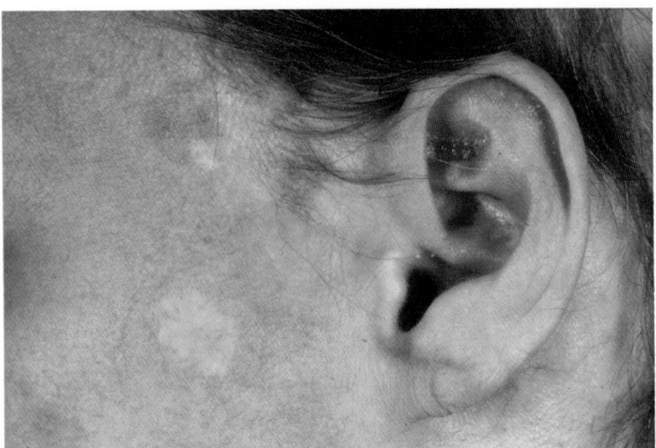

Figure 9.14 Discoid lupus erythematosus.

Discoid lupus erythematosus (DLE) is a photosensitive disorder in which well-defined erythematous lesions with atrophy, scaling and scarring occur on the face (Figure 9.14), scalp (alopecia, follicular plugging) and occasionally arms. This is a condition in which circulating antinuclear antibodies are very rare and only 5% of patients go on to develop SLE. DLE should be treated with potent and super-potent topical steroids to limit scarring.

Neonatal lupus erythematosus is caused by transplacental passage of maternal lupus antibodies (particularly Ro/La) to the neonate who may suffer skin lesions, which are characterised by annular scaly and inflammatory lesions on the face/scalp (Figure 9.15) and congenital heart block (which may require pacing). Skin lesions may require topical steroid but usually resolve spontaneously as the level of autoantibody depletes.

Treatment of SLE with threatened or actual involvement of organs is important. Prednisolone is usually required and sometimes immunosuppressant drugs such as azathioprine as well. Treatment of DLE is generally with topical steroids and sunscreen. Hydroxychloroquine 200 mg twice daily can be effective. Rarely hydroxychloroquine can cause ocular toxicity; however, patients should be asked to report any visual disturbance.

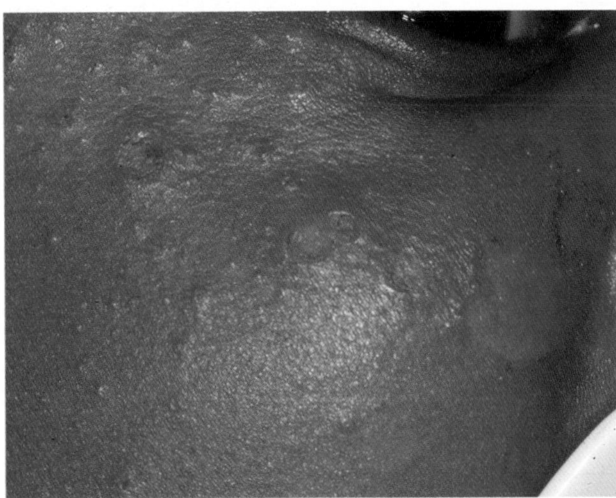

Figure 9.15 Neonatal lupus erythematosus.

Dermatomyositis

Dermatomyositis is a rare disorder that affects the skin, muscle and blood vessels. The cause is unknown but derangement of normal immune responses is observed. Evidence suggests that dermatomyositis may be mediated by damage to blood vessel walls triggered by a change in the humoral immune system, which leads to cytotoxic T-cell damage to skin and muscle. In the early stages, there is deposition of IgG, IgM and C3 at the dermoepidermal junction as well as a lymphocytic infiltrate with CD4+ cells and macrophages. Circulating immune complexes have been isolated in up to 70% of patients, and autoantibodies may be demonstrated. Dermatomyositis in adults may precede the diagnosis of an underlying tumour (most commonly breast, lung, ovary or gastrointestinal tract), and therefore patients should be investigated thoroughly.

Clinically, there is a rash in a mainly photosensitive distribution characterised by a purple hue (heliotrope) on the upper eyelids, cheeks and forehead. The anterior 'V' (Figure 9.16) and posterior aspect (shawl sign) of the neck are usually involved. The dorsal surface of the fingers may be affected by the erythematous eruption and purplish (Gottron's) papules may predominate over the dorsal finger joints (Figure 9.17). Ragged cuticles and dilated nail-fold capillaries may also be seen (Figure 9.18). There is a variable association with muscle discomfort and weakness, which is mainly in the proximal limbs but bulbar and respiratory muscles may be affected.

Investigations include creatine phosphokinase (CK), ESR, anti-Jo-1 antibody, and skin and muscle biopsy. Electromyography and MRI can help demonstrate myositis.

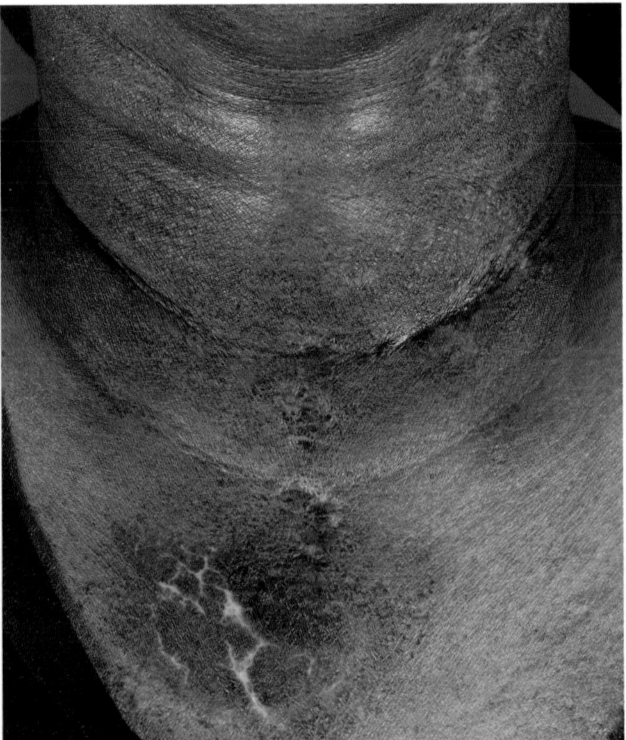

Figure 9.16 Dermatomyositis rash on the 'V' of the neck.

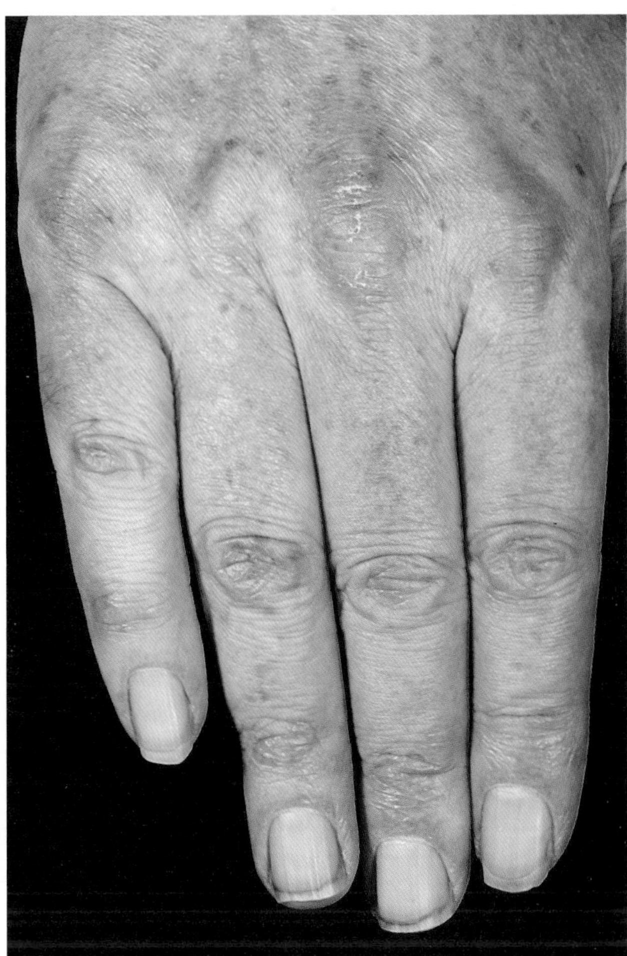

Figure 9.17 Dermatomyositis of the hands.

Treatment with high dose systemic corticosteroids (60–100 mg daily) or pulsed methyl prednisolone (1 g daily for 3 days) helps achieve rapid control of symptoms. Pulsed cyclophosphamide, azathioprine, methotrexate and mycophenolate mofetil may also be used to control the disease. Treatment of any underlying malignancy will usually lead to resolution of these skin signs.

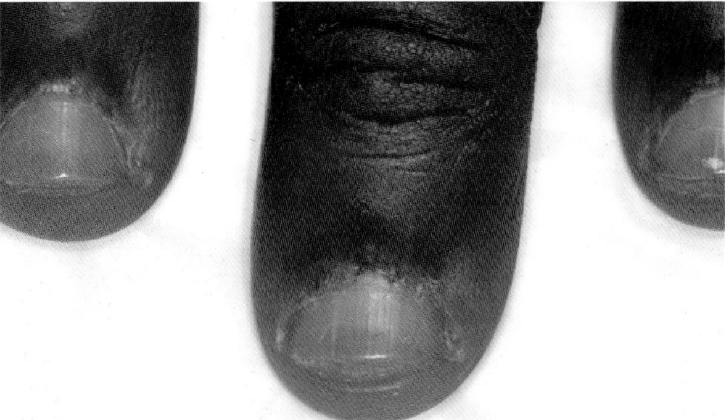

Figure 9.18 Dermatomyositis: ragged cuticles.

Mixed connective tissue disease (MCTD)

A group of patients with overlapping features of systemic lupus, scleroderma and myositis with characteristic autoantibodies have been diagnosed with so-called mixed connective tissue disease (MCTD). Although at first this group of mainly young women (age 15–25 years) seem difficult to characterise, clinically they usually have Raynaud's phenomenon, sclerodactyly/swollen hands, arthritis/arthralgia, Sjogren syndrome, myositis, malaise, oesophageal dysmotility, trigeminal neuralgia and pulmonary hypertension. Patients usually have positive antibodies to U1-ribonucleoprotein (RNP) and small nuclear ribonucleoprotein (snRNP). Treatment aims to reduce pain and maintain function, with the aim of trying to keep patients as active as possible. Traditional NSAIDs are used to reduce pain and inflammation and the newer cyclooxygenase 2 (COX-2) inhibitor celecoxib is increasingly used to help reduced arthritis and myositis. Hydroxychloroquine can also be used and for more refractory disease low dose oral corticosteroids and methotrexate.

Further reading

Edwards C. *Connective Tissue Disease in Clinical Practice*, Springer, New York, 2013.

Silver R and Denton C. *Case Studies in Systemic Sclerosis*, Springer, New York, 2011.

CHAPTER 10

The Skin and Systemic Disease

Rachael Morris-Jones

Dermatology Department, Kings College Hospital, London, UK

> **OVERVIEW**
> - Skin changes may be the first sign of an underlying systemic disease.
> - Widespread reactive rashes result from underlying infections, medications, connective tissue diseases and malignancy.
> - Characteristic skin reactions such as erythema multiforme and erythema nodosum are often associated with underlying diseases.
> - Reduced numbers of melanocytes can be genetic or associated with autoimmune disease or hormonal changes.
> - Increased pigment in the skin can be associated with hormonal changes or underlying neoplasia.
> - Generalised pruritus without a skin rash is a strong indicator of an underlying systemic disease – such as renal/hepatic dysfunction.
> - Gastrointestinal disease may be associated with skin conditions such as dermatitis herpetiformis and pyoderma gangrenosum.

Introduction

The skin is the window on underlying systemic diseases as it may give visible diagnostic clues to underlying disease (Box 10.1). Cutaneous manifestations of systemic diseases are numerous and may be one of the first indicators of an underlying illness. Therefore, recognition of these reaction patterns and classic lesions in the skin associated with systemic disease can a valuable aid to rapid and accurate diagnosis (Box 10.2). Systemic diseases may affect the skin in the same way that is affects other internal organs – such as connective tissue diseases (Chapter 9). However, underlying conditions may be associated with skin changes brought about by quite different processes, such as those seen in acanthosis nigricans (AN), dermatomyositis and erythema multiforme (EM).

> Box 10.1 **Clues to a possible underlying systemic disease**
>
> - Rash associated with other symptoms such as joint pains, weight loss, fever, weakness, breathlessness and altered bowel function.
> - Rash not responding to topical treatments.
> - Erythema of the skin due to inflammation around the blood vessels, which may be migratory or fixed.
> - Vasculitis, characterised by non-blanching often palpable purplish fixed lesions which may be painful and blistering.
> - Unusual changes in pigmentation or texture of the skin.
> - Palpable dermal lesions secondary to granulomas, metastases, lymphoma or deposits of amyloid, and so on.

> Box 10.2 **Characteristic rashes associated with underlying systemic disease**
>
> - Erythema multiforme – herpes simplex virus, mycoplasma pneumonia, hepatitis B/C, borelliosis, pneumococcus (medications).
> - Pyoderma gangrenosum – haematological malignancy, inflammatory bowel disease, rheumatoid arthritis, monoclonal gammopathy.
> - Erythema nodosum – streptococcal infection, TB, sarcoid, pregnancy, inflammatory bowel disease, Hodgkin's lymphoma, Behcet disease.
> - Vasculitis – hepatitis B/C, streptococcal infection, parvovirus B19, systemic lupus erythematosus (SLE), rheumatoid, inflammatory bowel disease, leukaemia, lymphoma.

Many widespread reactive cutaneous reactions are a result of medications taken and are manifested as toxic erythema (Chapter 7). The florid skin lesions associated with HIV vary from severe manifestations of common dermatoses to rare skin infections to exaggerated hypersensitivity reactions to drugs (Chapter 15). Drug rashes and manifestations of HIV are important topics and are addressed in detail in Chapters 7 and 15 respectively.

Skin reactions associated with infections

Toxic erythema is the term used for a widespread symmetrical reactive rash consisting of maculopapular erythema (Figure 10.1) which looks 'morbilliform' (which means measles-like). The rash usually starts on the trunk and then spreads to the limbs and is blanching and may be mildly itchy. Toxic erythema is most commonly triggered by viruses including measles, rubella, Epstein–Barr virus (glandular fever patients given amoxicillin classically develop a toxic erythema), parvovirus B19, West Nile virus, human herpes

ABC of Dermatology, Sixth Edition. Edited by Rachael Morris-Jones.

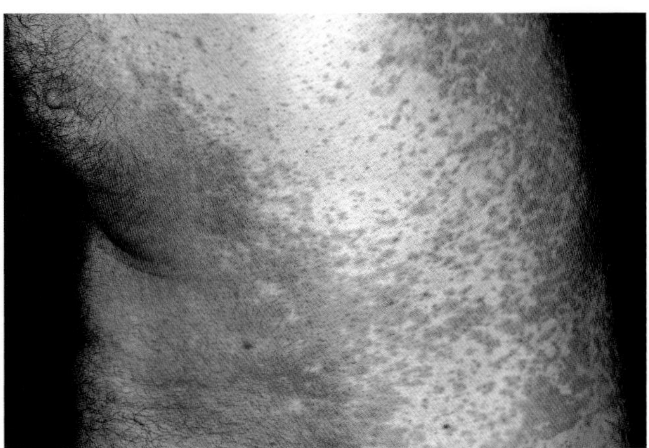

Figure 10.1 Toxic erythema reactive morbilliform rash.

virus 6 (roseola infantum), flavivirus (dengue), coxsackievirus 4/5 and typhus (*Salmonella typhi*); bacterial infections such as Scarlet fever (group A *Streptococcus*), Rickettsiosis (Rocky Mountain spotted fever) and parasitic infections (trypanosomiasis – sleeping sickness) can also result in this widespread reactive rash. No treatment is usually required for these toxic erythema rashes except an emollient and occasionally a mild topical steroid if symptomatic; what is required is management of the underlying disease.

EM consists of lesions that are erythematous macules that become raised and typically develop into characteristic 'target lesions' (Figure 10.2) in which there is a dusky red or purpuric/blistered centre with a pale indurated zone surrounded by an outer ring of erythema. The lesions are usually asymptomatic (occasionally painful) and may be few/multiple/diffuse and symmetrical, developing over a few days at acral sites (palms, soles, digits, elbows, knees and face). The rash is thought to result from an immunologically mediated hypersensitivity reaction. Systemic symptoms of the underlying infection usually precede the EM rash by 2–14 days. Involvement of mucous membranes (oral, conjunctival, genital) accompanies the classic cutaneous EM rash (<10% of body surface area) in the so-called EM Major. The most common infectious trigger is herpes simplex virus (HSV 1 or 2), which usually presents with a cold sore on the lip or sores/ulcers on the genitals or rarely herpetic whitlow. Other infectious triggers include *Mycoplasma pneumonia* (shortness of breath, cough, chest radiograph relatively normal), haemolytic *Streptococcus* (upper respiratory tract infection), adenovirus, coxsackievirus, Epstein–Barr virus, parvovirus B19, viral hepatitis, borreliosis and *Neisseria meningitides*. Adverse reactions to medications are also a common trigger for EM (Chapter 7). If possible, treat the underlying disease (e.g. aciclovir, penicillin) and apply topical steroid to skin lesions if painful or blistering; occasionally systemic steroids may be needed. EM can be recurrent with each reactivation of HSV, in which case patients may need secondary prophylaxis with aciclovir and possibly additional azathioprine.

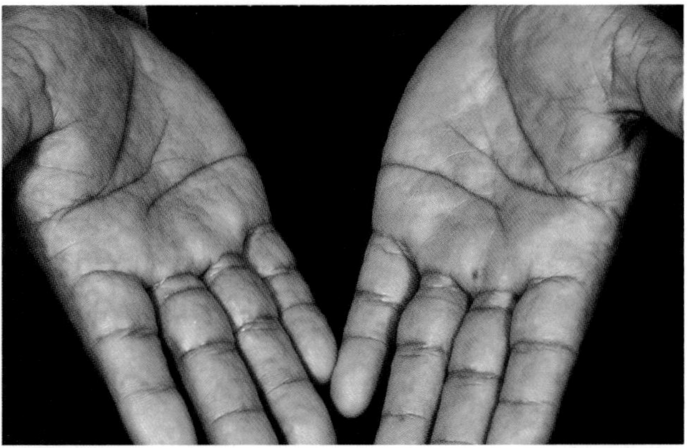

Figure 10.2 Erythema multiforme.

Gianotti–Crosti Syndrome (GCS) – papulovesicular acrodermatitis of childhood is a viral exanthema characterised by sheets of minute erythematous papules which may become vesicular in young children (age <12 years) that are distributed initially on the limbs (elbows/knees/feet/hands) and may affect the face (spares the trunk). Individual erythematous papules may coalesce into clusters of larger patches of erythema and may feel 'rough' like sandpaper and usually lasts for several weeks. Viral triggers include enteroviruses, echo virus, respiratory syncytial virus, rotavirus, rubella parvovirus B19, hepatitis B and Epstein–Barr virus. GCS may also be triggered by vaccinations (polio, diphtheria, hepatitis B, measles, influenza, pertussis, swine-flu H_1N_1). GCS is more common in children with atopic dermatitis (AD). The exanthema settles over a few weeks with simple emollients.

Erythema nodosum (EN) consists of tender/painful subcutaneous erythematous nodules on the shins secondary to a hypersensitivity reaction leading to inflammatory panniculitis (inflammation in the adipose tissue) (Figure 10.3). The lower leg lesions usually evolve over a few days following systemic symptoms such as fever and malaise and last for weeks or months depending on the trigger. Infectious causes of EN include *Streptococcus*, *Mycoplasma pneumoniae*, TB, histoplasmosis, coccidioidomycosis and blastomycosis. Other non-infectious triggers include medications, inflammatory bowel disease, sarcoidosis, pregnancy, Behcet and Hodgkin disease. In approximately 50% of cases there is no obvious cause determined. Management involves treating or removing the underlying cause, elevation and compression of the lower legs and nonsteroidal anti-inflammatory drugs (NSAIDs).

Erythema annulare centrifugum (EAC) consists of single/multiple erythematous expanding rings (annular/figurate/gyrate erythema) usually on the thighs or trunk which are asymptomatic. EAC lesions slowly enlarge to form incomplete/complete rings of palpable/macular erythema which may have a slight scale on the inner edge of the ring (Figure 10.4). A hypersensitivity reaction is the current thinking with triggers including Epstein–Barr virus, HIV, *Escherichia coli*, *Streptococcus*, *Trichophyton* fungal infections (tinea), *Candida albicans*, TB and pubic lice. Other non-infectious causes include underlying leukaemia/lymphoma, solid tumours (breast, ovarian, lung carcinoma), medications and other underlying systemic condition such as Graves' disease and sarcoid.

Erythema chronicum migrans is a migrating erythema that results from a cutaneous inflammatory response to infection caused by *Borrelia burgdorferi* (Lyme disease) (Chapter 17).

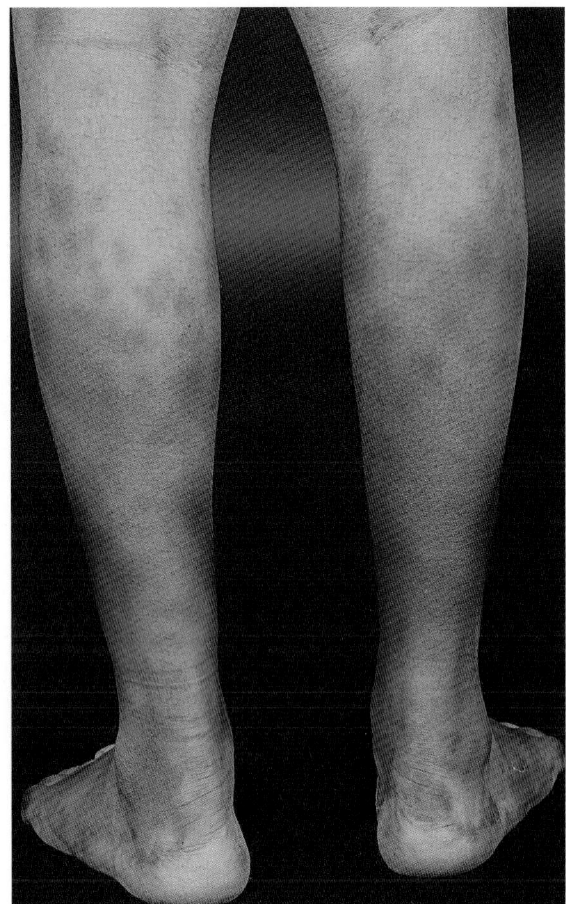

Figure 10.3 Erythema nodosum.

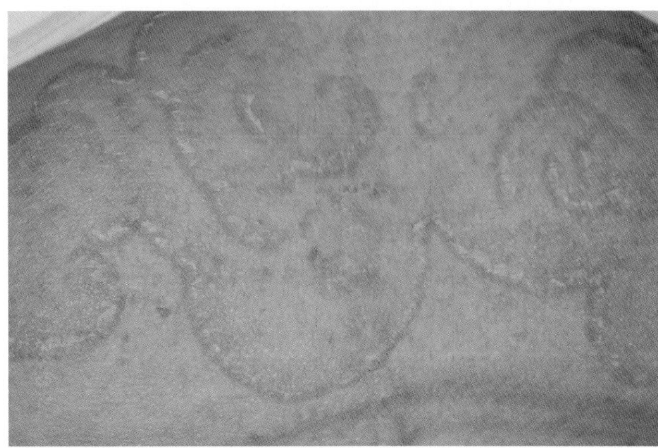

Figure 10.4 Annular erythema.

Sarcoidosis

The underlying aetiology of sarcoidosis remains unknown; however, there are increasing number of researchers who believe that an atypical mycobacterium may be the trigger. Pulmonary and other systemic manifestations of sarcoidosis may occur without cutaneous disease. However, skin disease is a common presenting sign of underlying sarcoidosis in about 40% of patients. The most common skin changes are

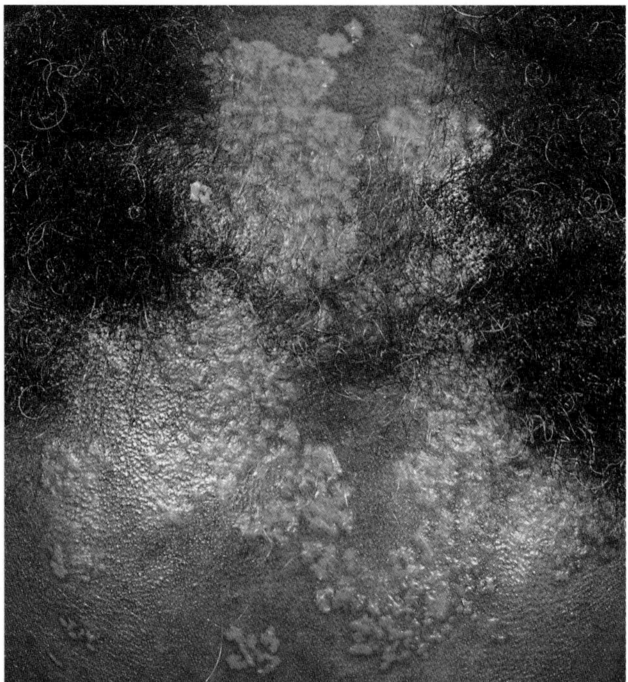

Figure 10.5 Nodular and plaque sarcoid.

- EN, which is often a feature of early pulmonary disease;
- papules, nodules, and plaques, which are associated with acute and subacute forms of the disease (Figure 10.5);
- scar sarcoidosis, with papules;
- lupus pernio with dusky red infiltrated lesions on the nose and fingers.

Skin changes associated with hormonal imbalance

Hyperpigmentation is an increase in circulating hormones with melanocyte-stimulating activity that occurs in hyperthyroidism, Addison's disease and acromegaly. In pregnancy or in those taking oral contraceptives there may be a localised increase in melanocytic pigmentation of the forehead and cheeks known as *melasma* (or *chloasma*) (Figure 10.6). It may fade slowly if ultraviolet light is excluded from the affected skin using daily sun block.

Hypopigmentation is a widespread partial loss of melanocyte functions with loss of skin colour seen in hypopituitarism and is caused by an absence of melanocyte-stimulating hormone.

Acanthosis nigricans AN is asymptomatic velvety thickening of the skin characteristically affecting the posterior and lateral aspects of the neck, axillae and arm flexures (Figure 10.7); it appears as dark symmetrical plaques. The most common association is obesity, and with weight reduction the AN resolves. Syndromic AN is subtyped into Type A, which is associated with insulin resistance in young black women with hirsutism and polycystic ovarian syndrome, and Type B, which is associated with autoimmune conditions such as diabetes, thyroid disease and lupus. Antibodies to insulin receptors may be detected in Type B. More extensive and rapidly evolving AN, particularly involving the lips/tongue/palms may herald underlying malignancy, particularly of the gastrointestinal (GI)

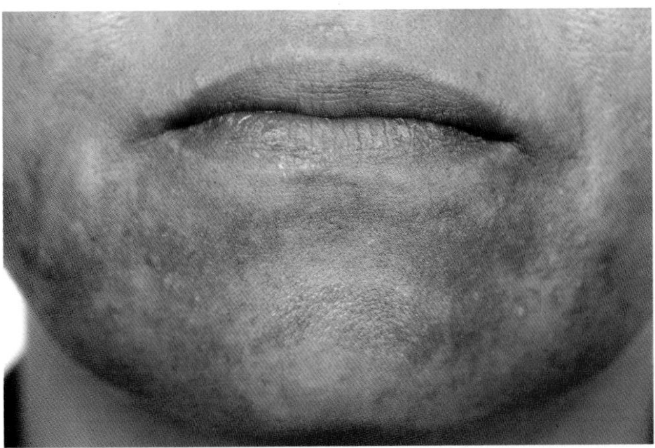

Figure 10.6 Melasma.

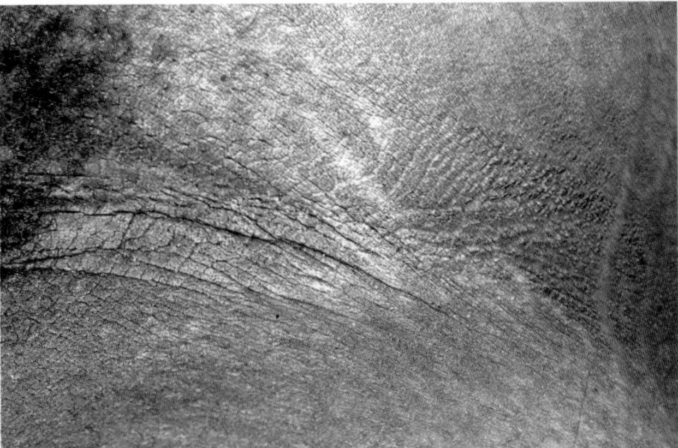

Figure 10.7 Acanthosis nigricans.

tract. When the underlying cause is treated, the skin signs of AN usually regress.

Diabetes leads to alteration of carbohydrate–lipid metabolism; small blood vessel lesions and neural involvement may be associated with skin lesions such as 'diabetic dermopathy' due to a microangiopathy, which consists of erythematous papules which slowly resolve to leave a scaling macule on the limbs. Atherosclerosis with impaired peripheral circulation is often associated with diabetes. Ulceration due to neuropathy (trophic ulcers) or impaired blood supply may occur, particularly on the feet. Diabetic patients have an increased susceptibility to cutaneous infections including staphylococcal, streptococcal, coliforms, *Pseudomonas* and *C. albicans*.

Necrobiosis lipoidica – between 40% and 60% of patients with this condition may develop diabetes, but it is actually uncommon in the diabetic population (0.3%), but checking of fasting glucose is recommended. Necrobiosis indicates necrosis of the underlying connective tissue with lymphocytic and granulomatous infiltrate. There is replacement of degenerating collagen fibres with lipid material. It usually occurs over the shin but may appear at any site (Figure 10.8).

Granuloma annulare usually presents with localised papular lesions on the hands/feet and limbs (Figure 10.9) but may occur elsewhere also. The lesions may be partly or wholly annular and

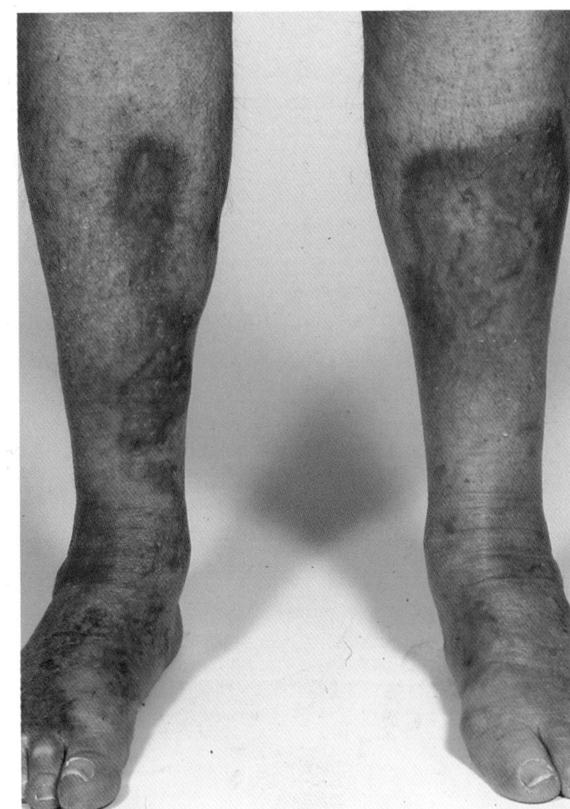

Figure 10.8 Necrobiosis lipoidica.

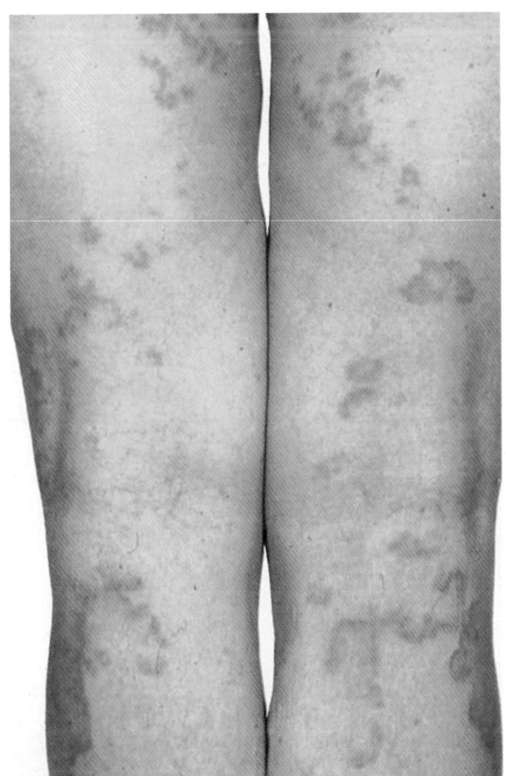

Figure 10.9 Granuloma annulare.

may be single or multiple. There is some degree of necrobiosis, with histiocytes forming 'palisades' as well as giant cells and lymphocytes. It is seen more commonly in women under the age of 30. There is an association with insulin-dependent diabetes. It may be pruritic or asymptomatic and is usually self-limiting but may recur.

Thyroid disease

Thyroid disease is associated with changes in the skin, hair and nails and may be among the earliest signs of underlying thyroid dysfunction (Table 10.1). Associated increases in thyroid-stimulating hormone concentration may lead to pretibial myxoedema (Figure 10.10). In autoimmune thyroid disease, vitiligo and other autoimmune conditions may be present.

Table 10.1 Clinical signs of thyroid disease.

Hypothyroidism	Hyperthyroidism
Dry skin	Soft, thickened skin
Oedema of eyelids and hands	Pretibial myxoedema
Absence of sweating	Increased sweating (palms and soles)
Coarse, thin hair; loss of pubic, axillary and eyebrow hair	Thinning of scalp hair Diffuse pigmentation
Pale 'ivory' skin	Rapidly growing nails Palmar erythema
Brittle poorly growing nails	Facial flushing
Purpura, bruising and telangiectasia	

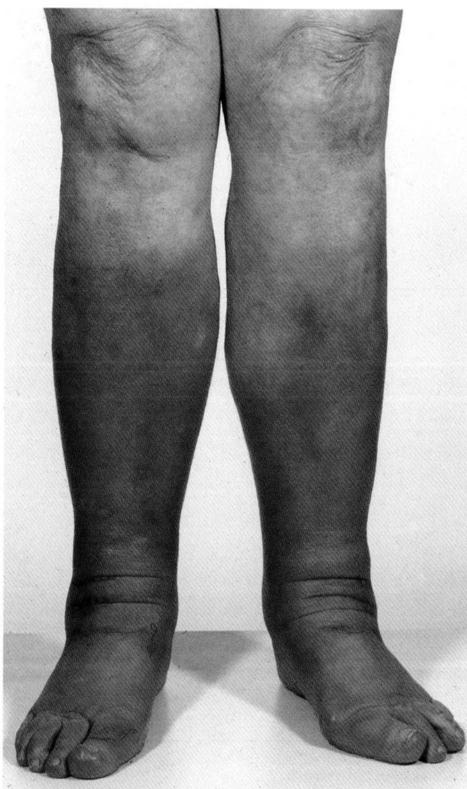

Figure 10.10 Pretibial myxoedema.

Skin changes associated with disorders of the gastrointestinal system and liver

Skin changes may occur as part of a systemic disease involving multiple organs such as vasculitis which may be associated with polyarteritis nodosa (medium vessel vasculitis) and connective tissue diseases (such as scleroderma) or as part of a metabolic disease such as porphyria, malabsorption/dietary deficiencies and inflammatory conditions.

Malabsorption can lead to deficiency of iron, zinc, vitamins, and so on, which can result in dry skin, asteatosis and pruritic skin, which can lead to superficial eczematous changes in a 'crazy paving' pattern. Increased pigmentation, brittle hair and nails may also be associated with malabsorption states.

Vitamin C deficiency (scurvy) occurs in those with malabsorption problems, those on a poor diet, the elderly and alcoholics and is manifested by fatigue, weakness, perifollicular hyperkeratotic papules which look similar to bruises usually on the legs, with corkscrew hairs. Bleeding and swollen gums may also be seen, and the majority of patients are also anaemic. Vitamin C supplementation of around 1 g is usually needed initially and then 0.5 g daily for a few weeks. Symptoms and signs will then recede as vitamin levels normalise.

Zinc deficiency (*acrodermatitis enteropathica*) is usually seen in neonates either as a genetic condition (defect in zinc transporter proteins) or as a result of breast milk deficient in zinc (i.e. mother may be zinc deficient) or malabsorption (breast/bottle fed/weaning). Skin changes usually appear within weeks of birth with erythematous inflamed scaly skin around the mouth, anus and eyes as well as acral sites (hands, feet, elbows and knees) (Figure 10.11). Patches may be confused with eczema, but this

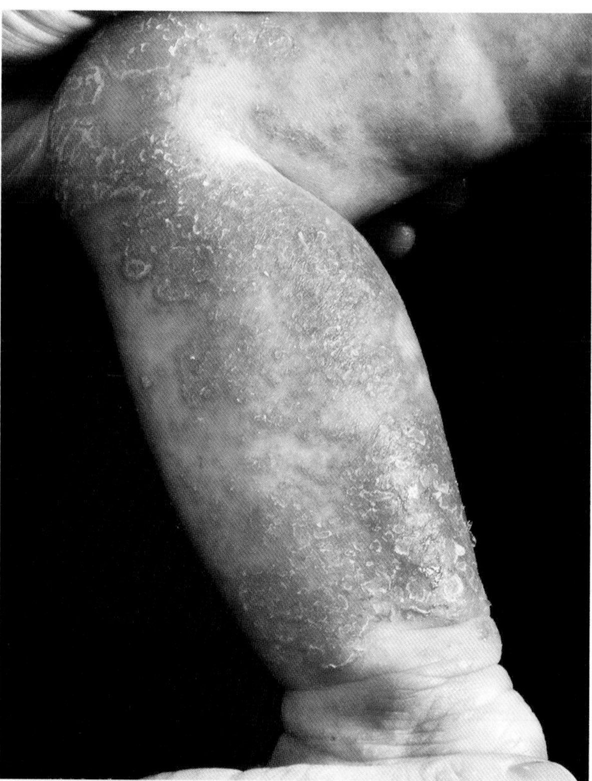

Figure 10.11 Zinc deficiency.

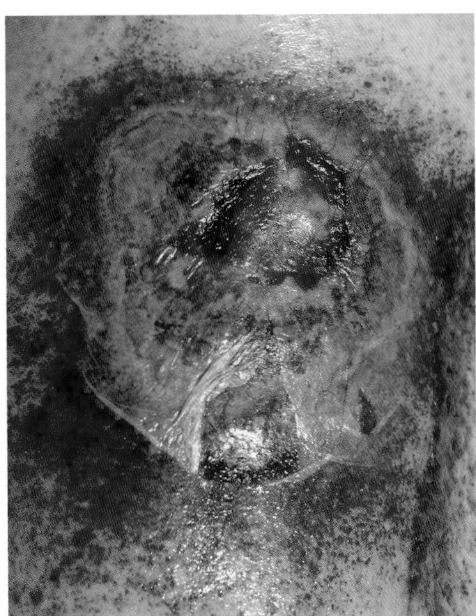

Figure 10.12 Pyoderma gangrenosum.

eruption is not itchy and is well demarcated at localised sites. If the condition is not recognised and treated promptly then the skin can become crusted, eroded and secondarily infected. Babies may become irritable, feed poorly, develop diarrhoea and fail to thrive. Serum zinc levels will be low. Zinc supplementation (1 mg/kg/day) should be continued until zinc levels normalise (or lifelong in inherited forms) – skin changes take several weeks to resolve.

Inflammatory conditions of the bowel may lead to skin breakdown and pruritic rashes.

Pyoderma gangrenosum is a rapid onset painful area of necrotic skin ulceration with characteristic hypertrophic undermined purplish margins (Figure 10.12). There is a strong association with ulcerative colitis and Crohn's disease, rheumatoid arthritis, abnormal gamma globulins and leukaemia (Box 10.3).

Box 10.3 **Associations of pyoderma gangrenosum**

- Ulcerative colitis
- Crohn's disease
- Rheumatoid arthritis
- Monoclonal gammopathy
- Leukaemia.

Crohn's disease (regional ileitis) causes patchy inflammation of the bowel (anywhere from lips to anus) and may be associated with erosions/ulceration and sinus formation in the mucous membranes/skin/ileostomy/colostomy sites. Glossitis and granulomatous thickening of the lips and oral mucosa and vasculitis may also be associated.

Dermatitis herpetiformis is an intensely itchy, chronic skin disorder characterised by erythematous and blistering papules, particularly on the elbows, knees and buttocks (Figure 10.13) and is usually associated with a gluten-sensitive enteropathy with some degree of villous atrophy. There is an associated risk of small bowel lymphoma.

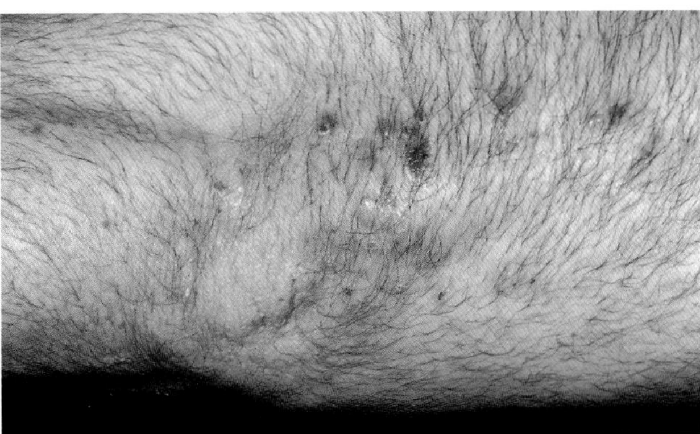

Figure 10.13 Dermatitis herpetiformis.

Congenital disorders of the bowel lead to various skin changes:

Peutz–Jeghers syndrome (hereditary intestinal polyposis syndrome) is an autosomal dominantly inherited condition characterised by the appearance in infancy of pigmented macules on the oral mucosal membranes, lips and face, hands/feet (differential diagnosis will include Addison's disease and McCune–Albright syndrome). Benign intestinal polyps, mainly in the ileum and jejunum, which rarely become malignant, are associated with the condition; however, carcinomas may develop in the liver, pancreas, breast, and so on.

Other conditions include congenital disorders with connective tissue and vascular abnormalities that affect the gut, such as Ehlers–Danlos syndrome and pseudoxanthoma elasticum (arterial GI bleeding), purpuric vasculitis (bleeding from GI lesions) and neurofibromatosis (intestinal neurofibromas).

Liver disease and the skin

Liver disease may affect the skin, hair and nails to a variable degree (Box 10.4). Obstructive jaundice is often associated with itching

Box 10.4 **Liver disease and the skin**

Obstructive

Jaundice
Pruritus.

Liver failure

Multiple spider naevi
Palmar erythema
White nails: hypoalbuminaemia
Porphyria cutanea tarda.

Cirrhosis

Xanthomas (primary biliary cirrhosis)
Asteatosis.

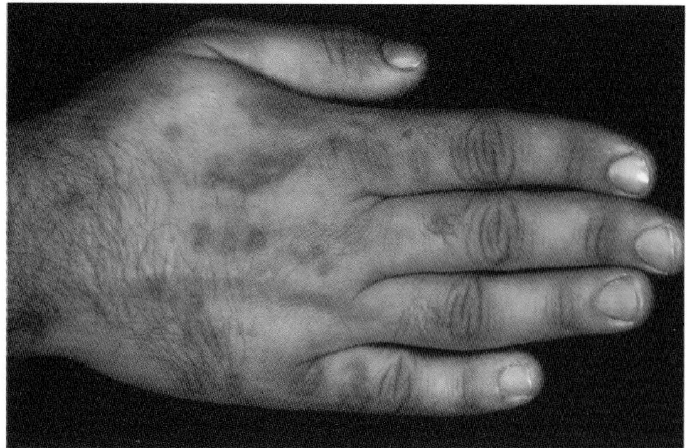

Figure 10.14 Porphyria cutanea tarda.

which is thought to be due to the deposition of bile salts in the skin. Evidence of this is the fact that drugs that combine with bile salts such as cholestyramine improve pruritus in some patients. Jaundice is the physical manifestation of bile salts in the skin.

Liver failure is characterised by a number of skin signs, particularly vascular changes causing multiple spider naevi and palmar erythema due to diffuse telangiectasia. It is not unusual to see spider naevi on the trunk in women but large numbers in men should raise suspicion of underlying hepatic disease.

Porphyria cutanea tarda (PCT) as a result of chronic liver disease produces bullae, scarring and hyperpigmentation in sun-exposed areas of the skin (Figure 10.14). PCT usually occurs in men, with a genetic predisposition, who have liver damage as a result of an excessive intake of alcohol. There is an underlying deficiency of uroporphyrinogen decarboxylase in the haem synthesis pathway that leads to skin fragility and photosensitivity, with blisters and erosions, photosensitivity on the face and dorsal hands. A condition called *pseudoporphyria* mimics PCT clinically but no porphyrins are found in urine/blood. Pseudoporphyria occurs in patients with chronic renal failure on haemodialysis, triggered by a number of medications (NSAIDs, diuretics, antibiotics and oral contraceptives) and relating to underlying liver disease.

Porphyrias may also result from the accumulation of intermediate metabolites in the metabolic pathway of haem synthesis. There are several types. In hepatic porphyrias there is skin fragility leading to blisters from exposure to the sun or minor trauma. In erythropoietic and erythrohepatic photoporphyrias, there is intense photosensitivity including sensitivity to long-wavelength ultraviolet light that penetrates window glass.

Xanthomas are lipid-laden macrophages deposited in the skin and may be associated with liver disease such as primary biliary cirrhosis and Alagille syndrome (Figure 10.15) and associated with hyperlipidaemia (either primary or secondary to diabetes, the nephrotic syndrome or hypothyroidism). Diabetes may be associated with an eruptive type of xanthoma.

Multiple spider naevi, with a central blood vessel and radiating branches, are most frequently seen in women (especially during pregnancy) and children (see Chapter 21). If they occur in large numbers, however, they may indicate underlying liver or connective tissue disease. Palmar erythema and yellow nails may also be present in liver failure.

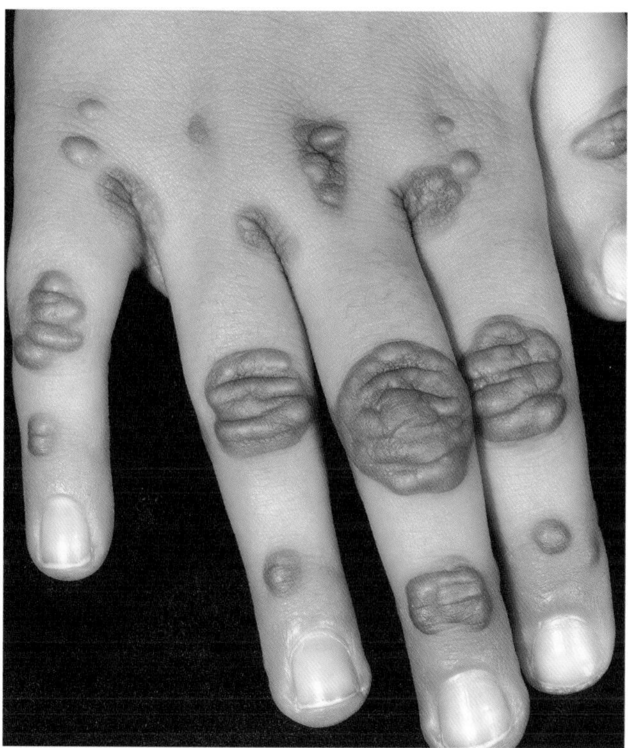

Figure 10.15 Xanthomas in Alagille syndrome.

Pigmentation disorders

Hypopigmentation

Albinism is inherited through a recessive gene and may manifest as diminished or loss of pigment in the skin, hair and eyes (see Chapter 6). Other genetic conditions with loss of skin pigment include piebaldism (Figure 10.16), phenylketonuria and tuberous sclerosis.

Localised depigmentation is most commonly seen in vitiligo; a family history of the condition is found in one-third of the patients. In the sharply demarcated, symmetrical macular lesions there is loss

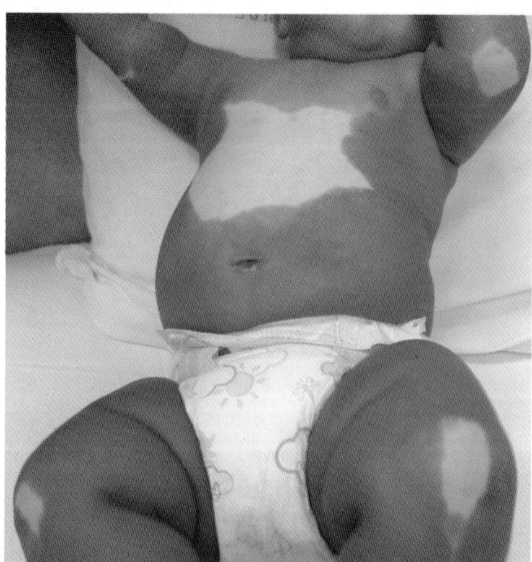

Figure 10.16 Piebaldism.

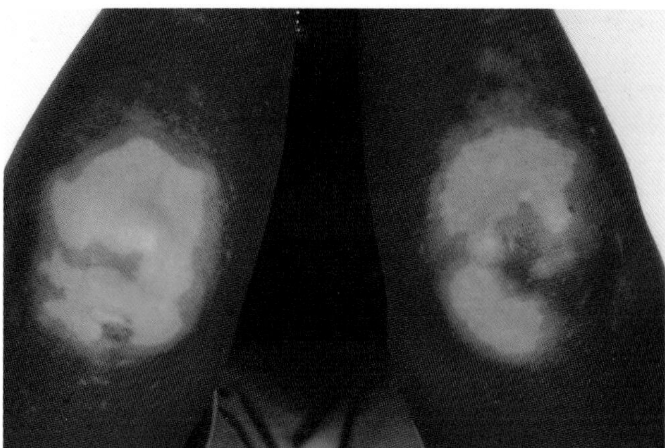

Figure 10.17 Vitiligo.

of melanocytes and melanin (Figure 10.17). There is an increased incidence of organ-specific antibodies and their associated diseases (Box 10.5).

Box 10.5 **Autoimmune associations with vitiligo**

- Thyroid disease
- Myasthenia gravis
- Pernicious anaemia
- Alopecia areata
- Hypoparathyroidism
- Halo naevus
- Addison's disease
- Morphoea and lichen sclerosus
- Diabetes.

Other causes of hypopigmented macules include post-inflammatory conditions such as psoriasis, eczema, lichen planus and lupus erythematosus; infections, for example, pityriasis versicolor and leprosy; chemicals, such as hydroquinones, hydroxychloroquine and arsenicals, reactions to pigmented naevi, seen in halo naevi (when the mole develops a pale ring around it) and genetic diseases, such as tuberous sclerosis ('ash leaf' macules).

Hyperpigmentation

There is wide variation in the pattern of normal pigmentation as a result of hereditary factors and exposure to the sun. Darkening of the skin may be due to an increase in the normal pigment melanin or to the deposition of bile salts from liver disease, iron salts (haemochromatosis) (Figure 10.18), drugs or metallic salts from ingestion. In agyria, ingested silver salts are deposited in the skin. Medications such as chlorpromazine, other phenothiazines and minocycline may cause an increased pigmentation in areas exposed to the sun. Phenytoin can cause local hyperpigmentation of the face and neck. AZT can cause cutaneous and nail hyperpigmentation.

AN is characterised by darkening and thickening of the skin of the axillae, neck, nipples and umbilicus (see above). Increased skin pigmentation may also be observed in patients with acromegaly who have an underlying pituitary tumour.

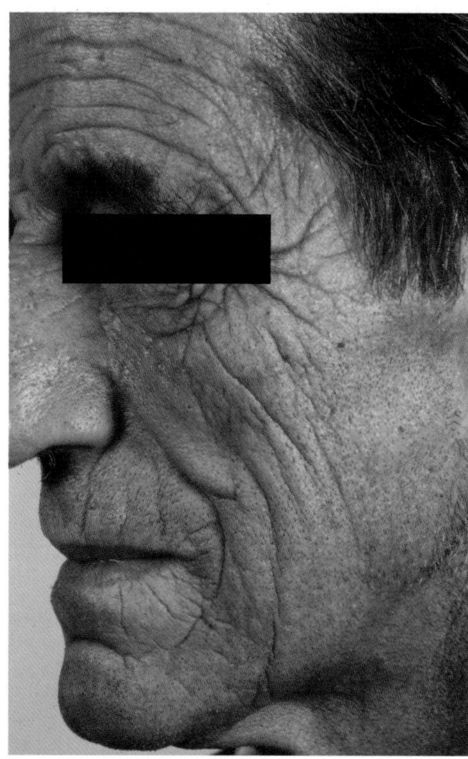

Figure 10.18 Haemachromatosis.

Post-inflammatory pigmentation is common, often after acute eczema, fixed drug eruptions and lichen planus. Areas of lichenification from rubbing the skin are usually darkened. In malabsorption syndromes, pellagra and scurvy, there is commonly increased skin pigmentation.

Skin manifestations of underlying malignancy

Underlying systemic malignancies may lead to characteristic patterns in the skin such as those seen in dermatomyositis or may present as a nodule of secondary deposits (metastases) (Boxes 10.6 and 10.7). Lymphomas can arise in or invade the skin. Pruritus may be associated with Hodgkin's disease.

Mycosis fungoides is a T-cell lymphoma of cutaneous origin. Initially, well-demarcated erythematous plaques usually develop over the trunk area, which may be mildly pruritic. In some cases,

Box 10.6 **Skin markers of internal malignancy**

- Acanthosis nigricans can be associated with gastric adenocarcinoma.
- Figurate erythemas can be associated with bronchial/oesophageal/breast carcinoma.
- Pruritus can be associated with lymphoma.
- Dermatomyositis can be associated with lung/breast/ovarian/testicular carcinomas.
- Acquired ichthyosis can be associated with Hodgkin's disease, sarcoma, lymphoma.

Box 10.7 **Non-specific skin changes associated with malignant disease**

- Secondary deposits
- Secondary hormonal effects
- Acne (adrenal tumours)
- Flushing (carcinoid)
- Pigmentation (pituitary tumours)
- Generalised pruritus (particularly lymphoma)
- Figurate erythema
- Superficial thrombophlebitis.

there is a gradual progression to infiltrated lesions, nodules and ulceration and occasionally erythroderma in Sezary syndrome (Figure 10.19) where there are atypical circulating Sezary cells. In others, the tumour may occur *de novo* or be preceded by generalised erythema. Primary cutaneous B-cell lymphoma can also rarely occur (Figure 10.20).

Parapsoriasis is a term used for well-defined erythematous scaly patches and plaques that slightly resemble psoriasis often in a 'digitate pattern' on the lateral borders of the trunk in middle/old age. Some cases undoubtedly develop into mycosis fungoides and a biopsy specimen should be taken from any fixed plaques that do not clear with topical steroids.

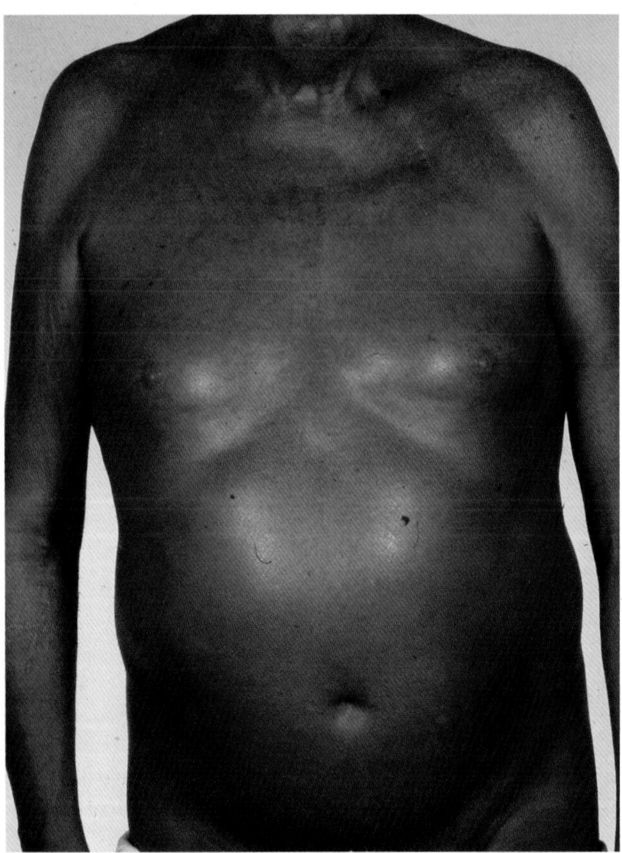

Figure 10.19 Sezary syndrome (erythroderma with abnormal circulating Sezary cells).

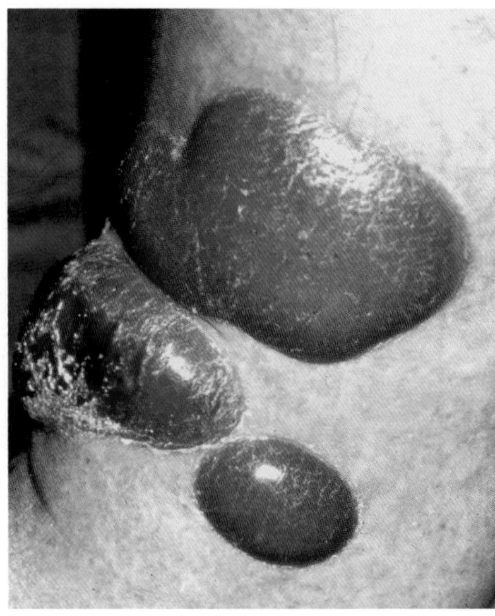

Figure 10.20 Cutaneous B-cell lymphoma.

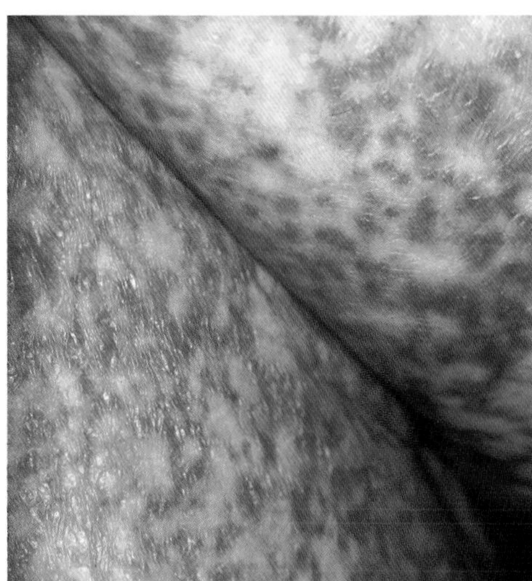

Figure 10.21 Poikiloderma.

Poikiloderma, in which there is telangiectasia, reticulate pigmentation (Figure 10.21), atrophy and loss of pigment, may precede mycosis fungoides, but it is also seen after radiotherapy and in association with connective tissue diseases.

Pregnancy and the skin

Pregnancy may be associated with pruritus, in which the skin appears normal in 15–20% of women (prurigo gestationis). It is generally more severe in the first trimester.

Polymorphous eruption of pregnancy (PEP) (previously named pruritic urticarial papules and plaques of pregnancy, PUPPP) (Figure 10.22) is a pruritic erythematous rash that usually starts in the striae of the abdomen during the third trimester and can become widespread. The condition does not affect the baby.

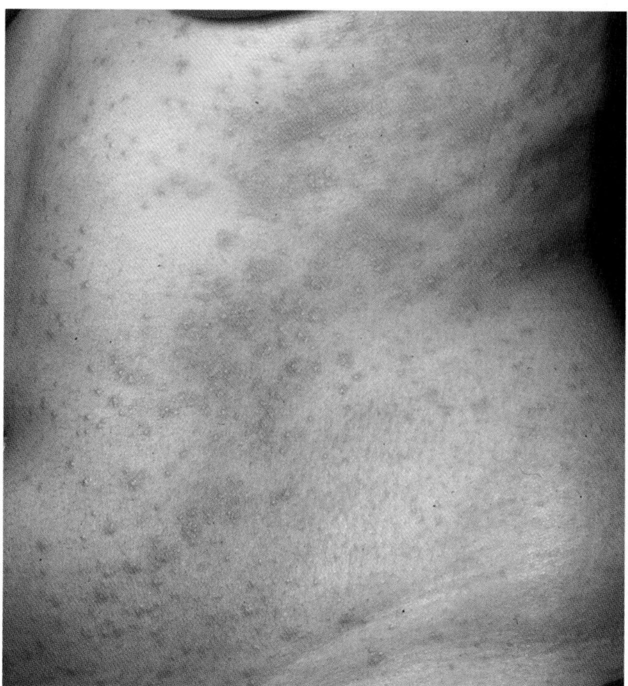

Figure 10.22 Polymorphous eruption of pregnancy (PEP).

It usually resolves post partum and rarely recurs in subsequent pregnancies with the same partner. Topical (and occasionally systemic) steroids usually provide symptomatic relief.

Pemphigoid gestationis (PG) is a rare disorder that may initially resemble PEP but develops pemphigoid-like vesicles, spreading over the abdomen and thighs (Figure 10.23). PG is an autoimmune disorder, in which cross-reactivity between placental tissues and the skin is thought to be important. It is strongly associated with HLA-DR3/4 and most patients develop anti-HLA antibodies. There is a greater prevalence of premature and small-for-dates babies and occasional mortality of the foetus.

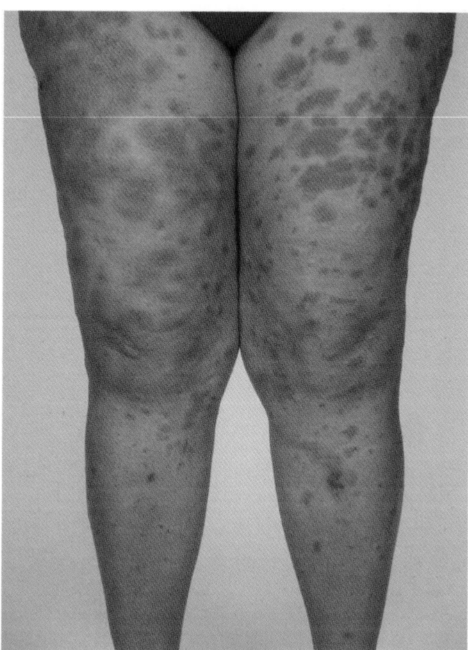

Figure 10.23 Pemphigoid gestationis.

Genetics and skin disease

An international project to sequence the human genome (3 billion base pairs) was completed in 2003. This human genome database will allow genetic researchers the opportunity to examine closely the specific genes that are of interest in relation to specific diseases. For example, those working in the field of genodermatoses can look at the structure, function, any detrimental mutations, interaction with other genes and other diseases mapped to that gene's location when undertaking research on a particular cutaneous disorder.

Cutaneous disorders that were originally classified according to clinical manifestations are now being more logically classified according to molecular defects at a genetic level (Table 10.2). Currently, around 500 single inheritance gene disorders with a significant cutaneous component have been identified at the molecular level. Although these disorders tend to be rare they can provide valuable information into the function of the particular protein or adhesion molecule, and so on, that is affected by the gene defect. In addition, this has led to a deeper understanding of inheritance patterns, more accurate diagnoses for neonates, where applicable prenatal diagnosis, and the hope for future treatments in the form of gene therapy.

As a general rule, common cutaneous disorders that run in families (familial), such as psoriasis, atopic eczema and acne, have more complex patterns of inheritance and are therefore more difficult to define genetically. These disorders are referred to as *multifactorial* as several genes are involved in the expression of the disease in addition to environmental modification (aeroallergens, food allergy, medication, infections).

Recent advances include the identification of two loss-of-function filaggrin gene defects that lead to dysregulation of keratohylin synthesis manifesting as *ichthyosis vulgaris* (*IV*) (which affects 1 in 250 individuals) (Figure 10.24), an inherited condition that affects skin barrier function. Filaggrin is an essential structure barrier function molecule in the stratum corneum. Abnormalities of filaggrin lead

Table 10.2 Abnormality underlying some inherited skin disorders.

Skin disorder	Abnormality
Ehlers–Danlos syndrome	Collagen and the extracellular matrix
Dystrophic epidermolysis bullosa	Type VII collagen
Pseudoxanthoma elasticum	Elastic tissue
Xeroderma pigmentosum	DNA repair
Simple epidermolysis bullosa	Keratins 5 and 14
Epidermolytic hyperkeratosis	Keratins 1 and 10
Palmo-plantar keratoderma	Keratins 9 and 16
Junctional epidermolysis bullosa	Laminins
X-linked recessive ichthyosis	Steroid sulphatase
Ichthyosis vulgaris	Filaggrin in stratum corneum
Darier's disease	Epidermal cell adhesion
Albinism (tyrosinase negative type)	Tyrosinase

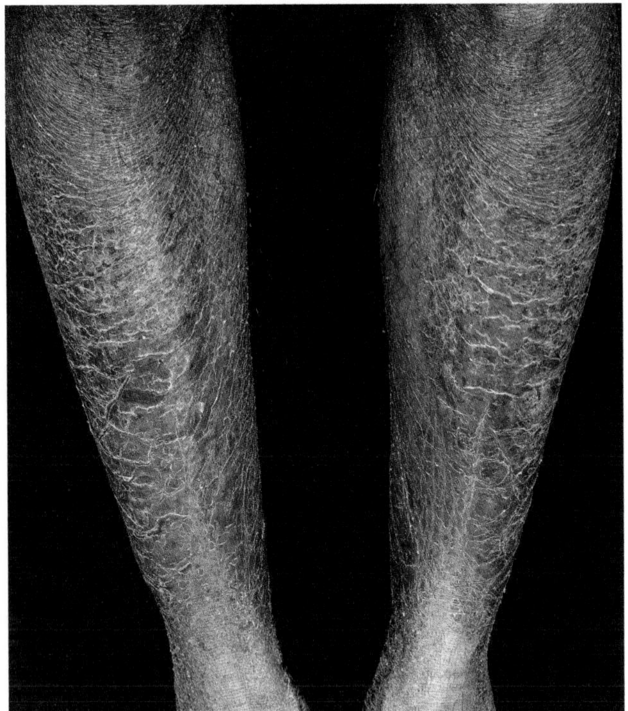

Figure 10.24 Ichthyosis vulgaris.

to increased levels of transepidermal water loss. Many patients with IV also suffer from AD, which leads to the discovery of similar filaggrin mutations in some patients with AD.

Gene therapy is an exciting future prospect in the management of gene defect associated disease. The accessibility of the skin as a therapeutic target is being exploited in developing novel treatments for the delivery of 'corrected genes' into skin tissues and beyond. Inherited blistering disorders such as epidermolysis bullosa could, in theory, be corrected by the delivery of corrective gene transfer. Novel techniques are moving away from the use of transfected viruses to transport genes into the skin and are focusing on nanoparticle technology such as spherical nucleic acid nanoparticle conjugates (SNA-NC). These comprise a gold core surrounded by a dense shell of small interfering ribonucleic acids (siRNAs) which penetrate the epidermis in an emollient vehicle.

Single gene disorders

These tend to be rare disorders that are inherited in a Mendelian pattern: autosomal recessive, autosomal dominant and X-linked recessive/dominant. Most of these disorders result from a single gene mutation that affects its protein product, which may in turn be increased, lost or modified. Not all these genetic disorders are evident at birth: many may present in later life such as neurofibromatosis type 2. The 'two-hit' principle is thought to be responsible for later presentations of genetic disorders when patients possess one mutant gene, but its counterpart is normal until a second event occurs later in life. When the second gene mutates the disease is expressed.

Single gene mutations may affect particular molecular structures in the skin such as the hemidesmosome (BP180), leading to one of the inherited types of junctional epidermolysis bullosa. However, the same BP180 protein may be targeted by acquired disorders such as bullous pemphigoid. Clinically, both conditions are characterised by skin fragility due to subepidermal splits.

Mosaicism refers to two or more cell populations that are genotypically different from each other but occur in the same individual. Cutaneous mosaicism may result from a mutation during development that is restricted to a few particular skin cells. This frequently results in linear abnormalities in the skin, usually present at birth. The mosaic defects often follow Blashko's lines (Figure 10.25), a bizarre pattern of lines and whorls which are thought to represent the developmental growth patterns in the skin (Figure 10.26).

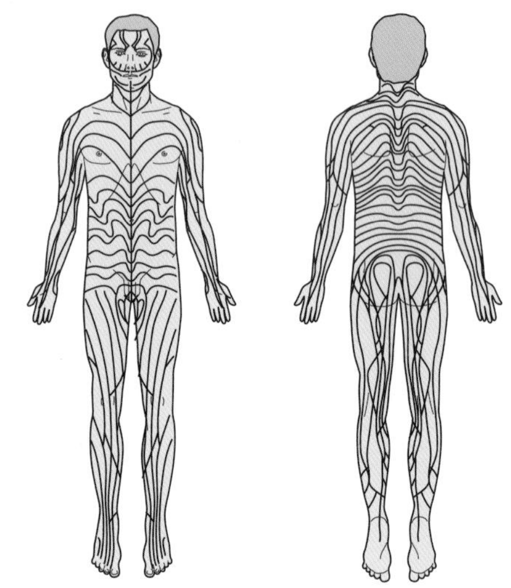

Figure 10.25 Blashko's lines.

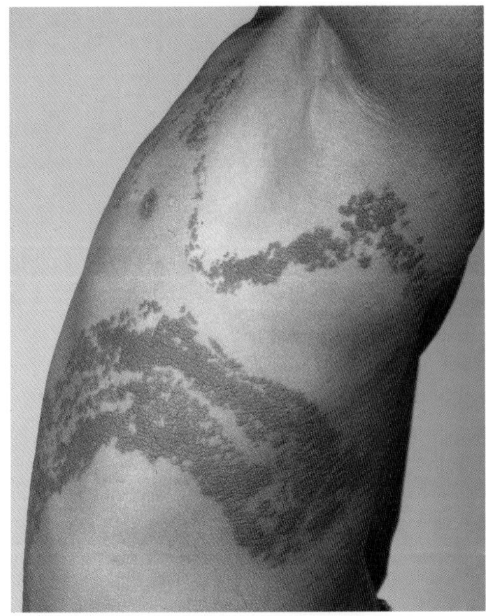

Figure 10.26 Epidermal naevus following Blashko's lines.

The genetic abnormalities found in localised mosaic cells may be identical to those found in generalised genodermatoses. For example, the same abnormalities in the genes controlling the production of keratins 1 and 10 can be responsible both for a generalised epidermolytic hyperkeratosis and for localised warty linear naevi.

Further reading

Lebwohl MG. *The Skin and Systemic Disease. A Colour Atlas and Text*, 2nd Edition, Churchill Livingstone, Oxford, 2003.

Sarzi-Puttini P, Doria A, Girolomoni G and Kuhn A. *The Skin in Systemic Autoimmune Disease*, Elsevier Science, Amsterdam, 2006.

Spitz JL. *Genodermatoses: A Clinical Guide to Genetic Skin Disorders*, 2nd Edition, Lippincott Williams and Wilkins, Philadelphia, 2004.

CHAPTER 11

Leg Ulcers

Rachael Morris-Jones

Dermatology Department, Kings College Hospital, London, UK

OVERVIEW

- The underlying cause of most ulcers is inadequate blood perfusion of the skin.
- The majority of leg ulcers arise due to oedema and raised pressure in the intercellular space, preventing capillary perfusion and causing back pressure in the venules.
- Risk factors for venous ulceration include increasing age, immobility, obesity, lower leg trauma, oedema, varicose veins and thrombosis.
- Risk factors for arterial ulcers include hypertension, atherosclerosis, peripheral vascular disease, polycythaemia, cryoglobulinaemia, vasculitis and connective tissue disease.
- Clinical features of venous ulcers: most commonly over medial malleolus; pitting oedema, dilated tortuous veins; ulcers have a well-defined, sloping edge and central slough.
- Clinical features of arterial ulcers: most commonly over shins, dorsal foot; painful, pale hairless legs, poor peripheral pulses, ulcers sharply defined with 'punched-out' edge.
- Management: correction of underlying cause if possible, clean ulcers, application of non-adherent dressings and appropriate compression bandages.

Introduction

The prevalence of leg ulceration is estimated to be between 0.3% and 1.0% of the general population, rising to 2% of those over the age of 80 years; however, with rising rates of obesity the incidence is expected to rise. Leg ulcers cause significant morbidity for those affected and the cost to the National Health Service in the UK is estimated to be £400 million per annum. Many patients have recurrent ulceration requiring repeated courses of bandages and dressings; 80% of patients are treated in the community. If the underlying cause of ulceration cannot be relieved by an operation or medical intervention, then the key worker will often be the specialist nurse who has considerable experience in assessing and facilitating the healing of difficult chronic ulcers.

Assessment of any ulcer should include consideration of the following parameters: site, size, edge, base, surrounding skin, leg shape, duration, symptoms, underlying systemic/cutaneous diseases, peripheral pulses/sensation, medication, and current and past ulcer treatments. Investigations may include ankle: brachial pressure indices (ABPI), venous and/or arterial duplex scanning, microbiology swabs, ulcer biopsy (usually through the edge) and patch testing.

A basic understanding of the underlying principles of ulceration is essential in reaching a clinical diagnosis and appreciating the different approaches to management. Most (95%) of ulcers are 'venous' (stasis) in nature (Figure 11.1) and therefore these are considered first in some detail.

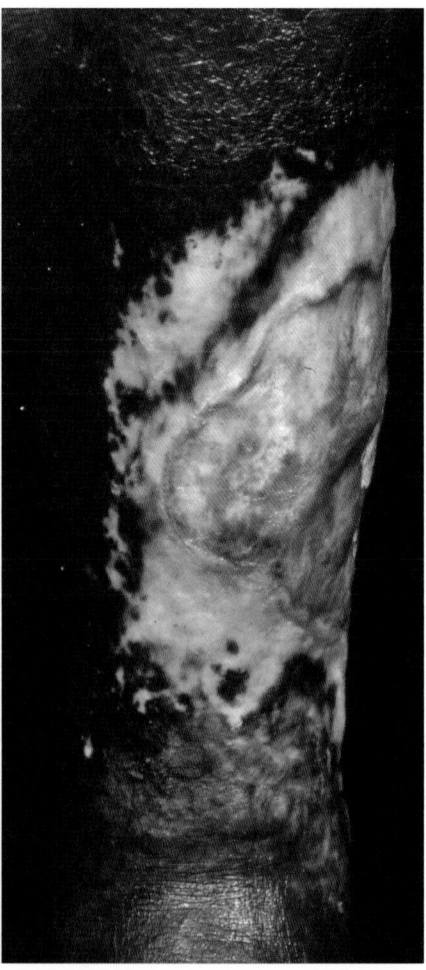

Figure 11.1 Venous leg ulcer.

ABC of Dermatology, Sixth Edition. Edited by Rachael Morris-Jones.

Venous ulcers

Pathology

The skin

Ulcers arise because the skin (epidermis and dermis) dies from inadequate provision of nutrients and oxygen. This occurs as a consequence of (a) oedema in the subcutaneous tissues with poor lymphatic and capillary drainage and (b) the extravascular accumulation of fibrinous material that has leaked from the blood vessels.

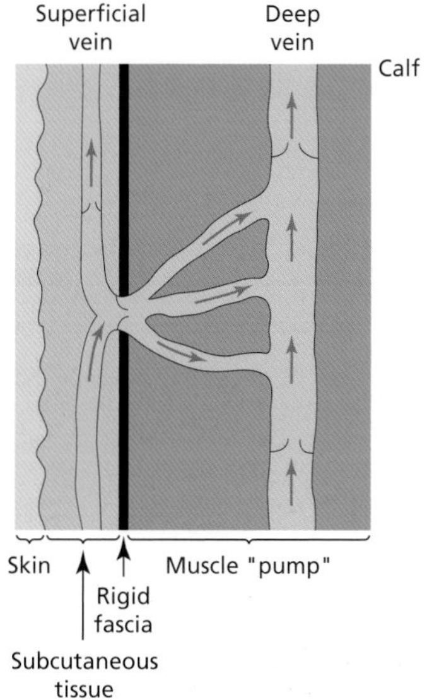

Figure 11.2 Healthy valves in legs.

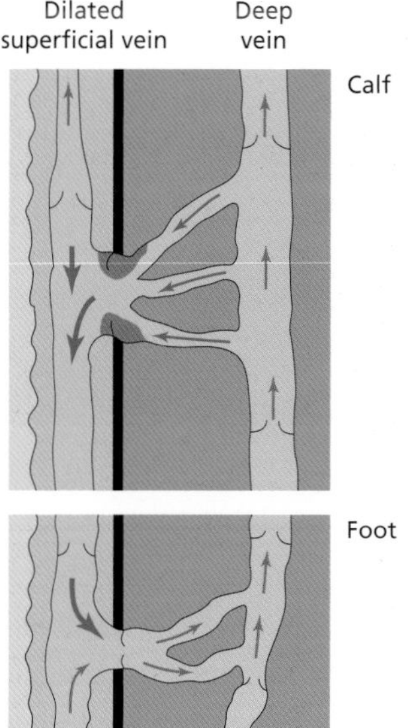

Figure 11.3 Incompetent valves in legs.

The result is a rigid cuff around the capillaries, which prevents diffusion of oxygen and nutrients through the vessel wall into the surrounding tissues with consequent fibrosis.

The blood vessels

Arterial perfusion of the leg is usually normal or increased, but stasis occurs in the venules. The lack of venous drainage is a consequence of incompetent valves between the superficial veins and the deeper large veins on which the calf muscle 'pump' acts. In the normal leg, there is a superficial low-pressure venous system and deep high-pressure veins (Figures 11.2 and 11.3). If the blood flow from superficial to deep veins is reversed, then the pressure in the superficial veins may increase to a level that prevents venous drainage (Figure 11.4). The resulting back pressure leads to varicose veins with stasis and oedema; consequently, there is diminished blood flow to the skin, causing ulceration. Chronic venous insufficiency and the resulting venous hypertension cause venous ulcers.

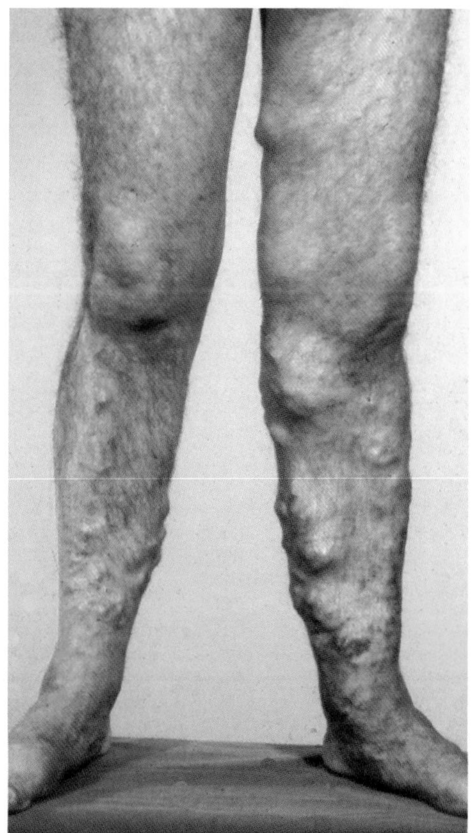

Figure 11.4 Varicose veins.

Incompetent valves

Incompetent valves leading to gravitational ulcers may be preceded by:

1 Deep vein thrombosis (DVT) associated with pregnancy, injury, immobilisation or infarction.
2 Primary long saphenous vein insufficiency.
3 Familial venous valve incompetence that presents at an earlier age (approximately 50% of patients).
4 Deep venous obstruction.

Risk factors for venous ulceration

Women are more at risk than men. Other risk factors are a family history of venous disease, increasing age, immobility, obesity, lower leg trauma, peripheral oedema, DVT, varicose veins and a previous history of venous leg ulceration. Patients may develop severe venous eczema prior to ulceration (Figure 11.5), which, if treated early and effectively, can prevent ulceration.

Clinical features

Venous ulcers occur around the ankle (gaiter area), most commonly over the medial malleolus. Patients frequently have swollen lower legs with marked pitting oedema. Chronic pitting oedema and fibrinous exudate often lead to fibrosis of the subcutaneous tissues, which may be associated with localised loss of pigment and dilated capillary loops, an appearance known as '*atrophie blanche*' (Figure 11.6). This occurs around the ankle with oedema

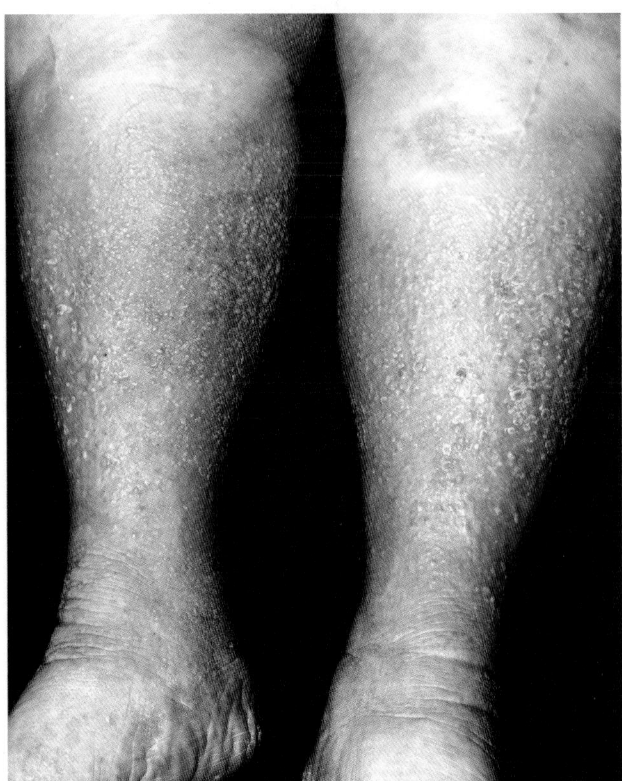

Figure 11.5 Varicose eczema.

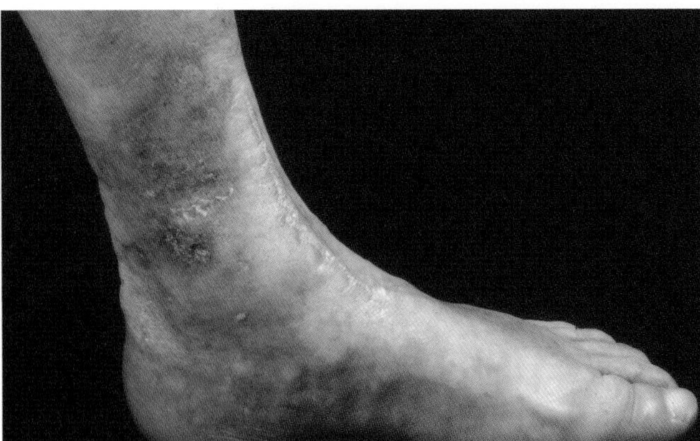

Figure 11.6 Atrophie blanche.

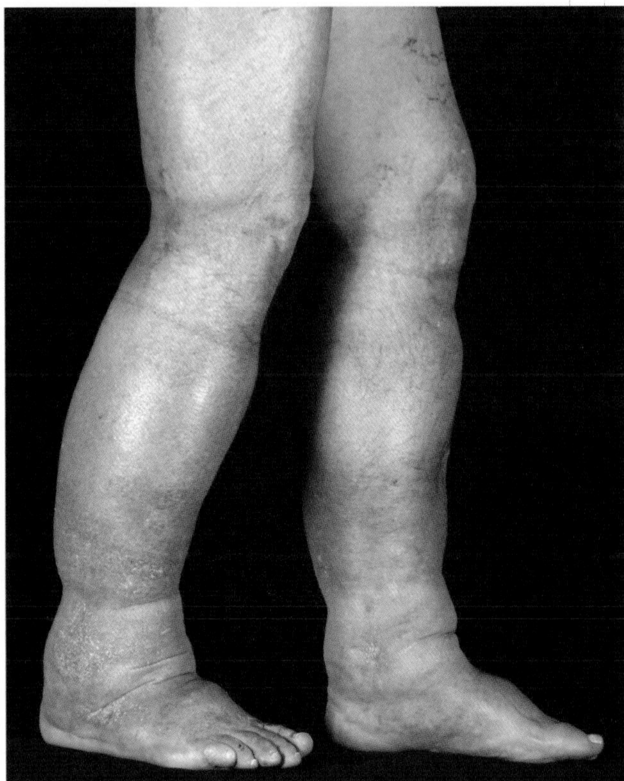

Figure 11.7 Lymphoedema.

and dilated tortuous superficial veins proximally and can lead to 'inverted champagne bottle'-shaped legs. Lymphoedema results from obliteration of the superficial lymphatics, with associated fibrosis (Figure 11.7). There is often hypertrophy of the overlying epidermis known as *lipodermatosclerosis*, which is a scleroderma-like hardening of the legs in patients with venous insufficiency characterised by induration, hyperpigmentation and depression of the skin (Figure 11.8).

Ulceration often occurs for the first time after a trivial injury. The ulcer margin is usually well defined with a shelving edge and central slough. The surrounding skin may be eczematous (erythematous, inflamed and itchy): the so-called *varicose eczema*. Venous ulcers

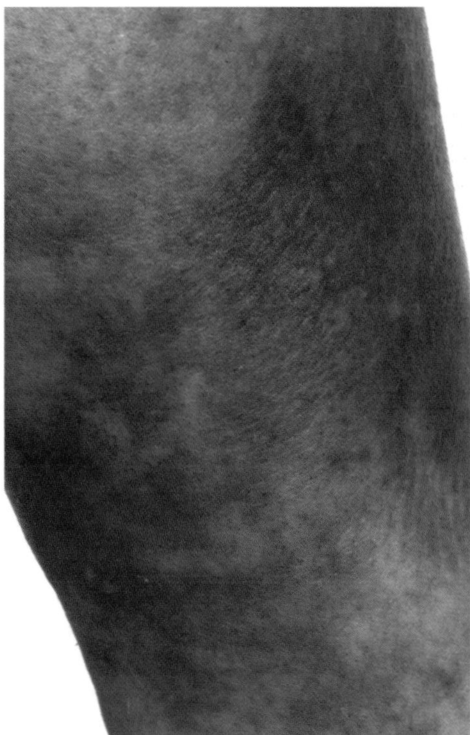

Figure 11.8 Lipodermatosclerosis.

may be mildly painful, may exude serous fluid and may become odorous from secondary infection.

It is important to check the pulses in the leg and foot as compression bandaging of a leg with impaired blood flow can cause ischaemia and necrosis. Long-standing ulcers can rarely undergo malignant change (Marjolin's ulcer) when the edge becomes heaped up and atypical because of transformation to squamous cell carcinoma.

Local/topical treatments

When new epidermis can grow across an ulcer it will, and the aim is to produce an environment in which this can take place. To this end several measures can be taken (Box 11.1).

> Box 11.1 **Treatment of venous leg ulcers**
>
> - Elevation of the leg and compression is the key to healing leg ulcers.
> - Never apply steroid preparations to the ulcer itself or it will not heal.
> - Beware of contact allergy developing to topical agents (antibiotics, steroids, dressings and bandages).
> - Antibiotics should only be given if there is clinical/microbiological evidence of infection (cellulitis).
> - A vascular 'flare' around the ankle and heel with varicose veins, sclerosis or oedema indicates a high risk of imminent ulceration.
> - Make sure arterial pulses are present. A Doppler apparatus can be used to measure ABPIs.

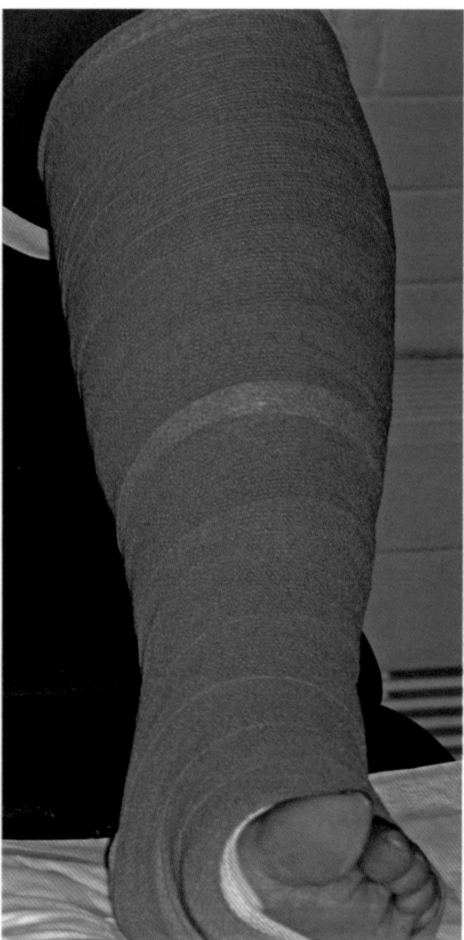

Figure 11.9 Compression bandaging.

- Try to eliminate oedema by means of: (a) diuretics; (b) keeping the legs elevated when sitting; (c) avoiding standing as far as possible; (d) walking helps through activation of the 'calf muscle pump'; (e) applying compression bandages with greater pressure at the ankle than the thigh (see Chapter 25) (Figure 11.9).
- Exudate and slough should be removed. Lotions can be used to clean the ulcer, such as 0.9% saline solution, sodium hypochlorite solution or 5% hydrogen peroxide (Figure 11.10). Modern dressings such as alginate, hydrocolloid and Hydrofiber® can efficiently absorb the exudate. There is some evidence that antiseptic solutions and chlorinated solutions delay collagen production and cause inflammation. Enzyme preparations may help by 'digesting' the slough. To prevent the formation of over-granulation tissue, use silver nitrate 0.25% compresses, a silver nitrate 'stick' for more exuberant tissue and curettage, if necessary.
- The dressings applied to the ulcer can consist of (a) simple non-stick, paraffin gauze dressings (an allergy may develop to those with an antibiotic); (b) wet compresses with saline or silver nitrate solutions for exudative lesions; (c) silver sulphadiazine (Flamazine) or hydrogen peroxide creams (Hioxyl and Crystacide); (d) absorbent dressings, consisting of hydrocolloid patches or powder, which are helpful for smaller ulcers (see Chapter 25) and (e) try to ensure patients sleep in a bed at night rather than a chair.

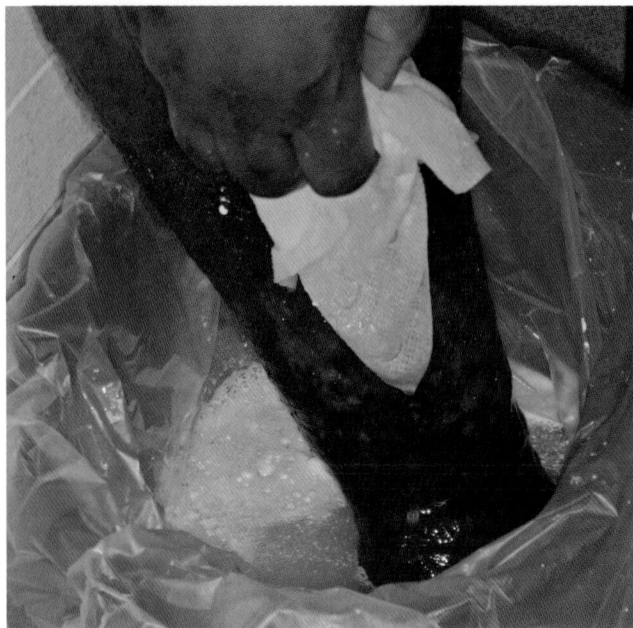

Figure 11.10 Cleaning leg ulcers.

- Paste bandages, impregnated with zinc oxide and antiseptics or ichthammol, help to keep dressings in place and provide protection. They may, however, traumatise the skin, and allergic reactions to their constituents are not uncommon.
- Treatment of infection is less often necessary than is commonly supposed. All ulcers are colonised by bacteria to some extent, usually coincidental staphylococci. A purulent exudate is an indication for a broad-spectrum antibiotic and a swab for bacteriology. Erythema, oedema and tenderness around the ulcers suggest a β-haemolytic streptococcal infection, which may require longer courses of antibiotic treatment. Soaking the leg in a bucket containing potassium permanganate can be a very effective antiseptic and can help reduce exudate and slough. A swab for culture and sensitivity helps keep track of organisms colonising the area.
- Surrounding eczematous changes should be treated with moderate-strength topical steroids avoiding the ulcer itself. Ichthammol 1% in 15% zinc oxide and white soft paraffin or Ichthopaste bandages can be used as a protective layer, and topical antibiotics can be used if necessary. It is important to remember that any of the commonly used topical preparations can cause an allergic reaction: neomycin, lanolin, formaldehyde, tars and clioquinol (the 'C' of many proprietary steroids).
- Skin grafting can be very effective. There must be a healthy viable base for the graft, with an adequate blood supply; natural re-epithelialisation from the edges of the ulcer is a good indication that a graft will be supported. Pinch grafts or partial-thickness grafts can be used. However, autologous keratinocyte suspensions harvested from the patients healthy skin may ultimately become the preferred surgical approach.
- Maintaining general health, with adequate nutrition and weight reduction, is important.
- Corrective surgery can be done for associated venous abnormalities.

Additional manoeuvers in the management of venous ulcers:

1. Modern 'active' dressings have been shown to heal over 80% of wounds that have previously failed to respond to conventional approaches. These active dressings may contain growth-promoting factors such as platelet or fibroblast-derived growth factors (see Chapter 25).
2. Some units are using low-intensity ultrasonic stimulation to help heal wounds through local activation of angiogenesis, leukocyte adhesion and production of growth factors.
3. Studies using intermittent pneumatic compression have shown good efficacy in treating chronic venous ulcers and may be a viable alternative to conventional compression bandaging.

Arterial ulcers

Ulcers on the leg also occur as a result of (a) atherosclerosis with poor peripheral circulation, particularly in older patients; (b) vasculitis affecting the larger subcutaneous arteries; and (c) arterial obstruction in macroglobulinaemia, cryoglobulinaemia, polycythaemia and 'collagen' disease, particularly rheumatoid arthritis.

Arterial ulcers are sharply defined and accompanied by pain, which may be very severe, especially at night. The pretibial area of the lower leg, dorsal foot and toes are most commonly affected. In patients with hypertension, a very tender ulcer can develop posteriorly (Martorelli's ulcer). The legs may be hairless and pale with poor peripheral pulses (Figure 11.11). Adequate control of the patient's hypertension is essential to facilitate ulcer healing.

Simple or magnetic resonance angiography may be needed to map the arterial tree and look for obstructions and narrowing.

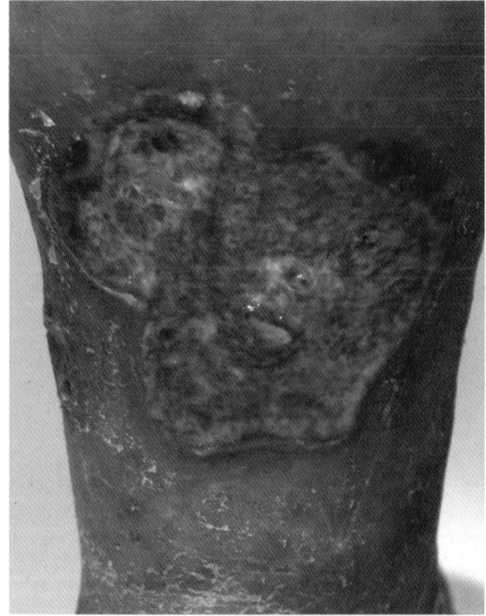

Figure 11.11 Arterial ulcer.

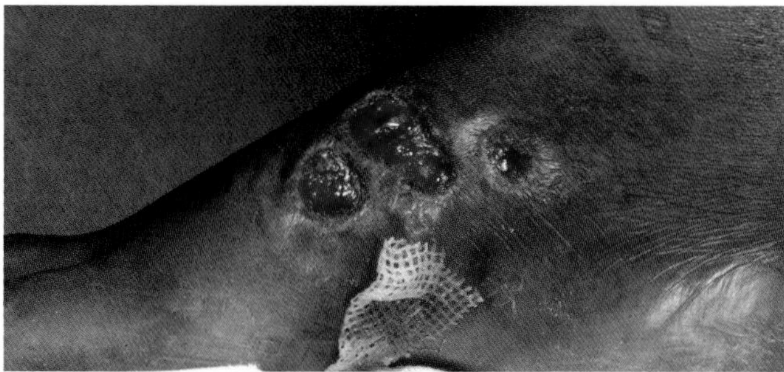

Figure 11.12 Ulcers in diabetic foot.

As mentioned above, compression bandaging will make arterial ulcers worse and may lead to ischaemia of the leg.

Diabetic/neuropathic ulcers

Up to 15% of patients with diabetes will develop a foot/leg ulcer at some stage during their lifetime; a significant proportion will recur following initial healing and leading to a higher risk ultimately of amputation. Diabetics suffer from peripheral vascular disease and peripheral neuropathy. The loss of or reduction in peripheral sensation leads to damage to the skin and subcutaneous tissue. Much of the trauma is minor and unnoticed, particularly over pressure points, but nonetheless resulting in ulceration. Poorly fitting shoes and extremes of heat or cold can also result in significant damage. Diabetic ulcers are usually well defined and 'punched-out', occasionally with deep sinus tracts that can be explored with a sterile probe (Figure 11.12). Assessment of the patient's arterial system can be crudely assessed by feeling the dorsalis pedis pulse (on the dorsal aspect of the foot just lateral to extensor hallucis longus tendon). More sophisticated measurements of the haemodynamic state of the lower leg can be made using plethysmography, which determines pulse volume recordings. ABPI measurements can be inaccurate in diabetic patients who are more likely to have calcified blood vessels which may result in falsely raised readings. Management of diabetic ulcers usually requires taking the pressure off the ulcerated area sometimes by making specialised footwear or limiting weight-bearing for a period of time. Cleaning wound and non-adherent dressings need to be used just as for the management of venous ulcers in the text outlined above.

Inflammatory conditions

Ulcers of the lower legs may occur in polyarteritis nodosa and vasculitis (Figure 11.13). Pyoderma gangrenosum (Figure 11.14), a rapidly developing necrotic ulcer with surrounding induration, may occur in association with ulcerative colitis or rheumatoid vasculitis (Figures 11.13 & 11.14). In severe cases of pyoderma gangrenosum, systemic corticosteroids are usually required often with additional ciclosporin and even infusions of Infliximab may be needed in recalcitrant cases. An underlying cause for the pyoderma gangrenosum should be sought.

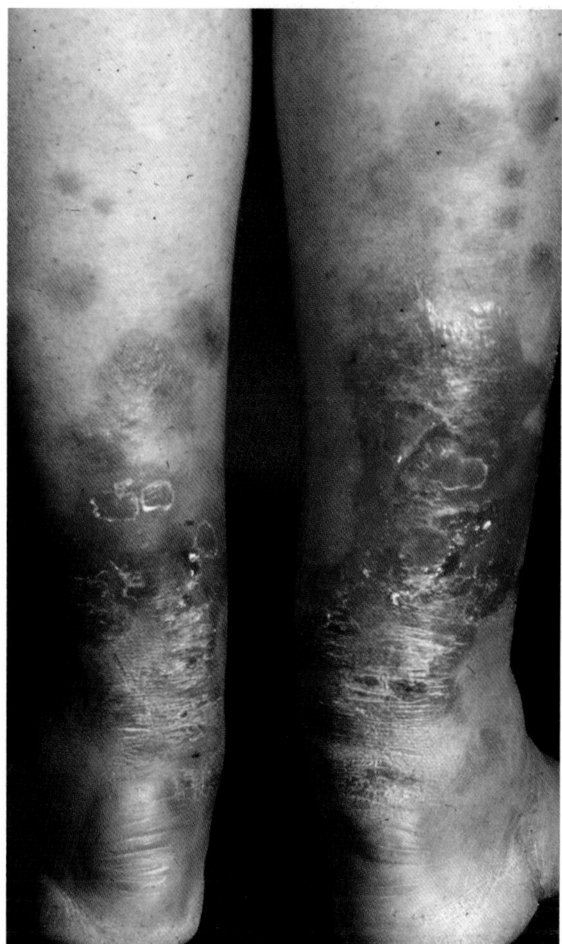

Figure 11.13 Vasculitis and perniosis pre-ulceration.

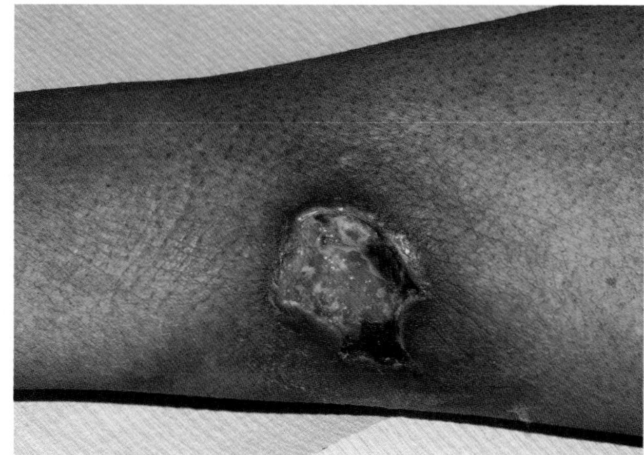

Figure 11.14 Pyoderma gangrenosum.

Infectious ulcers

Infections that cause ulcers include staphylococcal or streptococcal infections, tuberculosis (which is rare in the UK but may be seen

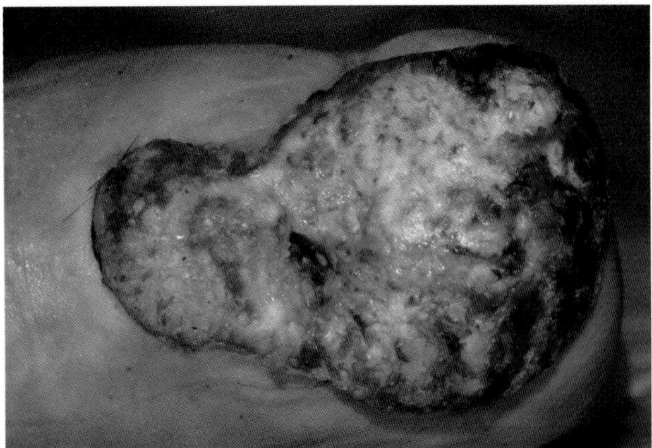

Figure 11.15 Squamous cell carcinoma in a chronic diabetic ulcer.

in recent immigrants and may be associated with tuberculous osteomyelitis) and anthrax. Leishmaniasis may present with an ulcer at the cutaneous site of a sandfly bite (see Chapter 18).

Malignant diseases

Squamous cell carcinoma may present as an ulcer or, rarely, develop in a pre-existing usually long-standing ulcer (Marjolin's ulcer) (Figure 11.15). Basal cell carcinoma and melanoma may develop into ulcers, as may Kaposi's sarcoma.

Trauma

Patients with diabetic or other types of neuropathy are at risk of developing trophic ulcers. Rarely, ulcers may be self-inflicted: 'dermatitis artefacta' where patients damage their own skin, leading to erosions and ulceration (Figure 11.16).

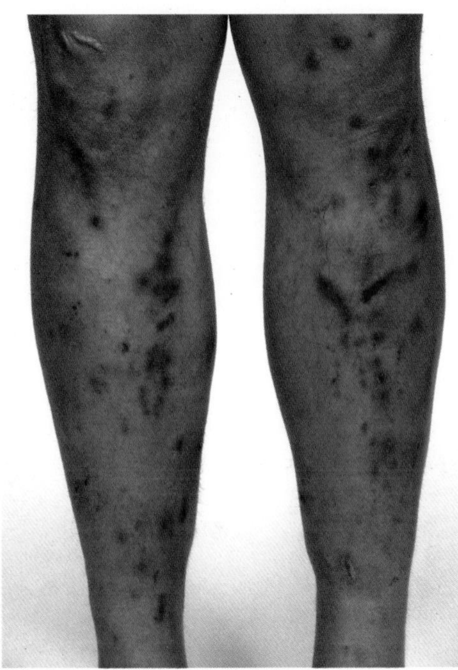

Figure 11.16 Dermatitis artefacta.

Further Reading

Morison M, Moffatt C and Franks P. Leg Ulcers: *A Problem-Based Learning Approach*, Elsevier Health Sciences, Edinburgh, 2007.

Ryan K. Nursing and Health Survival Guide: Wound Care, Pearson, Harlow, 2013.

CHAPTER 12

Acne and Rosacea

Rachael Morris-Jones

Dermatology Department, Kings College Hospital, London, UK

OVERVIEW

- 80% of people living in developed countries suffer from acne at some stage in their lives.
- Acne lesions can be pustular and painful leading to scarring and psychological/emotional upset.
- Androgenic hormones increase sebum secretion and the numbers of *Propionibacterium acnes*.
- Exposure to oils/pomades, tar, agricultural chemicals and topical steroids can promote acne.
- Increased levels of oestrogen, testosterone, cortisol and growth hormone can trigger acne.
- Medications implicated in promoting acne include steroids, oral contraceptives, phenytoin, isoniazid, ciclosporin and lithium.
- Rosacea is characterised by facial flushing, persistent erythema, telangiectasia, inflammatory papules, pustules and oedema.
- Unlike acne, rosacea tends to start in adult life.
- Conjunctivitis, blepharitis and eyelid oedema may be associated with rosacea.
- Chronic oedema in rosacea can lead to gross thickening and hypertrophy of the nose called rhinophyma.

Introduction

Most adolescents in developed countries suffer from acne leading many to conclude that acne is a 'normal'. However, the significant morbidity associated with it means it frequently has a negative impact on people's lives. Acne, from the Greek word 'acme' meaning 'prime of life', suggests a disorder mainly during adolescence; however, this is somewhat misleading as acne can affect young infants through to individuals in their 40s and 50s. Indeed, over the past two decades the number of individuals who suffer from acne in later life has been increasing. Estimates show that 5% of the population over the age of 45 years still suffers from acne. Acne can have a significant psychological impact on patients regardless of its severity. Nonetheless, severe acne may, in addition, also be very painful, may cause irreversible scarring and may be associated with systemic symptoms including fever, joint pains and malaise.

ABC of Dermatology, Sixth Edition. Edited by Rachael Morris-Jones.

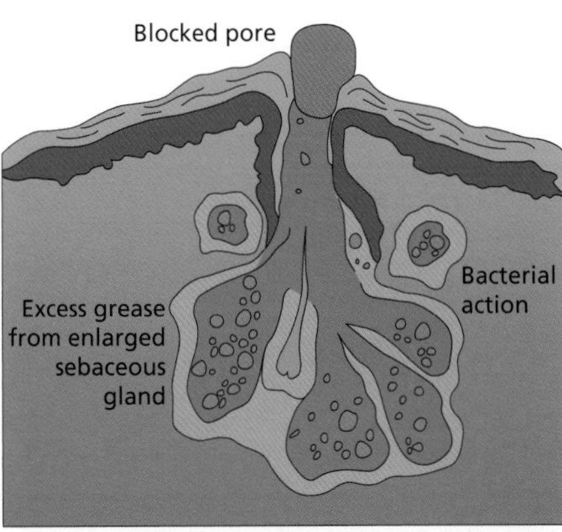

(a)

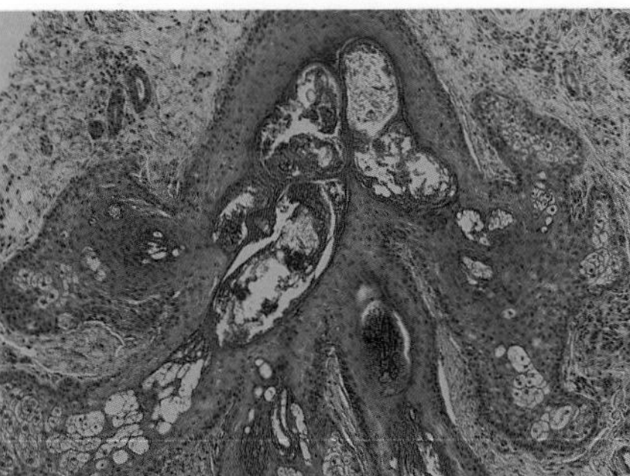

(b)

Figure 12.1 (a) Sebaceous gland: pathology in acne. (b) Histology of acne.

What is acne?

Acne lesions develop from the sebaceous glands associated with hair follicles: face, back, chest and anogenital area (Figure 12.1). (Sebaceous glands are also found on the eyelids and mucosa, prepuce and cervix; however, they are not associated with hair follicles.) The sebaceous gland contains holocrine cells that secrete triglycerides, fatty acids, wax esters and sterols as 'sebum'. The main changes in acne include

- thickening of the keratin lining and subsequent obstruction of the sebaceous duct resulting in closed comedones ('whiteheads') (Figure 12.2) or open comedones ('blackheads' whose colour is due to melanin, not dirt) (Figure 12.3). Acne cannot be diagnosed

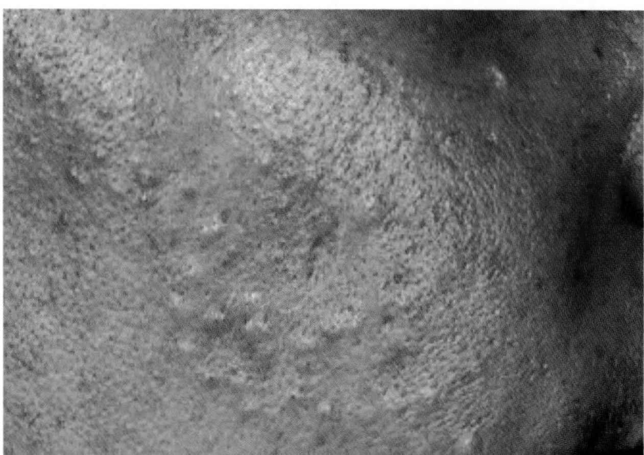

Figure 12.2 Acne with closed comedones.

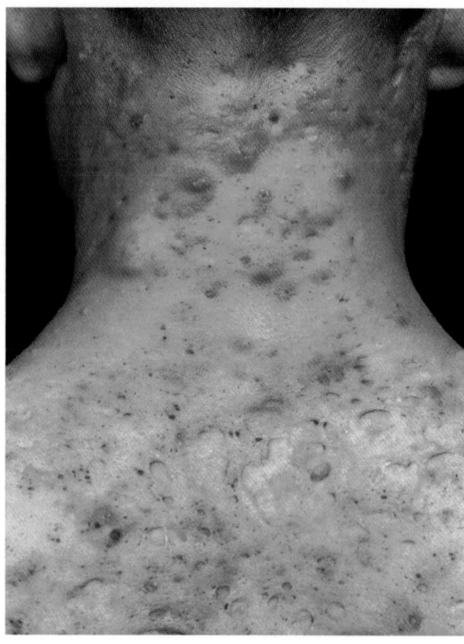

Figure 12.3 Acne with open comedones, cysts and scars.

without the presence of comedones (there are no comedones seen in rosacea).

- an increase in sebum secretion.
- an increase in *Propionibacterium acnes* bacteria within the duct.
- inflammation around the sebaceous gland.

Underlying causes

There are various underlying causes of these changes (Box 12.1).

Hormones

Androgenic hormones increase the size of sebaceous glands and the amount of sebum in both male and female adolescents. Although androgen levels may be normal there is thought to be an increased sensitivity of the glands to androgen hormones. In some women with acne, there is a lowered sex hormone-binding globulin concentration with a consequent increase in free testosterone levels. This change in the hormone balance is mimicked by many combined oral contraceptive pills (OCPs) resulting in increased acne. Oral contraceptives containing more than 50 μg ethinyloestradiol can also make acne worse. Oestrogens have the opposite effect in prepubertal boys and eunuchs. Infantile acne occurs in the first few months of life. It can rarely be caused by congenital adrenal hyperplasia or virilising tumours, but is most commonly due to transplacental stimulation of the adrenal gland by maternal hormones causing increased adrenal androgens.

Box 12.1 **Factors causing acne**

Intrinsic factors

Hormones

- Polycystic ovary syndrome.
- Virilising tumours.
- Congenital adrenal hyperplasia.
- Increased cortisol (Cushing's syndrome).
- Increased growth hormone (acromegaly).

Medications

- Topical and systemic steroids.
- Oral contraceptive pill (higher androgen content).
- Phenytoin.
- Barbiturates.
- Isoniazid.
- Ciclosporin.
- Lithium.

Extrinsic factors

- Oils/pomades.
- Coal and tar.
- Chlorinated phenols.
- DDT and weed killers.

Fluid retention

Premenstrual exacerbation of acne is thought to be due to fluid retention leading to increased hydration and swelling of the sebaceous duct. Sweating also makes acne worse, possibly by the same mechanism.

Stress

It has long been observed by patients that stress leads to a worsening of their acne. Now there is evidence to back up the clinical observation. Stress induces inflammation in the pilosebaceous unit leading to acne or acne exacerbation. There is evidence that within sebocytes is a complete corticotropin-releasing hormone system that leads to increased lipid and steroid synthesis and an interaction with testosterone and growth hormone.

Diet

Many patients believe their acne is exacerbated by eating certain foods. Most commonly implicated foods include dairy products, chocolate, nuts, coffee and fizzy drinks. Some epidemiological studies have suggested that a Westernised diet of high levels of refined sugars and starch may explain striking differences in the prevalence of acne amongst different populations that are not thought to be explained by genetic factors or weight differences. However, during studies when Westerners were fed a low glycaemic diet, there was no significant improvement in their acne.

Seasons

Acne often improves with natural sunlight. Phototherapy with artificial light sources using visible blue light alone or in combination with red light has been shown in several clinical trials to be an effective treatment for acne in a proportion of patients.

External factors

Oils, whether vegetable oils in the case of cooks in hot kitchens or mineral oils in engineering, can cause 'oil folliculitis', leading to acne-like lesions through contact with the skin. Other acnegenic substances include coal tar, dicophane (DDT), cutting oils and halogenated hydrocarbons. Cosmetic acne is seen in adult women who have used cosmetics containing comedogenic oils over many years. Individuals who use rich oils in the scalp can suffer from 'pomade acne', which occurs close to the hairline.

Iatrogenic factors

Corticosteroids, both topical and systemic, can cause increased keratinisation of the pilosebaceous duct resulting in acne. Androgens, gonadotrophins and corticotrophin can induce acne in adolescence. OCPs of the combined type and antiepileptic drugs may also cause acne. However, an OCP with a high oestrogen combined with low androgen can actually be used to treat acne in women. Some patients develop perioral dermatitis (Figure 12.4) after application of topical steroids to the face, which is characterised by papules and pustules around the mouth and eyes that may mimic acne but there are no comedones. The topical steroid should be stopped and the patient treated with oral tetracycline or erythromycin for 6 weeks.

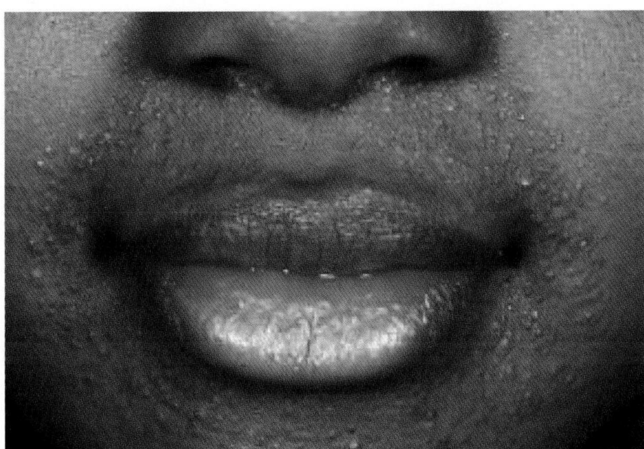

Figure 12.4 Perioral dermatitis.

Types of acne

Acne vulgaris

Acne vulgaris, the common type of acne, occurs during puberty and affects the comedogenic areas of the face, back and chest. There may be a familial tendency to acne. Acne vulgaris is more common in boys, 30–40% of whom develop acne between the ages of 18 and 19 (Figure 12.5). In girls, the peak incidence is between 16 and 18 years. Adult acne is a variant affecting 3% of men and 5% of women over the age of 40. Acne keloidalis is a type of scarring acne seen particularly on the neck in men (Figure 12.6; Box 12.2).

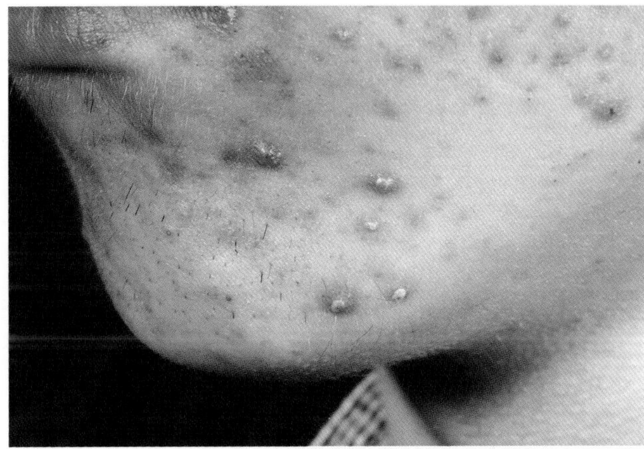

Figure 12.5 Acne vulgaris with inflammatory papules and pustules.

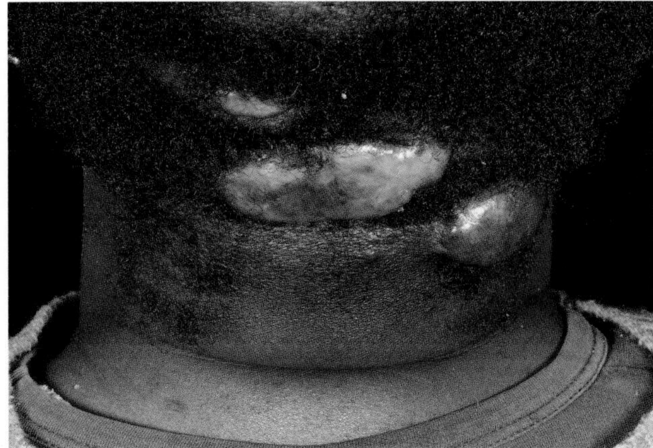

Figure 12.6 Acne keloidalis nuchae.

Box 12.2 **Ladder of treatment for rosacea**

Avoid exacerbators:

- Avoid harsh soaps, strong sunlight, oil-based make-up and hot showers.
- Avoid alcohol and spicy food.

Topical treatment:

- Water-based emollient.
- Metronidazole gel or cream.
- Azelaic acid.
- Tacrolimus/pimecrolimus cream.

Systemic treatment:

- Tetracycline antibiotics (minocycline 100 mg MR once daily (OD), lymecycline 408 mg OD,
- Low dose Isotretinoin.

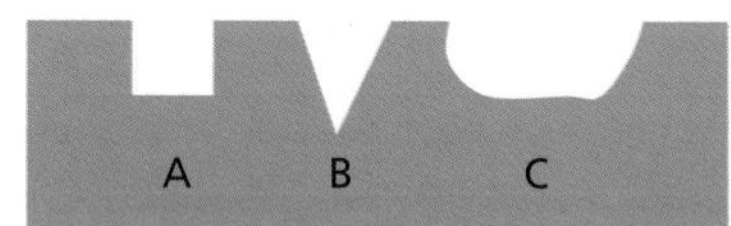

Figure 12.7 Types of atrophic acne scars. (Notes: A, Boxcar; B, icepick and C, rolling).

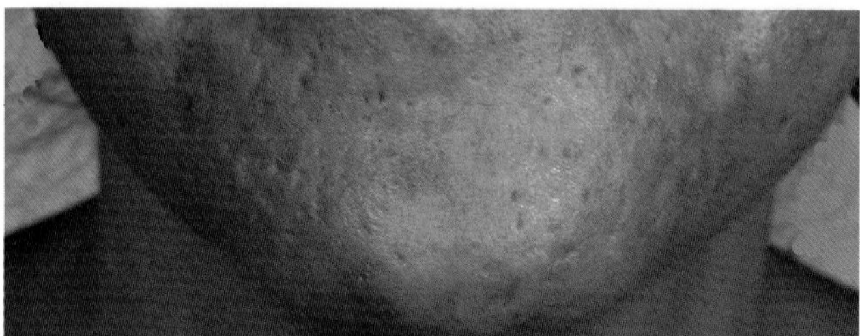

Figure 12.8 'Ice-pick' scars.

Patients with acne often complain of excessive greasiness of the skin, with 'spots', 'blackheads' or 'pimples'. These may be associated with inflammatory papules and pustules developing into larger cysts and nodules. Resolving lesions leave post-inflammatory pigment changes and scarring. Scars (Figure 12.7) may be atrophic and pitted, deep, ('ice pick') (Figure 12.8), rolling and boxcar or they may be more hypertrophic or even keloid (Figure 12.9). Scars may also be hyper/hypopigmented and erythematous.

Treatment of acne scarring does depend on the severity and scar type. Generally, more superficial procedures are used to improve the appearance of shallow acne scars (chemical peel, dermabrasion and fillers) whereas deeper scars may require more aggressive therapy (dermaroller, punch excision, spot fractional resurfacing, fraxel and intense pulsed light).

Acne excoriée

In this variant of acne, the patient picks at the skin producing disfiguring erosions (Figure 12.10). The acne itself is usually mild but tends to be persistent as it is often very difficult to help the patient break this habit.

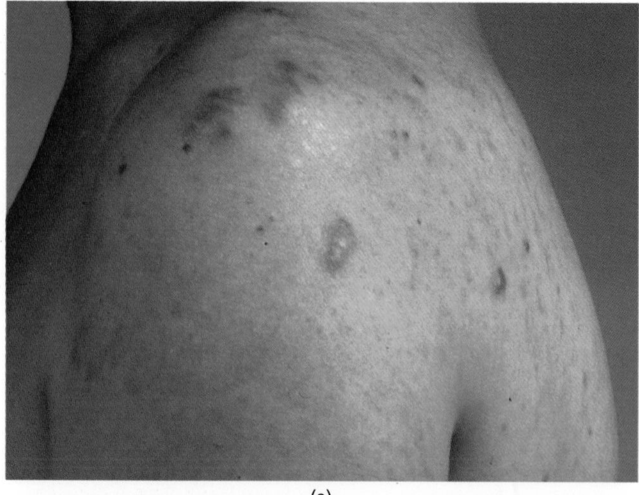

(a)

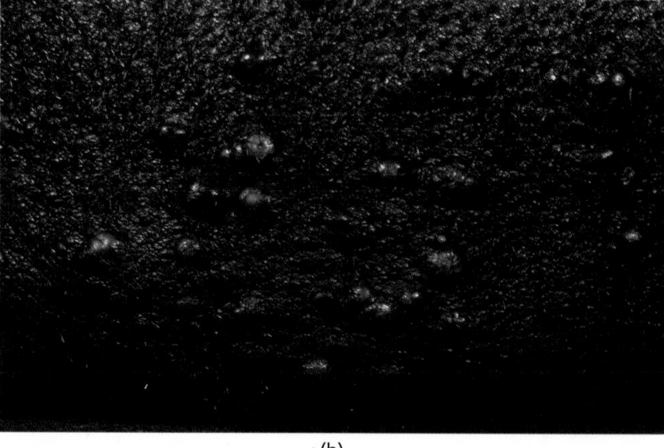

(b)

Figure 12.9 Keloid scars.

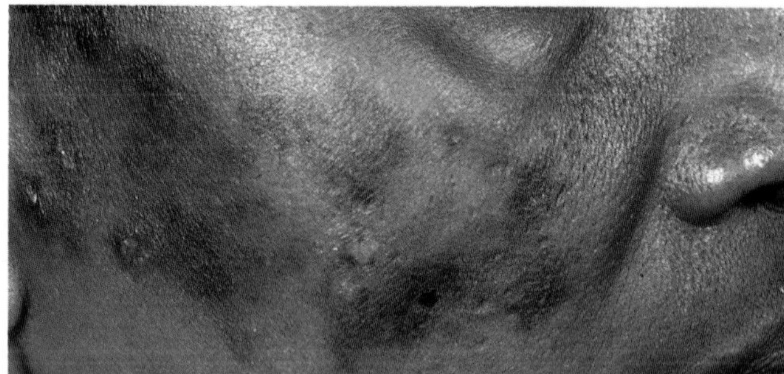

Figure 12.10 Acne excoriée.

Infantile acne

Localised acne lesions occur on the face in the first few months of life. Infantile acne may require topical or systemic therapy as although it will resolve spontaneously it may last up to 5 years and can cause scarring. There is an association with severe adolescent acne.

Acne conglobata/fulminans

This is a severe form of acne, more common in boys and in tropical climates. There is extensive, nodulocystic acne and

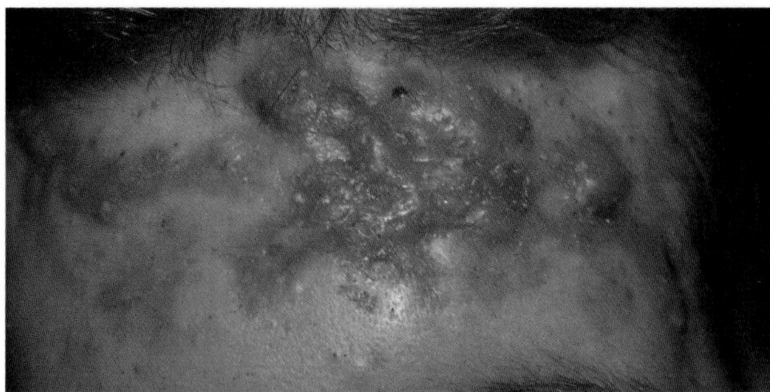

Figure 12.11 Acne conglobata.

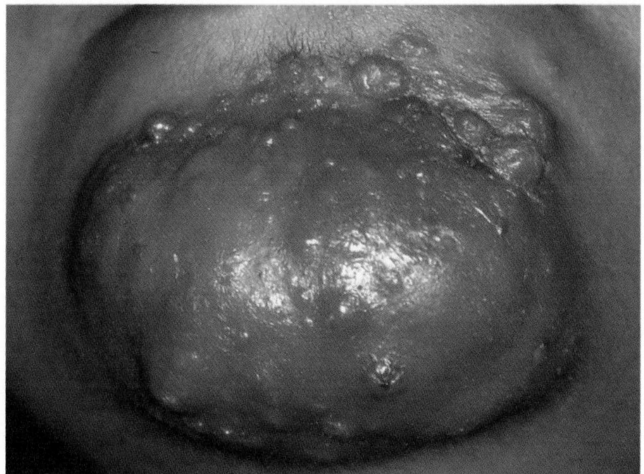

Figure 12.12 Acne fulminans.

abscess formation affecting particularly the trunk, face and limbs (Figure 12.11). Acne fulminans is similarly severe but is associated with systemic symptoms of malaise, fever and joint pains (Figure 12.12). It appears to be associated with a hypersensitivity to *Propionibacterium acnes*. Another variant is pyoderma faciale, which produces erythematous and necrotic lesions and occurs mainly in adult women.

Gram-negative folliculitis occurs with a proliferation of organisms such as *Klebsiella*, *Proteus*, *Pseudomonas* and *Escherichia coli*.

Treatment of acne

Although acne can be very painful and may result in pigment change and scarring it is the psychological impact of the condition that is often the most debilitating for those affected. In the past some medical practitioners have underestimated the effect acne has on patients' lives and consequently patients were often dismissed with no treatment on the assumption they would 'grow out of it'. Although most acne will settle with time early intervention for those seeking medical advice results in a significant improvement in their quality of life scores as determined by DLQI (dermatology life quality index which is a validated questionnaire to assess the impact of skin disease on quality of life). DLQI scores for acne are similar to those for psoriasis. Early intervention can also help reduce the likelihood of permanent scars and post-inflammatory pigment changes (Table 12.1).

When choosing a topical formulation to prescribe for a patient with acne it is worth bearing in mind the patient's skin type: for dry/sensitive skin, prescribe creams; for oily skin, use solutions or gels; and for combination skin and hair-bearing sites, lotions are well tolerated.

When treating patients with acne it is important to warn them that they may not see any improvement in their acne for several months and that treatment may need to continue for months or years.

Cleansers

Mild acne may respond well to simple measures such as cleansing the skin with proprietary keratolytics; these dissolve the keratin plug of the comedones. Cleansers need to be used with care as they can cause considerable dryness and scaling of the skin.

Topical treatments

Benzoyl peroxide has been available for the treatment of acne for many years; it has bacteriostatic effects against *P. acnes* and is mildly comedolytic. It is available with or without prescription at concentrations ranging from 1% to 10% in numerous formulations including lotions, creams, gels and washes. Mild irritant dermatitis may result, particularly if the patient is using additional anti-acne treatments. Bleaching of clothing and bedding may occur.

Salicylic acid promotes desquamation of follicular epithelium and therefore inhibits the formation of comedones. It is available over the counter at concentrations between 0.5% and 2% in cream and lotion formulations to be used twice daily.

Azelaic acid appears to be effective through its antikeratinising and antibacterial effects. Twenty percent azelaic acid cream is

Table 12.1 Treatment of acne.

Treatment	Comedones	Inflammatory papules/pustules	Mixed picture	Nodulocystic
First line	Topical retinoid Azelaic acid Salicylic acid	Benzoyl peroxide	Topical retinoid ± topical antibiotic ± benzoyl peroxide Combination of all three	Oral antibiotic + topical retinoid
Second line	Physical comedone extraction	Oral antibiotic Oral contraceptive pill (high oestrogen, low androgen, e.g. Yasmin®)	Azelaic acid + benzoyl peroxide ± topical antibiotic	Oral isotretinoin A short course of systemic steroids may be given initially with the isotretinoin
Third line		Anti-androgens e.g. co-cypindiol (Dianette®) Different oral antibiotic	Hormone therapy Oral antibiotic Oral isotretinoin	Triamcinolone injections to unresponsive lesions

available on prescription and can be used twice daily for up to 6 months. Mild skin irritation can result in approximately 5% of patients. Azelaic acid can cause depigmentation of the skin and therefore should be used with care.

Topical retinoids are vitamin A derivatives that are anti-inflammatory and comedolytic. Treatments currently available include tretinoin, adapalene and tazarotene. Topical retinoids are available in cream and gel formulations and are usually applied once daily at night (as they can cause photosensitivity). The main side-effect is skin irritation that results in erythema and desquamation; if this occurs patients may be able to tolerate alternate night applications. Tolerance to the irritation usually appears with continued use. Occasionally, an initial acne flare may occur with the use of topical retinoids; this is not, however, an indication to stop treatment as it usually heralds accelerated resolution of the acne.

Topical antibiotics are effective through their bactericidal activity against *P. acnes* and consequent anti-inflammatory effects. The most commonly prescribed antibiotics include erythromycin and clindamycin either alone or in combination with other agents such as zinc or benzoyl peroxide. Preparations are usually applied twice daily. Antibiotic resistance has been reported more commonly with antibiotics used alone than in combination.

Phototherapy with ultraviolet or visible light is an alternative therapy that may be helpful in those unresponsive to or unable to tolerate conventional treatments. Photodynamic therapy has been shown to be superior to blue-red light treatment for mild to moderate acne. However, new hand-held blue-light devices (2 J/cm^2/day and 29 J/cm^2/day) are available for use at home with reported reduction in acne lesions about 70% at 8 weeks after daily treatment to the whole face.

Systemic treatments

Hormone therapies. These include certain types of OCPs that increase sex hormone-binding globulin and consequently reduce free testosterone levels. These are generally OCPs that have higher oestrogen and lower androgen potential (such as Yasmin®). *Antiandrogen* treatment alone can be teratogenic and therefore is given to women in the form of a contraceptive that contains cyproterone acetate with ethinyloestradiol (Dianette®). Long-term safety data are available up to 5 years. Dianette® may also help diminish mild hirsutism.

Oral antibiotics. Tetracyclines remain the mainstay of treatment in those over the age of 12 years (below this age, they may cause dental hypoplasia and staining of teeth). Once-daily preparations (lymecycline 408 mg, minocycline 100 mg (MR) and doxycycline 40 mg) are more convenient to use than twice-daily preparations (tetracycline and oxytetracycline) and are equally well tolerated. Tetracyclines should be avoided in pregnancy/breastfeeding and children <12 years. Erythromycin and trimethoprim are good alternatives. Treatment benefits may not be seen for the first 6–8 weeks of therapy. An adequate treatment course should last approximately 6–12 months, depending on severity and response.

Oral retinoids. Isotretinoin has revolutionised the treatment of severe acne, but it is usually reserved for resistant disease unresponsive to other oral therapies. This is because of its side-effect profile including teratogenesis (90% risk of birth defects) and its ability to cause a rise in liver enzymes and lipids. Blood testing before initiation is essential and during therapy as indicated clinically. Female patients of child-bearing age will need to use a robust form of contraception while taking isotretinoin and for 1 month following its cessation. Pregnancy testing is usually undertaken before release of prescriptions for females.

All patients will experience some drying of the lips (Figure 12.13) and skin (Figure 12.14), and it is this side-effect that may limit the dose of isotretinoin tolerated, at least initially. Mood change and depression have been suggested as a possible side-effect of isotretinoin and consequently some practitioners preclude its use in those with a history of mental illness. All patients and their carers

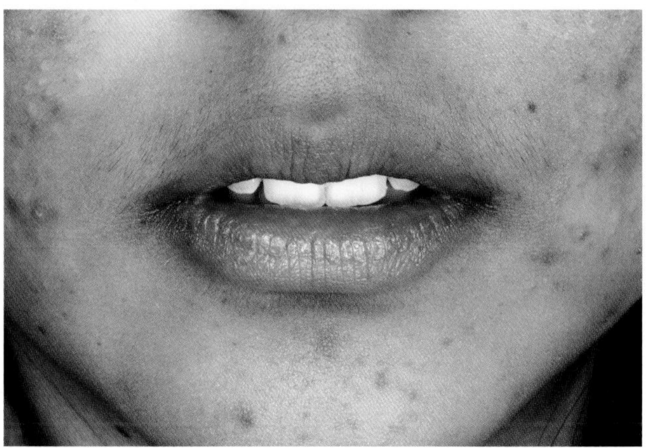

Figure 12.13 Dry lips as a result of oral Isotretinoin.

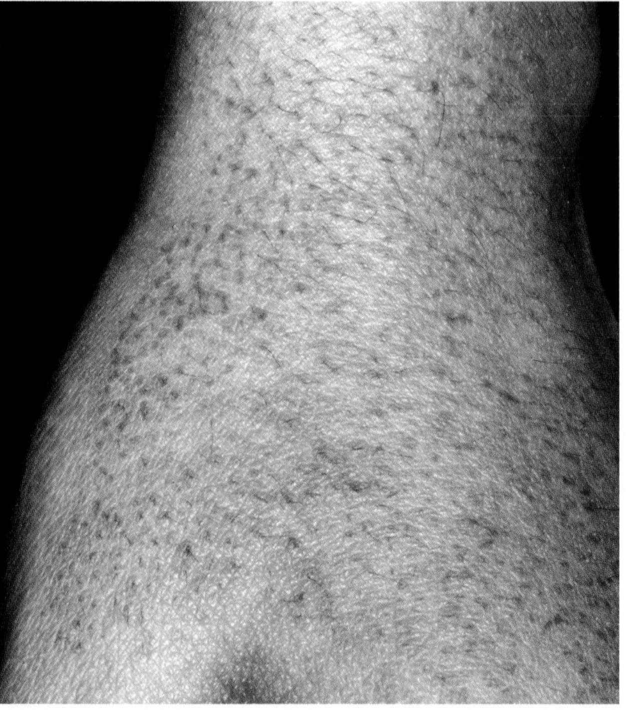

Figure 12.14 Classic rash on the dorsal hand secondary to taking oral Isotretinoin.

should be warned that there is a potential risk of mood swings and depression and to stop the medication immediately if they experience problems. A modern approach to isotretinoin dosing is to begin patients on a low dose for the first 1–2 months (20–40 mg daily) and then increase to 1 mg/kg/day to minimise initial xerosis. The cumulative target dosage for isotretinoin is 120–150 mg/kg based on studies showing that acne is likely to be 'cured' if a full treatment course is taken. Occasionally, patients require a second or even third course of isotretinoin treatment, and some patients (particularly males with very severe acne/seborrhoea) may require long-term treatment with very low doses such as 20 mg/week.

Residual lesions, keloid scars, cysts and persistent nodules can be treated by injection with triamcinolone, topical retinoids, chemical dermabrasion, carbon dioxide laser resurfacing and collagen injections. For severe atrophic boxcar and 'ice-pick' scarring punch biopsies can be used to remove scars from the face and pinch grafts applied to the areas (harvested from behind the ear). When healing is complete dermabrasion can then be used for resurfacing with good cosmetic results. For milder scarring chemical peels or dermaroller treatments may be considered.

Rosacea

Rosacea is characterised by facial flushing, persistent erythema, telangiectasia, inflammatory papules, pustules and oedema (Figure 12.15); in some patients the changes may be localised to one cheek or the nose (Figure 12.16). In chronic rosacea the nasal skin can become coarse in texture, eventually resulting in gross thickening and hypertrophy – known as rhinophyma (Figure 12.17) (from the Greek, 'rhis' nose, 'phyma' growth). Conjunctivitis, blepharitis (Figure 12.18) and eyelid oedema may be associated. Facial flushing and erythema are frequently exacerbated by heat, exercise, hot food/drinks, spicy food, emotion, alcohol and sunlight. Eventually, facial erythema can become permanent due to multiple dilated blood vessels – telangiectasia.

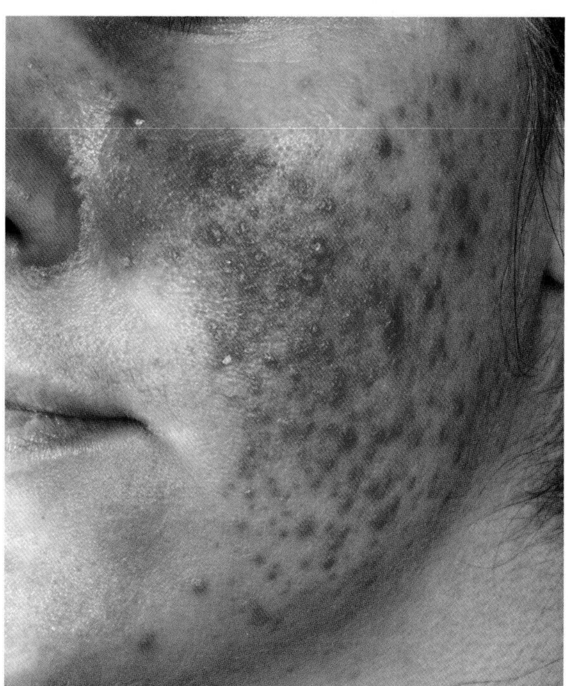

Figure 12.15 Rosacea.

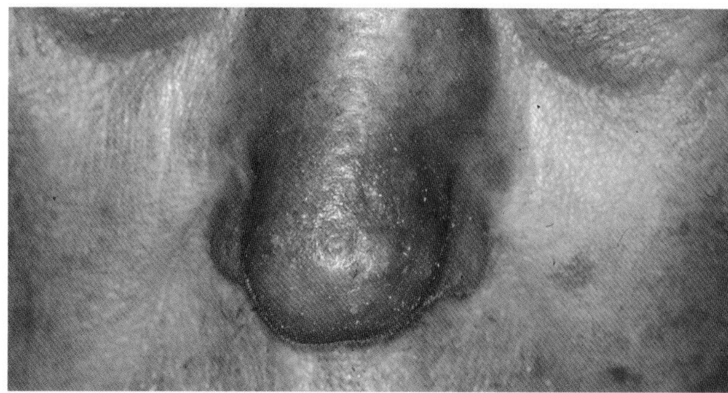

Figure 12.16 Rosacea localised to the nose.

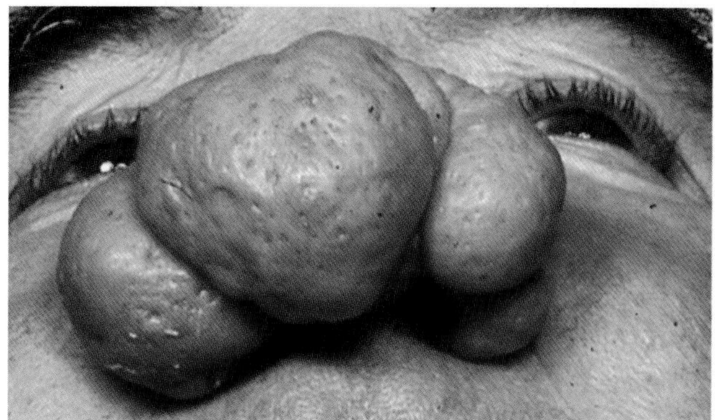

Figure 12.17 Rhinophyma.

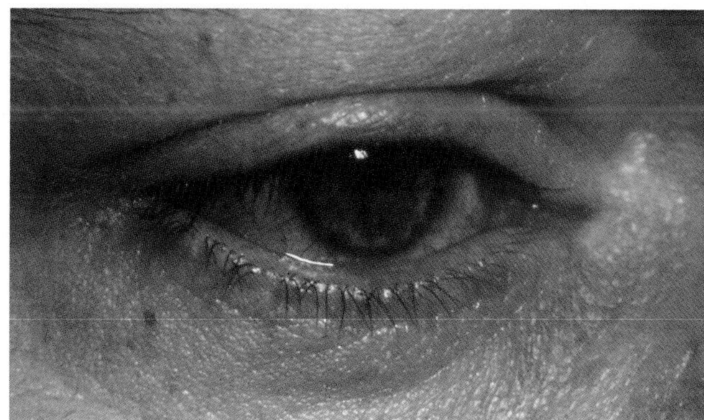

Figure 12.18 Blepharitis.

Differential diagnosis of rosacea

- Acne, in which there are comedones, a wider distribution and improvement with sunlight. (Acne may however coexist with rosacea – hence the older term 'acne rosacea'.)
- Seborrhoeic eczema, in which there are no pustules and eczematous changes are present. (However, an overlap syndrome is now recognised.)

- Dermatomyositis, where there may be periorbital and upper eyelid swelling and erythema.
- Lupus erythematosus, which shows light sensitivity, erythema and scarring, but no pustules.
- Perioral dermatitis, which occurs in women with pustules and erythema around the mouth and chin (Figure 12.4). This may be precipitated by the use of potent topical steroids; some patients experience a premenstrual exacerbation. Treatment is to stop the topical steroids and prescribe oral tetracyclines.

Management

Trigger factors should be identified and ideally avoided. All patients should be encouraged to avoid using skin irritants such as soaps or astringent cleansers. There is evidence that regular use of a broad-spectrum sunscreen can be helpful.

Topical metronidazole can be helpful in the treatment of mild disease; however, benefits may not be apparent for several months. Gel and cream formulations of metronidazole 0.75–1% should be used twice daily to the affected skin. Fifteen percent azelaic acid in a gel formulation is now also available for the treatment of rosacea. Topical preparations seem to be more effective at treating the papules and pustules than the erythema and flushing. However, α-adrenoreceptor agonists have recently been evaluated for treatment of diffuse facial erythema because of their ability to reversibly constrict peripheral vasculature with some promising results. Oxymetazoline/xylometazoline (0.05% solutions once daily), both α1-agonists, and brimonidine tartrate (0.5% gel once daily), α2-agonsist, have been shown to reduce diffuse facial erythema for up to 12 h; however, larger studies are ongoing and there is the theoretical risk of tachyphylaxis and rebound once the applications are stopped.

Oral antibiotics including tetracycline, doxycycline, erythromycin and minocycline have all been used to effectively treat rosacea. Patients should be warned that there may be no visible clinical improvement for several weeks, and treatment courses may need to continue for many months.

The use of low-dose oral isotretinoin for between 3 and 9 months has been shown to be effective in those with refractory disease.

Laser ablation of dilated telangiectatic vessels with a pulsed dye laser can be undertaken once the inflammatory component has been treated. An average of three treatments 6–8 weeks apart is usually required to achieve significant improvement. Intense pulsed light (IPL) can also be effective for reducing erythema, telangiectasia and papules. One study delivered IPL every 3 weeks for an average of seven treatments, which led to 70% of patients reporting reduced flushing and improved skin texture. Carbon dioxide laser or shave removal with a scalpel blade of excess skin from the nose can significantly improve the appearance of rhinophyma.

Further reading

Goldberg DJ. *Acne and Rosacea. Epidemiology, Diagnosis and Treatment*, Manson Publishing, London, 2011.

Zouboulis CC, Katsambas AD and Kligman AM. *Pathogenesis and Treatment of Acne and Rosacea*, Springer, New York, 2014.

CHAPTER 13

Bacterial Infections

Rachael Morris-Jones

Dermatology Department, Kings College Hospital, London, UK

OVERVIEW

- Damage to the epidermis/dermis results in reduced barrier function, which enables bacteria to invade the skin.
- Cutaneous bacterial infections produce signs of acute inflammation: erythema, swelling/oedema, heat/warmth and pain/discomfort.
- Localised superficial skin infections can be managed with antiseptic washes and topical antibiotics.
- Systemic antibiotics are needed for widespread, deep and persistent bacterial skin infections.
- Clinical signs of bacterial infections include folliculitis, boils/abscesses, blistering, crusting, erosions, ulcers and cellulitis.
- Mycobacterial skin infections most commonly arise from implantation/trauma and are usually localised in immunocompetent patients.
- Atypical mycobacteria can result in localised supurative lesions, persistent granulomas and sporotrichoid spread via lymphatics.

Introduction

Intact skin forms a highly effective barrier against invading pathogenic bacteria. Many micro-organisms come into contact with the skin and some live there as part of the normal skin flora, but they rarely cause disease. Normal skin flora consists of coagulase-negative *Staphylococcus*, *Corynebacterium*, diphtheroids and α-haemolytic *Streptococci* in the epidermis, and *Propionibacterium* in the pilosebaceous unit. Normal flora competes with invading pathogenic micro-organisms, thereby acting as a 'biological shield'. However, if the host immune system weakens or there is a change in the micro-environment (such as an underlying skin disease) this may allow such bacteria to become pathogenic.

Bacterial skin infections may be acquired from the external environment (from plants, soil, fomites, animals or other humans) by implantation, direct contact, aerosols or water-borne transmission. Bacteria most frequently invade a traumatic break in the skin, follicular openings and mucous membranes where host barriers are more vulnerable.

ABC of Dermatology, Sixth Edition. Edited by Rachael Morris-Jones.

Bacterial skin infections vary from the very minor to life-threatening and overwhelming. It is often tempting to assume a single organism is responsible for any particular cutaneous infection, but often the contrary is true. Synergistic microbial invasion is frequently present in cutaneous wounds. See Table 13.1 for a summary of the common patterns of bacterial infection in the skin.

Clinical presentation

Patients with a bacterial skin infection may recall an episode of trauma to the skin such as a graze, laceration, insect bite or implantation of foreign material, or they may have a history of ongoing skin disease. A more detailed history may reveal contact with potentially contaminated water via bathing, animal contact, travel abroad or other family members/close contacts similarly affected. However, many patients will not have any obvious source from the history alone.

Acute bacterial infections in the skin generally produce some or all of the classical characteristics of acute inflammation: erythema, swelling/oedema, heat/warmth and pain/discomfort. Patients may develop systemic symptoms such as fever and malaise. Many cutaneous infections start as an isolated lesion that then spreads to involve the surrounding previously uninvolved skin. Multiple lesions may be present in a follicular distribution.

Bacterial investigations

Taking bacterial swabs for microscopy and culture can be very useful in managing patients with probable cutaneous infections. Microbiological testing can identify the bacterial species, antibiotic resistance/sensitivity patterns and bacterial toxin production. This information allows medical practitioners to make informed decisions regarding patient management. Lesional skin and carrier sites can be swabbed. Nasal swabs may identify *Staphylococcus aureus* carriers who can suffer from recurrent infections because of bacterial shedding from the nose. When taking swabs they should be moistened in the transport media before contact with the skin and each surface of the swab should be rotated on the infected skin surface. Methicillin-resistant *S. aureus* (MRSA) may be community or hospital acquired. Panton Valentine Leukocidin (PVL) is a toxin produced by some strains of *S. aureus* which cause the bacteria to be highly virulent and highly transmissible. Patients with

Table 13.1 Common patterns of bacterial infection in the skin.

Infection	Clinical photograph	Clinical presentation	Organisms	Management
Infected eczema		Background inflammatory atopic dermatitis with excoriations and marked crusting and exudate	*Staphylococcus aureus* *Streptococcus pyogenes*	Antiseptic wash Topical antibiotic/steroid combination cream. Oral flucloxacillin or erythromycin
Impetigo		Mainly children, especially face and limbs. Highly contagious. Yellow crusted lesions surrounded by normal skin	*S. aureus* *S. pyogenes*	Antiseptic wash Topical antibiotic Oral flucloxacillin or erythromycin
Bullous impetigo		Children and adults. Face, limbs and flexures affected. Erythema with bullae which rupture leaving superficial erosions and crusts	*S. aureus* with exfoliative toxins A/B (may become generalised – staphylococcal scalded skin syndrome)	Oral flucloxacillin or erythromycin
Boils (abscesses)		Tender, inflamed indurated nodules with central pus may be single or multiple. If recurrent and recalcitrant consider toxin producing bacteria	*S. aureus* Consider Panton valentine leukocidin Toxin producing *S. aureus*	Antiseptic wash Oral flucloxacillin or erythromycin If PVL positive give nasal bactroban and consider giving clindamycin plus rifampicin for 4–6 weeks
Bacterial folliculitis		Hair-bearing sites particularly legs, beard area and scalp. May result from shaving damage to skin. In recurrent infections look for *S. aureus* nasal carriage	*S. aureus* *Pseudomonas aeruginosa* (differential diagnosis *Malassezia* spp)	Topical antibiotics Acetic acid cream EarCalm® for *P. aeruginosa* Oral flucloxacillin or erythromycin Avoid shaving if possible
Ecthyma		Children, the elderly/debilitated. Mainly on the legs. Initially small bullae with necrotic dry adherent crust and underlying ulceration Heal slowly with scarring	*S. pyogenes* *S. aureus*	Antiseptic wash Oral penicillin V or erythromycin
Erysipelas		Face or lower leg. Portal of entry is broken skin (trauma and tinea pedis) well-demarcated bright erythema	*S. pyogenes* (group A *Strep.* but also B, C, G) *S. aureus* (less common)	Intravenous benzyl penicillin or erythromycin

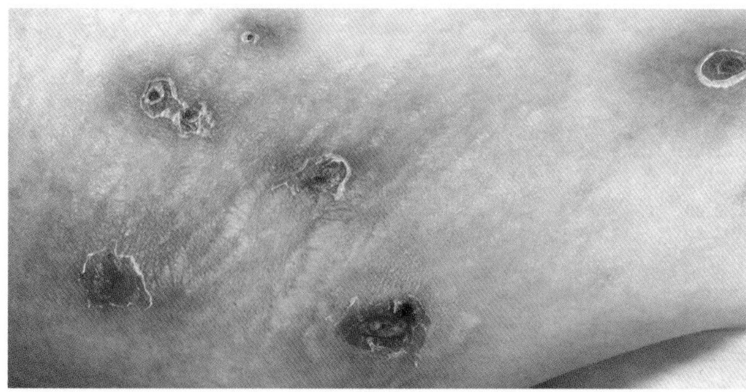

Figure 13.1 Mulitple abscesses due to PVL *Staphylococcus aureus* infection.

PVL-positive *S. aureus* often present with multiple/recurrent boils not settling with short courses of flucloxacillin (Figure 13.1). Often other family members are similarly affected. Request PVL testing when sending swabs to microbiology. In severe skin infections or when you suspect mycobacterial infections, take a skin biopsy for culture and polymerase chain reaction (PCR).

General approach to management

The treatment approach depends on the extent and the severity of the cutaneous infection.

Antiseptic skin washes or creams containing chlorhexidine hydrochloride can be helpful in removing superficial bacteria, and many of the novel formulations are suitable for use in patients with sensitive skin such as atopic eczema. Potassium permanganate soaks or diluted bleach can be very effective at treating any cutaneous infections, particularly on the lower legs, which may be submersed in a solution. The skin should be washed daily whenever possible to remove adherent infected crusts.

Topical antibiotics applied twice daily can be used alone to treat mild localised infections. Fusidic acid, mupirocin, neomycin, polymyxins, retapamulin, silver sulphadiazine and metronidazole are all available in topical formulations. Prolonged exposure to topical antibiotics leads to the selection of resistant organisms and rarely contact dermatitis (neomycin most commonly). Topical antibiotic/steroid combinations are useful in treating infection and inflammation simultaneously.

Systemic antibiotics are needed for more extensive cutaneous bacterial infections.

Staphylococcal cover is provided by flucloxacillin, erythromycin, clarithromycin, azithromycin, co-fluampicil (contains flucloxacillin and ampicillin), co-amoxiclav, clindamycin, fusidic acid, ciprofloxacin, cefuroxime, dicloxacillin, cloxacillin, linezolid, pristinamycin and roxithromycin. For MRSA, use vancomycin, nafcillin, daptomycin or tigecycline.

Streptococcal cover is provided by penicillin V, amoxicillin, flucloxacillin, erythromycin, clarithromycin, azithromycin, co-amoxiclav, cefuroxime, ceftazidime, clindamycin, pristinamycin, roxithromycin, vancomycin and levofloxacin.

Superficial infections

Impetigo is usually caused by *S. aureus* or *Streptococcus pyogenes* and is highly contagious between close contacts and develops rapidly into clusters of pustules and vesicles which break down into the classic golden crusts (Figure 13.2). Bullous lesions are more likely to occur with *Staphylococcal* infections which produce epidermolytic toxins A/B (Figure 13.3). *Streptococcus* is more likely to be the causative organism if there is associated regional lymphadenopathy, but many patients will have a mixed infection. Several family members may be affected simultaneously, particularly in conditions of poor hygiene in hot humid climates. There may be an association with minor trauma such as insect bites. Secondary impetigo may co-exist with any pre-existing skin lesion. Topical treatment includes antiseptic washes, fusidic acid, mupirocin and polymyxins. Oral antibiotics most frequently used include flucloxacillin and erythromycin.

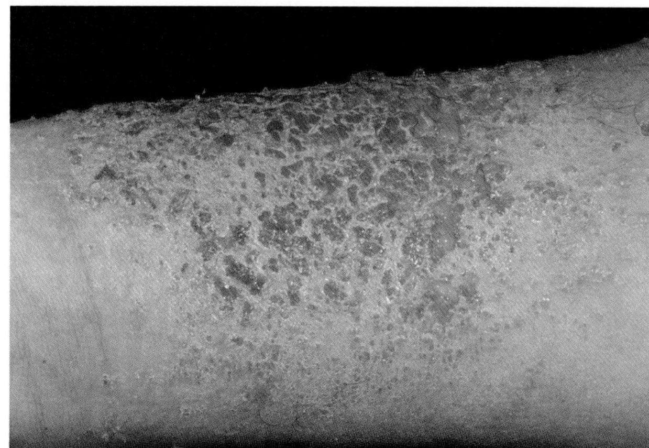

Figure 13.2 Impetigo with golden crusting.

Bacterial folliculitis is defined as infection in the hair follicles which may be superficial and/or deep and is usually caused by *S. aureus*. The majority of those affected by folliculitis never

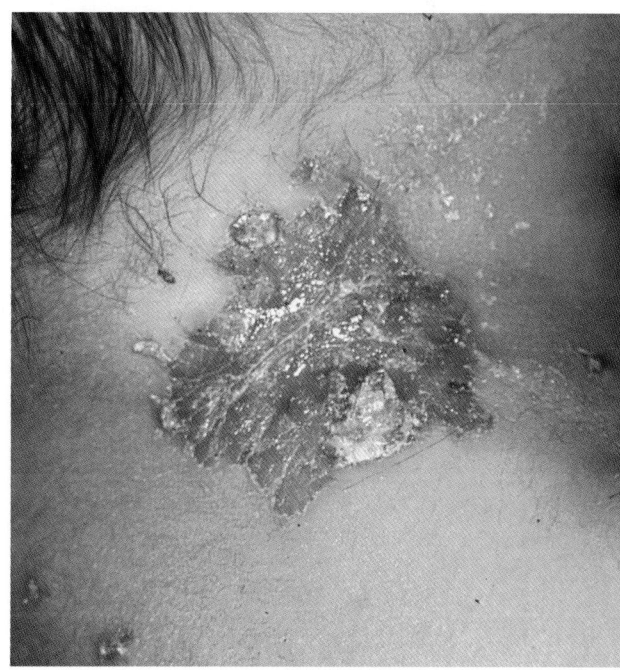

Figure 13.3 Impetigo with bullae and erosions.

seek medical advice as these infections are frequently mild and self-limiting. Clinically, there is a pustule and erythema around the follicular orifice which may be associated with mild irritation (Figure 13.4). Folliculitis may result from minor trauma such as hair removal by shaving or waxing.

Deeper follicular infections are characterised by abscess formation (which is termed *sycosis barbae* in the beard area), boils and furunculosis. When several furuncles coalesce they form a carbuncle. Hot-tub folliculitis caused by *Pseudomonas aeruginosa* appears within 2 days of exposure to contaminated water or water accessories (such as loofahs and wet-suits).

Pseudofolliculitis has a similar clinical appearance but this is caused by occlusion of the follicular openings by heavy emollients rather than bacterial infection. In pseudofolliculitis the lesions are all at the same stage of development and are clinically very monomorphic, and the pustules are sterile (Figure 13.5).

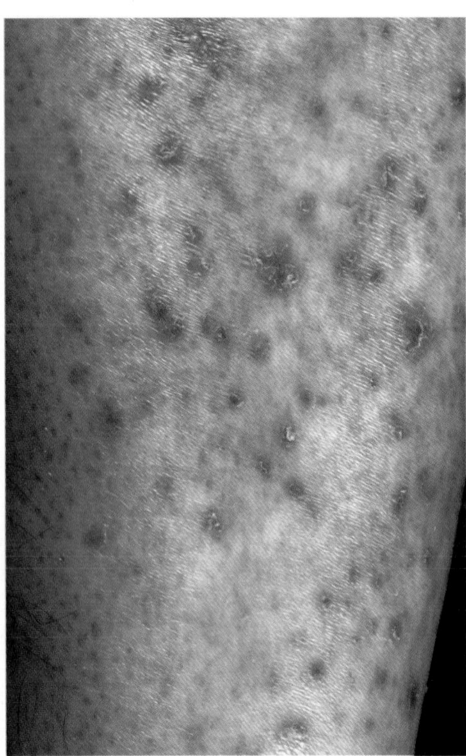

Figure 13.4 Bacterial folliculitis.

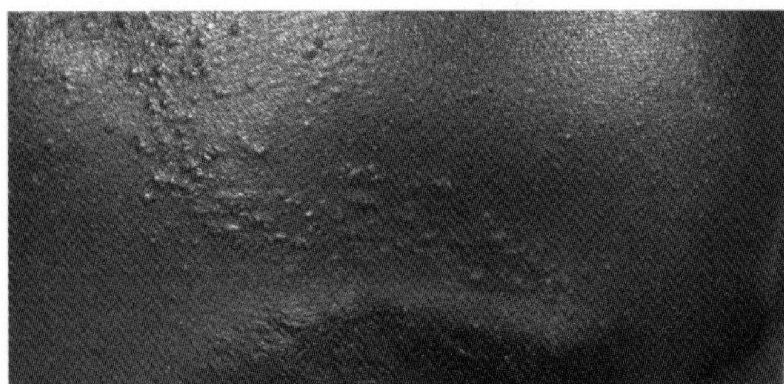

Figure 13.5 Pseudofolliculitis: forehead.

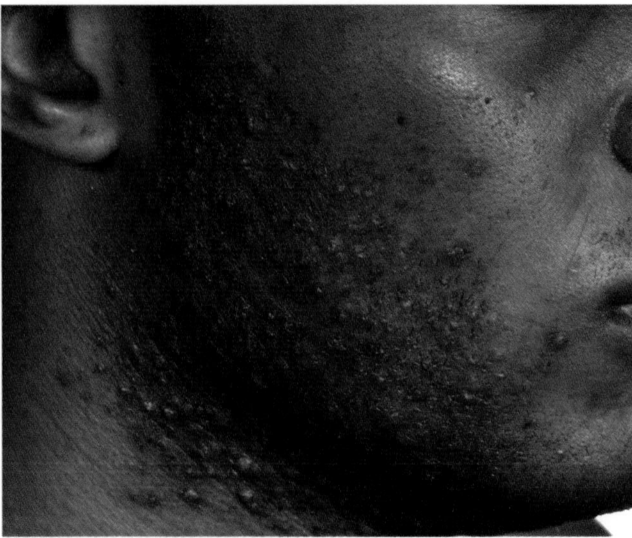

Figure 13.6 Acne keloidalis.

Pseudofolliculitis barbae in the beard area has a similar clinical appearance but is in fact a perifolliculitis. Coarse curly hair punctures the skin adjacent to the hair follicle (from which it has arisen) resulting in a foreign body reaction with inflammation which can become chronic and lead to scarring.

In the occipital area of the scalp *acne keloidalis nuchae* results from folliculitis and perifolliculitis with resultant alopecia and keloid scarring from chronic inflammation. A similar appearance is seen in the beard area (Figure 13.6). The cause is unknown but it occurs almost exclusively in black males who shave their hair very short.

Erythrasma usually affects the flexural skin sites, particularly the axilla and groin. There is superficial scaling and mild inflammation, often with a reddish-brown discolouration (Figure 13.7). It is frequently mistaken for a fungal infection so isolation of the causative bacterium *Corynebacterium minutissimum* from skin scraping can be useful. Under Wood's ultraviolet light the affected skin

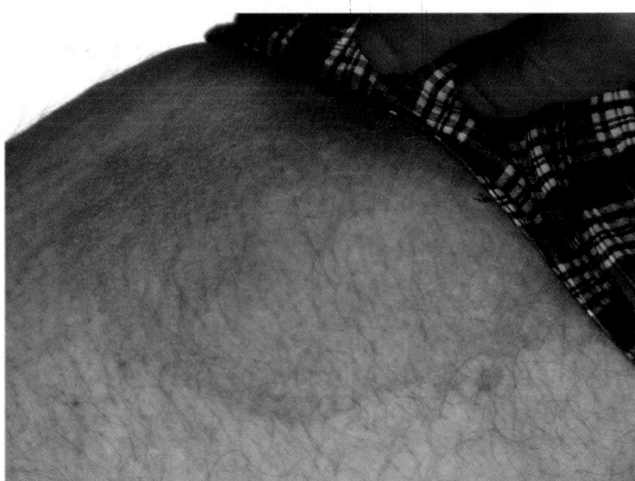

Figure 13.7 Erythrasma.

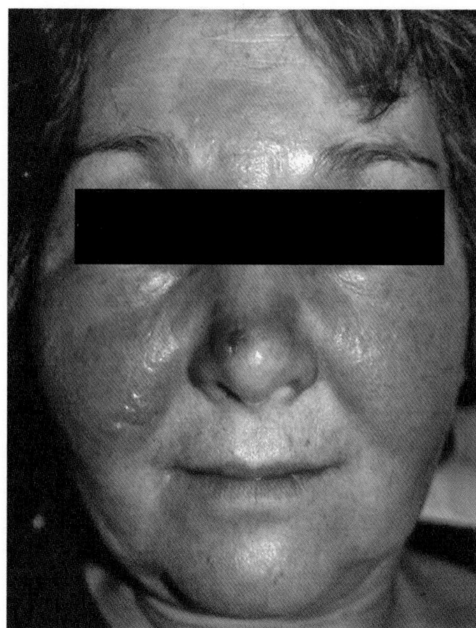

Figure 13.8 Erysipelas.

(bacteria) fluoresces pink. First-line treatment is usually oral erythromycin (250 mg QDS for 7–14 days), but if topical treatment is preferred, then clotrimazole, miconazole, fusidic acid or neomycin can be effective.

Deeper infections

Erysipelas is caused by a *Streptococcus* infection. Over approximately 48 h the inflammation spreads across the skin with a characteristic red, shiny, raised, spreading plaque with a well-demarcated edge (Figure 13.8). Occasionally, blistering may occur at the active edge; patients may have fever and malaise. The face (*S. pyogenes* from throat colonisation) and lower legs are most frequently affected. Differential diagnosis of erysipelas on the face includes contact dermatitis, photodermatitis, rosacea, systemic lupus erythematosus and fifth disease or 'slapped cheek'.

The *Streptococcus* organisms invade the dermis and penetrate the lymphatics, which clinically is well demarcated; this contrasts with the clinical appearance of cellulitis (infection in the deeper layers), which is poorly demarcated. There may be a minor skin laceration or tinea pedis (look between the toes) as the portal of entry. If the infection is severe, treat with intravenous benzylpenicillin or orally with amoxicillin, roxithromycin or pristinamycin for 1–2 weeks. Recurrent attacks are reported in 20% of patients with predisposing conditions; these individuals may require long-term secondary prophylaxis (Penicillin V 500 mg daily).

Erysipelas is the local manifestation of a group A Streptococcal infection; however, the same organism through the production of toxins or superantigens can cause other skin lesions such as (a) the rash of scarlet fever; (b) erythema nodosum; (c) guttate psoriasis and (d) an acute generalised vasculitis.

Cellulitis develops more slowly than erysipelas and has a poorly defined margin and marked regional lymphadenopathy. Patients may have fever and general malaise. In cellulitis, *S. pyogenes* (also groups C/G β-haemolytic *Streptococcus*, or rarely *S. aureus*) organisms invade deeper tissues than those found in erysipelas. The lower leg is the most common site affected (Figure 13.9). Patients may have underlying dermatoses such as a diabetic foot ulcer, tinea pedis or stasis dermatitis which act as a portal of entry for the Streptococcal bacteria. In severe infections intravenous benzylpenicillin may be needed for up to a week as the infection settles slowly.

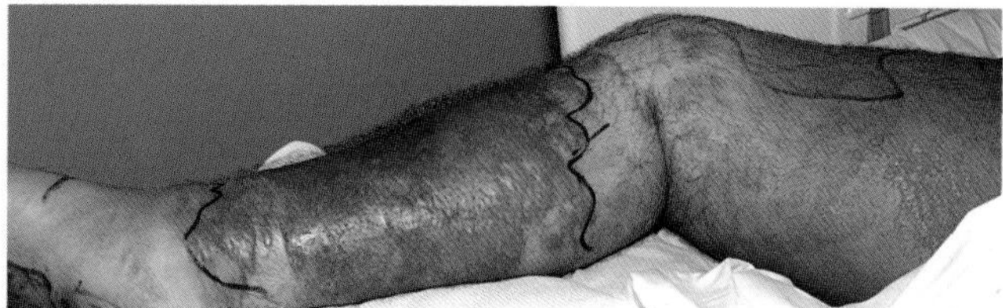

Figure 13.9 Extending cellulitis.

Necrotising fasciitis is characterised by dusky purplish erythema associated with extensive life-threatening necrosis of the deeper tissue because of rapidly progressive mixed (anaerobic and aerobic bacteria) infection of the deep fascia leading to gas formation in the subcutaneous tissues. Patients often have a history of recent trauma or surgery. There is usually severe pain initially at the site followed by anaesthesia. Patients appear very unwell – often disproportionately to the clinical picture. Dusky erythema associated with necrosis at the skin surface is usually the tip of the iceberg with much more extensive life-threatening necrosis of the deeper tissues. Urgent surgical debridement and broad spectrum antibiotics are indicated.

Staphylococcus scalded skin syndrome (*SSSS*) is caused by strains of *S. aureus* that produce exfoliative toxins A/B resulting in intraepidermal splitting (the target is desmoglein 1 which is responsible for keratinocyte adhesion). A localised form of the disease is called *bullous impetigo*. The clinical presentation in children below 5 years of age is usually with conjunctivitis, otitis media or a nasopharyngeal infection, with fever, malaise and red tender skin. Generalised cutaneous erythema is followed by widespread superficial blistering (Nikolsky sign positive) and exfoliation which may be most striking in the flexures (Figure 13.10). Although most children are not unwell there is a 4% mortality rate for generalised SSSS. Give systemic antibiotics to treat *Staphylococcus*. If patients fail to respond, then consider treating for MRSA which has a higher mortality rate.

Ecthyma is often referred to as a deeper form of impetigo as the group A β-haemolytic Streptococci (*S. pyogenes*) invade the dermis leading to superficial ulcers. Lesions start as small pustules that have adherent crust and underlying ulceration, and most commonly occur on the lower legs of children and elderly people who live in humid climates. Lesions usually heal slowly with scarring (Figure 13.11).

Mycobacterial disease

Clinical manifestations of mycobacterial infections are largely determined by the ability of the host to mount an immune

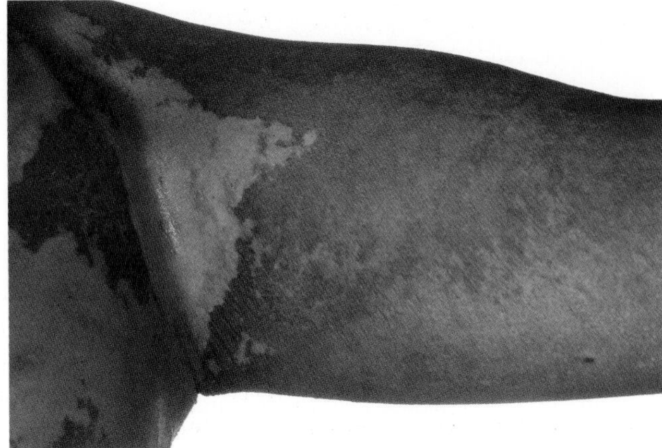

Figure 13.10 *Staphylococcus* scalded skin syndrome.

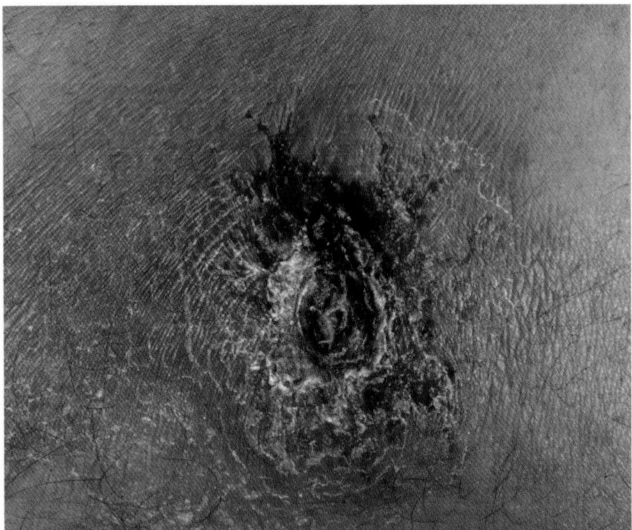

Figure 13.11 Ecthyma.

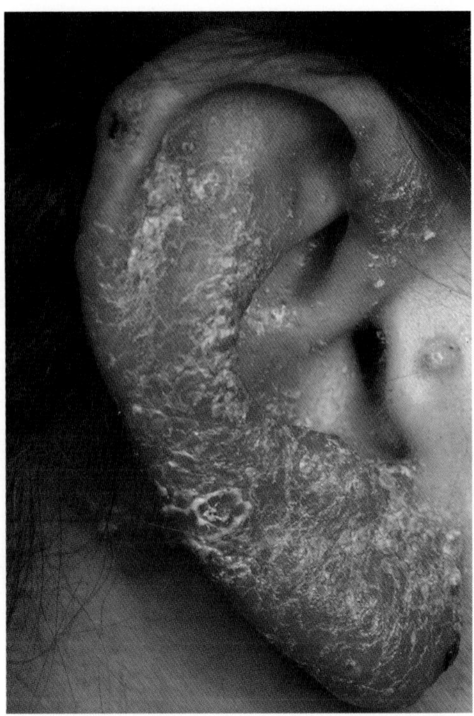

Figure 13.12 Lupus vulgaris.

response. Disease spectrums therefore range from dissemination to mild localised lesions; for example, *Mycobacterium tuberculosis* may present with miliary TB or lupus vulgaris, and *Mycobacterium leprae* may present with lepromatous (multibacillary) or more tuberculoid (paucibacillary) phenotypes (see Chapter 18).

Cutaneous *M. tuberculosis* (TB) is rare even in endemic areas. TB in the skin usually occurs as a secondary manifestation of disease with its primary focus in the respiratory tract. The most common manifestation is lupus vulgaris which usually presents on the head and neck. Lesions appear as slowly growing well-demarcated red-brown papules that coalesce to form indolent plaques of a gelatinous nature: the so-called '*apple-jelly nodules*' (Figure 13.12). A number of mechanisms are thought to cause clinical lupus vulgaris, including spread of TB to the skin from lymphatics or blood, and direct extension of TB from underlying tissues (scrofuloderma) from primary cutaneous inoculation or spread from a BCG vaccination site.

Allergic-type hypersensitivity reactions called *tuberculids* can occur in the skin of patients with underlying TB. Tuberculids are thought to represent hypersensitivity reactions to antigenic fragments of dead bacilli deposited in the skin via haematogenous spread. Recent studies have demonstrated TB DNA in the affected skin in 25–75% of cases. Tuberculids include erythema induratum (Bazin's disease) where patients present with tender nodules and plaques that ulcerate and heal with scarring on the lower legs. Papulonecrotic tuberculid (which some authors believe to be a more superficial form of Bazin's disease) (Figure 13.13) and lichen scrofulosorum (very small lichenoid papules over the trunk and limbs in young patients).

Atypical mycobacteria (*ATM*) are usually found in the environment in vegetation and water. Fast-growing *Mycobacterium chelonae complex*/*M. abscessus* may be associated with boil-like skin lesions from traumatic implantation. *M. avium complex* (MAC) is associated with lymphadenitis in children and disseminated disease (including papular skin lesions) in HIV patients. Immunocompromised patients are most frequently affected in addition to those with underlying systemic diseases such as diabetes, chronic renal failure, connective tissue disease and malignancy. Patients require treatment with clarithromycin ± rifampicin for 4–6 months or 6–8 weeks past clinical cure in immunocompromised patients.

Mycobacterium marinum or 'fish tank' or 'swimming pool granuloma' usually occurs because of contact with infected tropical fish or contaminated water. The hand or fingers are most frequently

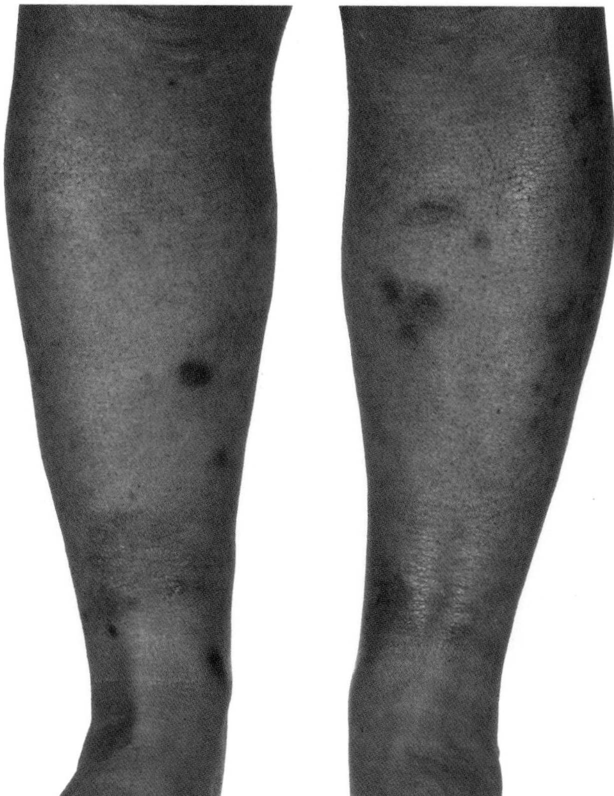

Figure 13.13 Erythema induratum (Bazin's disease).

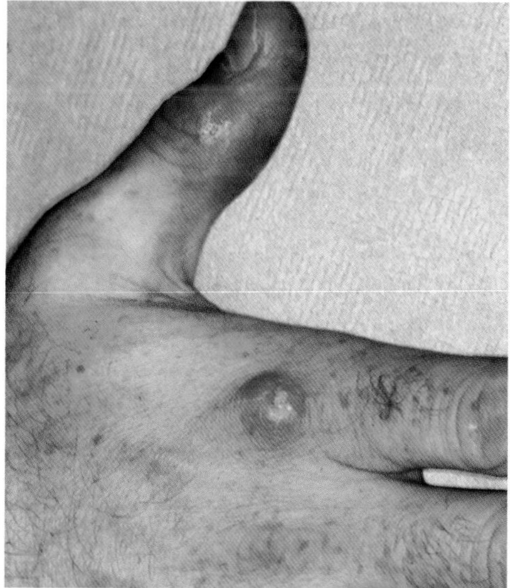

Figure 13.14 Sporotrichoid spread of *Mycobacterium marinum*.

affected; initially, a single warty nodular and occasionally pustular lesion appears with subsequent sporotricoid spread along local lymphatics, forming a chain of nodules (Figure 13.14). Patients should be treated with clarithromycin for several months.

Mycobacterium ulcerans causes extensive non-painful ulceration (buruli ulcer) usually on the limbs in children/young adults living in tropical humid areas associated with minor skin trauma and contact with the mycobacterium in standing water.

Other infections

Bacillary angiomatosis caused by *Bartonella henselae and Bartonella quintana* infections presents in HIV patients with multiple small haemangioma-like papules. Clinical manifestations are most commonly seen in the skin and mucous membranes, but underlying visceral disease (especially liver) may occur simultaneously. Patients usually present with multiple small cherry-like haemangiomas on the skin which appear over weeks to months (Figure 13.15). Serology rather than culture is usually used to confirm the diagnosis (indirect fluorescent assay or ELISA IgG >1:64 indicates likely current infection). Erythromycin 500 mg qds for up to 12 weeks is recommended, or 4–6 weeks of azithromycin 500 mg daily.

Cat-scratch disease is caused by the bacterium *B. henselae*. Crusted nodules appear within 3–12 days at the site of a scratch (usually by a kitten) associated with the development of regional painful lymphadenopathy 1 or 2 months later. The disease usually undergoes spontaneous remission within 2–4 months. A 5-day course of azithromycin can speed up recovery.

Rickettsial organisms are a diverse group of slow-growing small gram-negative bacteria that are mainly transmitted by ticks and mites. Rocky Mountain spotted fever (RMSF) is one of the most common rickettsial infections (*Rickettsia rickettsii*) in the USA and has a 4% mortality rate. The most common vector of RMSF is the dog tick. Within a week of the bite patients present with high fever, headache, myalgia and a petechial rash which characteristically appears on the palms and soles but may spread to the trunk (Figure 13.16). There may be a necrotic lesion (tache noire) at the site of the tick bite. Treat adults with doxycycline 100 mg twice daily for approximately 1 week and children with azithromycin for 5 days.

Syphilis is caused by the spirochete bacterium *Treponema pallidum* which is transmitted through sexual intercourse, transplacental spread and via unscreened blood transfusions. The incidence

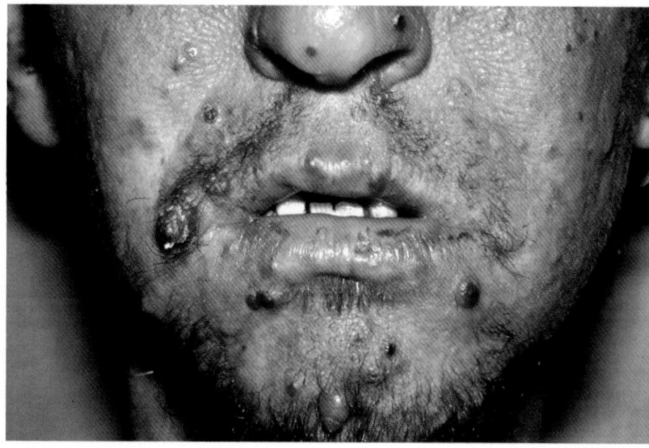

Figure 13.15 Bacillary angiomatosis.

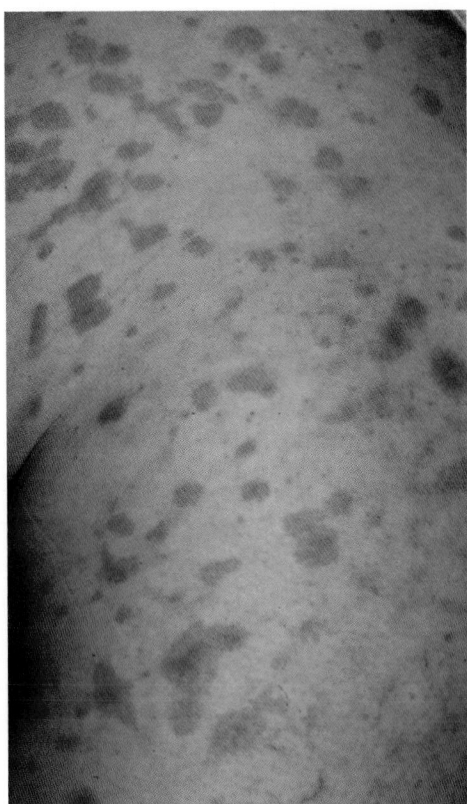

Figure 13.16 Rocky mountain spotted fever.

of syphilis is steadily increasing due to co-infection with human immunodeficiency virus (HIV) (see Chapter 15 for more details). Primary syphilis manifests as a painless genital ulcer at the site of inoculation. Cutaneous manifestations of secondary syphilis are characterised by a widespread eruption of red-brown scaly patches and macules that affects the trunk and limbs (particularly palms and soles) (Figure 13.17). In patients with HIV the rash may be florid with marked crusting. Serology is needed to know whether patients have previous or current infection, which will subsequently guide management and contact tracing.

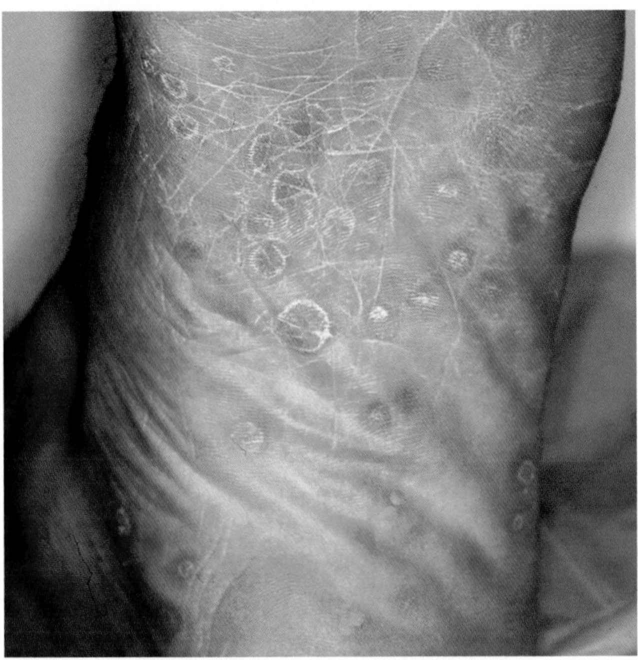

Figure 13.17 Secondary syphilis.

Further Reading

Hall BJ and Hall JC. *Skin Infections: Diagnosis and Treatment*, Cambridge University Press, 2009.

Weber CG. Wound care and skin infections 2013 (The clinical medicine series). www.ClinicalMedConsult.com. Primary Care Software, 2013.

CHAPTER 14

Viral Infections

Rachael Morris-Jones

Dermatology Department, Kings College Hospital, London, UK

OVERVIEW

- Viruses are obligate parasites able to make important changes in cellular function and immune responses of the host.
- As well as modifying genetic material of the host cell, the viral genome itself undergoes changes – shift and drift.
- RNA viruses are unstable, undergoing multiple mutations and causing systemic disease (measles).
- DNA viruses are more stable and cause local infections (human papilloma virus warts, molluscum).
- Herpes simplex infections are acquired by local contact and reactivate at the inoculation site, usually mucosae (lips and genitals).
- Herpes zoster (shingles) is due to reactivation of previously acquired varicella zoster virus (chicken pox).
- Specific antiviral medications are few and therefore the current primary strategy for reducing viral infections is vaccination.

Introduction

The term *virus* comes from Latin, meaning poison or toxin. Most modern medical practitioners think of viruses as micro-organisms rather than toxins, but some experts argue that viruses are not living organisms as they do not fulfill all the necessary criteria. Viruses do not have cell structures and they require host cells to replicate and synthesise new products. This spontaneous self-assembly within the host cells has been likened to the autonomous growth of crystals. Viral self-assembly has also been used to strengthen the hypothesis that the 'origins of life' started from self-assembling organic molecules. Nonetheless, viruses do possess genes, cause disease, trigger immune responses and evolve through natural selection; so, from a practitioner's point of view, living or otherwise, they have an enormous impact on human health.

The inability of viruses to grow or replicate outside the host cell means they have become masters at persistence within the host. Viruses persist within the host cell because they are often able to replicate without killing the host cells, their gene expression can be restricted, they can mimic host molecules, down-regulate host immunity and directly infect the host's immune cells. Viruses continuously change, either gradually (called '*drift*') where they accumulate minor mutations, or suddenly (called '*shift*') following major changes during recombination of the viral genome.

RNA viruses such as measles and human immunodeficiency virus (HIV) are unstable, undergoing immense drift and shift with up to 2% of their genome altered each year through multiple mutations. These viruses tend to cause systemic disease in humans, leading to generalised cutaneous eruptions such as a 'viral exanthem'. In contrast, DNA viruses such as human papillomavirus (HPV), molluscum contagiosum, herpes simplex virus (HSV), and varicella zoster virus (VZV) are more stable. They are frequently inoculated directly into the skin and replicate in epidermal cells.

Viruses can be transmitted by direct contact from skin to skin, through aerosols, transplacental spread, blood products, contaminated needles and via the faecal–oral route. Once inside the host, viruses can spread directly from cell to cell, via the blood, or central nervous system by axonal transport. Many viruses demonstrate tropism (in other words a predilection for a certain host cell) via virus attachment to protein-specific cell surface receptors. HPV, for example, has tropism for keratinocytes.

The behaviour of different viruses therefore determines the type of disease they cause with resultant localised or widespread reactive skin disorders. Common viral infections of the skin are usually easily identified by pattern recognition through the characteristic skin or mucous membrane site affected and/or typical lesions.

Herpes viruses

Herpes simplex

HSV is spread by direct contact – 'shedding' from one host to another. Two viral subtypes exist: type I is associated mainly with facial lesions although the fingers (Figure 14.1) and genitals may be affected. Type II is associated almost entirely with genital infections. HSV remains within the host for life, remaining latent in the sensory nerve ganglia leading to recurrent reactivation.

Primary herpes simplex (type I) infection usually occurs in or around the mouth/nose, with variable involvement of the face (Figure 14.2). Lesions consist of small vesicles (Figure 14.3) which crust over and are associated with regional lymphadenopathy. HSV type II infects the external genitalia; the initial vesicle or vesicles rapidly break down into painful ulcers (Box 14.1).

ABC of Dermatology, Sixth Edition. Edited by Rachael Morris-Jones.

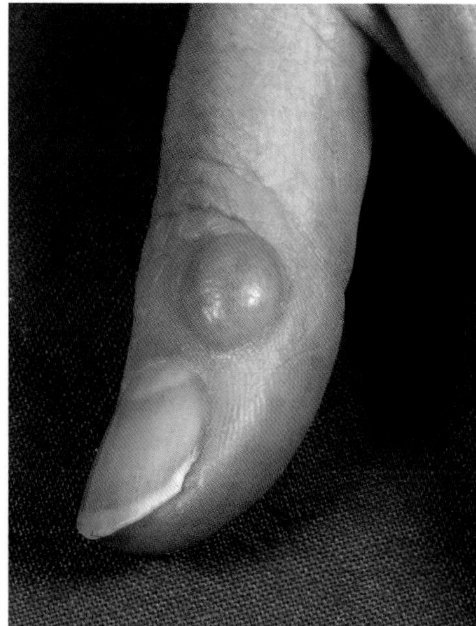

Figure 14.1 Inoculation herpes.

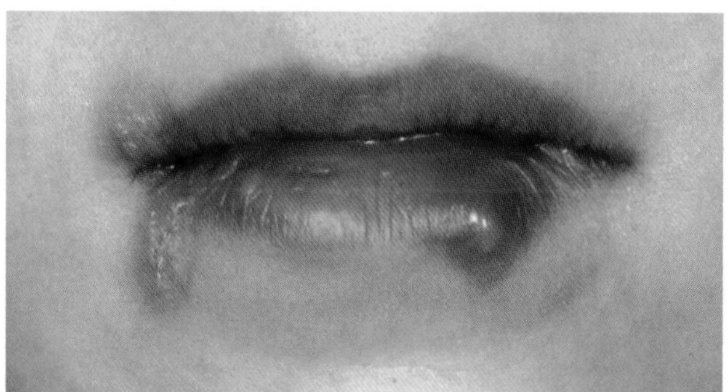

Figure 14.2 Herpes 'cold sore'.

Box 14.1 **Herpes simplex – points to note**

- Genital vesicles may not be visualised as they rapidly ulcerate.
- Prodrome symptoms consist of itching, tingling and tenderness.
- Rapid viral detection from scraping the vesicle/ulcer base using electron microscopy, immunofluorescence or PCR.
- Genital herpes in pregnancy carries a risk of ophthalmic infection of the infant. Caesarean section may be indicated.
- 'Eczema herpeticum' occurs in patients with atopic eczema where the HSV disseminates across abnormal skin (Figure 14.4).

Episodes of reactivation of HSV may be triggered by the cold ('cold sore'), bright sunlight, trauma, immunosuppression or intercurrent illnesses. There is frequently a prodrome of tingling or itching before the appearance of the vesicles, which occur in the distribution of a sensory nerve. Topical aciclovir/penciclovir/idoxuridine cream can be used to treat mild labial herpes. Severe infections should be treated with oral aciclovir 200–400 mg five times daily for 5 days. Secondary prophylaxis

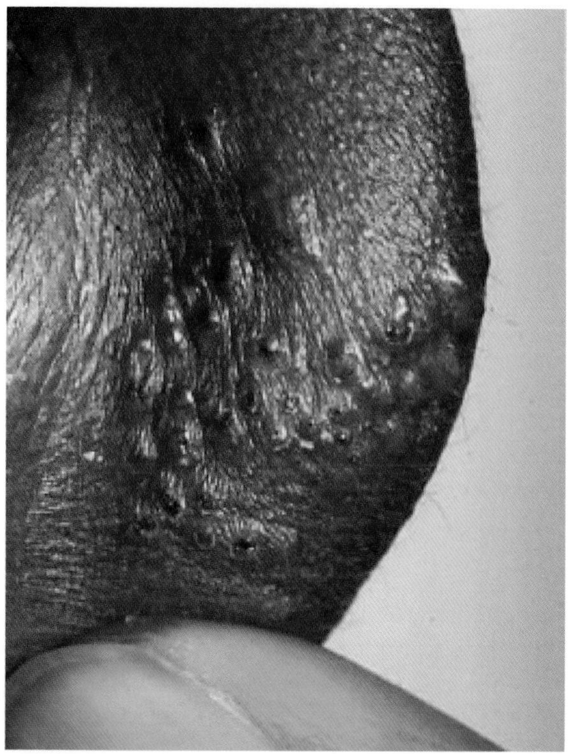

Figure 14.3 Herpes simplex vesicles on posterior pinna.

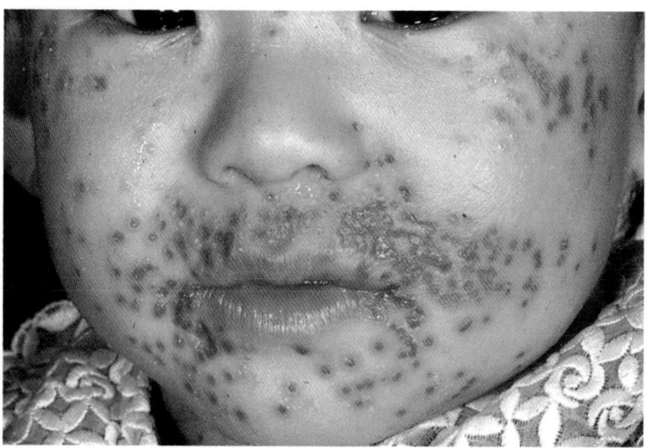

Figure 14.4 Eczema herpeticum.

for frequent reactivation can be given as 400 mg once or twice daily. Higher doses are needed in immunocompromised patients. Valaciclovir (HSV 500 mg twice daily for 5 days, VZV 1 g three times daily for 7 days) and famciclovir (genital HSV 250 mg three times daily for 7 days, VZV 750 mg daily for 7 days) are alternatives that are taken less frequently. Brisk inflammatory responses to genital HSV can be seen in patients with HIV whose immune system is reconstituting once they start their HAART (highly active antiretroviral therapy) – the so-called *immune reconstitution inflammatory syndrome* (IRIS). Clinically, this is seen as deteriorating signs and symptoms of HSV disease and may warrant aggressive treatment of the HSV and occasionally a reduction in the HAART medication.

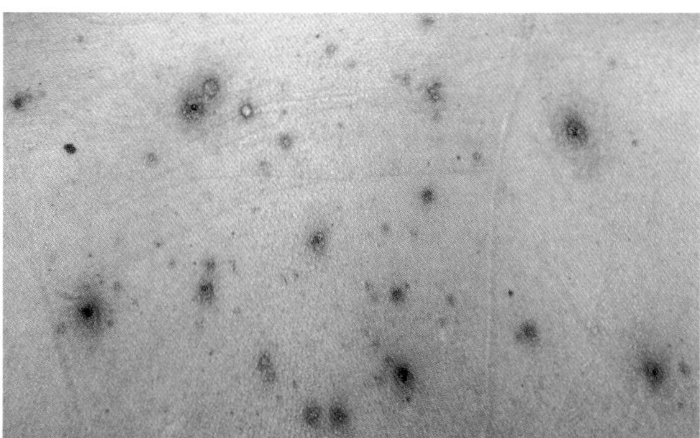

Figure 14.5 Varicella zoster virus chicken pox infection in an adult.

Varicella zoster virus

VZV is a herpes virus that causes chicken pox (the primary illness), which is characterised by a prodromal illness for about 2 days followed by crops of papular-vesicular lesions (Figure 14.5) that eventually crust over and heal. Subsequently shingles (reactivation) may occur as the virus remains latent in the sensory nerve ganglia (Box 14.2). The thoracic nerves are most commonly affected. In shingles, pain, fever and malaise may precede the rash which is characterised usually by its dermatomal distribution (Figure 14.6); however, adjacent dermatomes may be affected (Figure 14.7). Erythematous papules usually precede vesicles which develop over several days, crusting as they resolve, often with secondary bacterial colonisation. Occasionally, peripheral motor neuropathy can result and a proportion of patients develop severe chronic postherpetic neuralgia. Skin lesions of shingles and nasopharyngeal secretions can transmit chicken pox to susceptible individuals.

Box 14.2 **Shingles – points to note**

- Trigeminal shingles may affect.
  - the ophthalmic nerve (causing severe conjunctivitis).
  - the maxillary nerve (causing vesicles on the uvula or tonsils).
  - the mandibular nerve (causing vesicles on the floor of the mouth and on the tongue) (Figure 14.8).
- Shingles affecting the facial nerve presents with lesions in the external auditory canal (Ramsay Hunt syndrome).
- Disseminated shingles may present with widespread cutaneous and visceral lesions.
- In the context of HIV, shingles lesions may be multi-dermatomal, extensive and haemorrhagic.

Patients ideally should receive high-dose aciclovir (800 mg five times daily for 7 days) within 72 h of the onset of the eruption. If the eye is affected or there is nerve compression, then intravenous aciclovir (5 mg/kg every 8 h for 5 days) should be considered and patients may require systemic steroids (prednisolone 40–60 mg daily) to prevent nerve paralysis in severe cases. Greasy emollient should be applied to the affected skin regularly to prevent cracking and reduce pain as lesions heal. Topical antibiotic ointments can be used to treat secondary bacterial infections (mupirocin, fusidic acid and polymyxin). Post-herpetic neuralgia may respond to gabapentin or carbamazepine. Preliminary studies using a topical 8% capsaicin patch applied for 1 h reduced pain by >30% in 40% of shingles patients for up to 8 weeks.

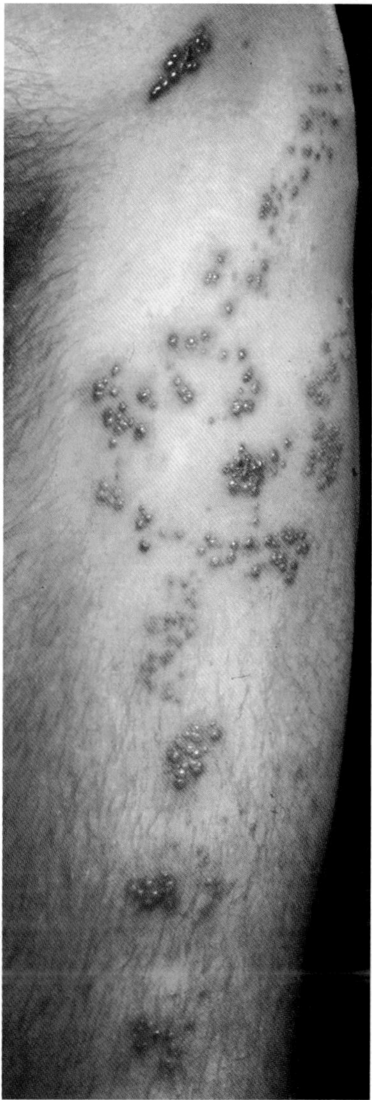

Figure 14.6 Herpes zoster in a dermatome (shingles).

Pityriasis rosea (PR) has been thought recently to be triggered by an upper respiratory tract infection with human herpes virus type 6 or 7. The evidence for this is not conclusive but for the ease of categorisation PR is described here. PR classically presents with an initial single annular erythematous patch with a collarette of scale – the herald patch (Figure 14.9a), so called because it heralds the onset of the rest of the rash within 5–8 days, which consists of multiple smaller scaly patches on the trunk (Figure 14.9b) and upper arms and thighs (old-fashioned bathing suit distribution). On the back, the lesions may follow the angle of the ribs in a 'Christmas tree pattern'. Patients may have experienced corysal symptoms before the onset of the rash as part of the viral illness. Patients mainly present in spring and autumn and there may be clustering

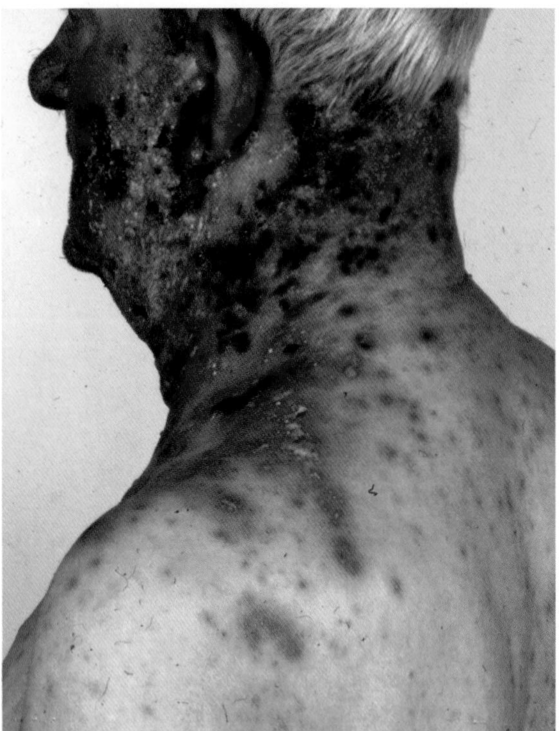

Figure 14.7 Multidermatomal varicella zoster virus (shingles).

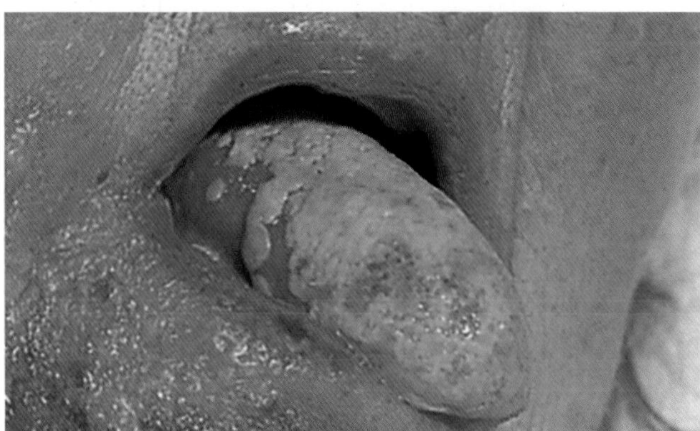

Figure 14.8 Mandibular nerve zoster.

of cases. The rash settles spontaneously over about 4–6 weeks, but a mild topical steroid and emollient can be given if the rash if pruritic or inflammatory.

Poxviruses

The poxviruses are large DNA viruses, with a predilection for the epidermis. Variola (smallpox), once a disease with high mortality, has been eliminated (last reported case of smallpox occurred in Somalia in 1977) by vaccination with modified vaccinia (cowpox) virus. Vaccination of the general population is no longer required due to the eradication of the virus, but some military and front-line medical personnel are being vaccinated due to the theoretical threat of biological attack with smallpox.

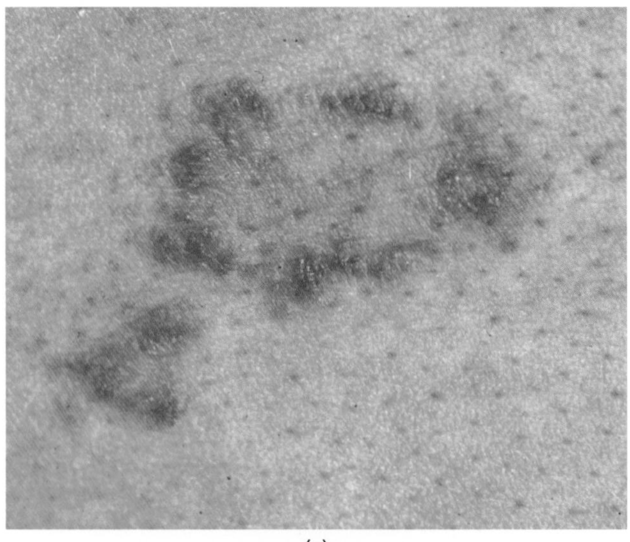

(a)

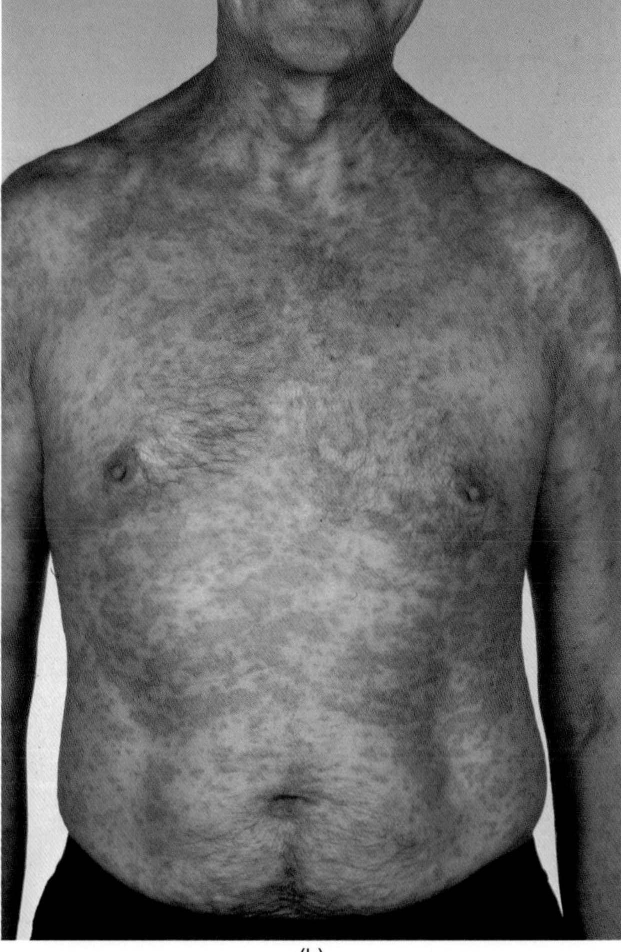

(b)

Figure 14.9 (a) Herald patch of pityriasis rosea. (b) Rash of pityriasis rosea.

Molluscum contagiosum

The commonest poxvirus skin infection is usually acquired in childhood. It is highly contagious and is spread by direct contact often within families or schools. The incubation period is

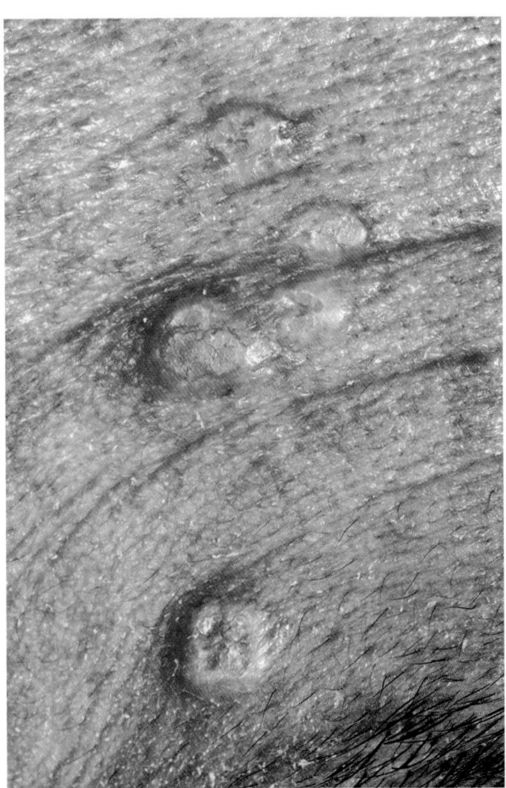

Figure 14.10 Molluscum contagiosum.

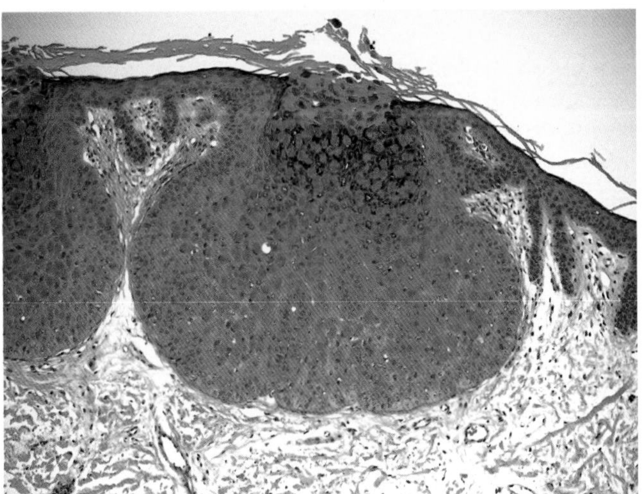

Figure 14.11 Histology showing molluscum bodies.

variable, between 14 days and 6 months. In adults florid molluscum may be an indication of underlying immunodeficiency such as HIV. Flesh-coloured, umbilicated papules are characteristic (Figures 14.10 and 14.11). Large solitary lesions (giant molluscus) and infected lesions may look atypical. Resolving lesions may be surrounded by a small patch of inflammation; this is usually a sign that the lesions may soon resolve because of activation of the immune system.

Parents may be keen for their children with molluscum to be treated. However, most lesions will resolve spontaneously, leaving no marks on the skin. Therefore, painful and scarring treatments should be avoided if possible. Topical hydrogen peroxide (Crystacide) and cryotherapy can be used to cause local inflammation and speed up resolution in non-cosmetically vulnerable sites. Daily 5% imiquimod cream can be used in immunocompromised patients not responding to destructive methods.

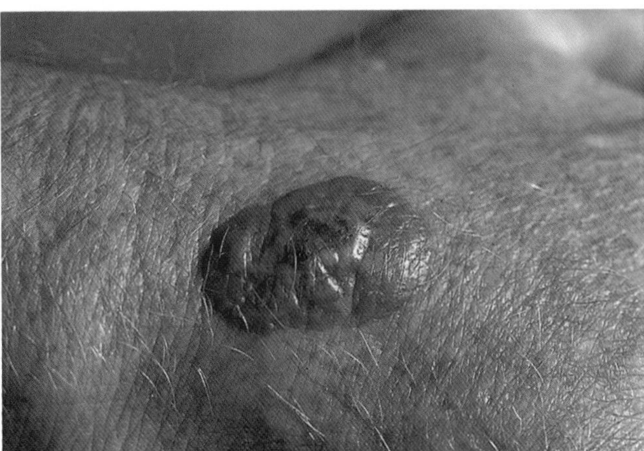

Figure 14.12 Orf.

Orf is usually recognised in rural areas. It is seen mainly in early spring as a result of contact with infected lambs. A single papule or group of lesions develops on the fingers or hands with purple papules developing into bullae (Figure 14.12). These rupture to leave annular lesions 1–3 cm in diameter with a necrotic centre and surrounding inflammation. The incubation period is a few days and the lesions last 2–3 weeks with spontaneous healing. Associated erythema multiforme and widespread rashes are occasionally seen. Lifelong immunity does not result from infections.

Wart viruses

More than 100 different subtypes of HPV have currently been identified. HPV subtypes 6 and 11 are responsible for the majority of genital warts and subtypes 16/18 with the development of cervical/anal/vulval/vaginal/oral carcinomas. This discovery led to the production of two vaccines against HPV (Cervarix against 16, 18 and Gardasil against 6, 11, 16, 18) which are administered in three doses mainly to teenage girls. It is thought, however, that HPV infection alone does not cause malignant transformation and identified cofactors include smoking, UV light, folate deficiency and immunosuppression. Vaccinated women should still have regular cervical smears.

Warts are classified as anogenital/mucosal, non-genital cutaneous and epidermodysplasia verruciformis (EV). The latter is a rare condition associated with a defect of specific immunity to wart virus. Genital HPV infections are also described as symptomatic (latent, i.e. viral DNA detected), subclinical (detected with acetic acid under magnification) or clinical (warts easily seen).

HPV only infects humans and is spread by direct contact, usually through a small break in the skin/mucous membrane. Viral warts can have a varied clinical appearance from filiform (Figure 14.13) to hyperkaratotic periungal (Figure 14.14). HPV can remain viable

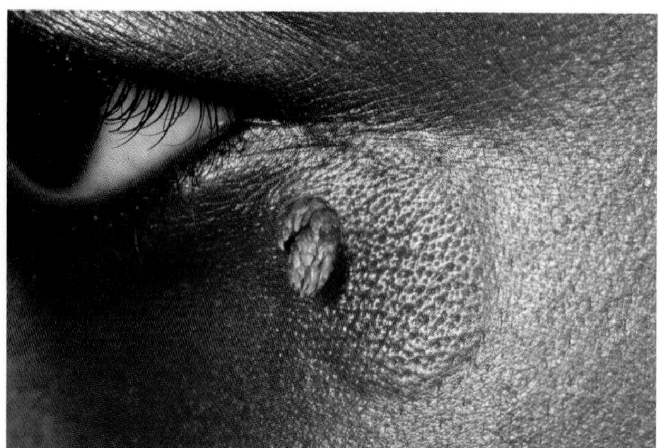

Figure 14.13 Filiform HPV wart.

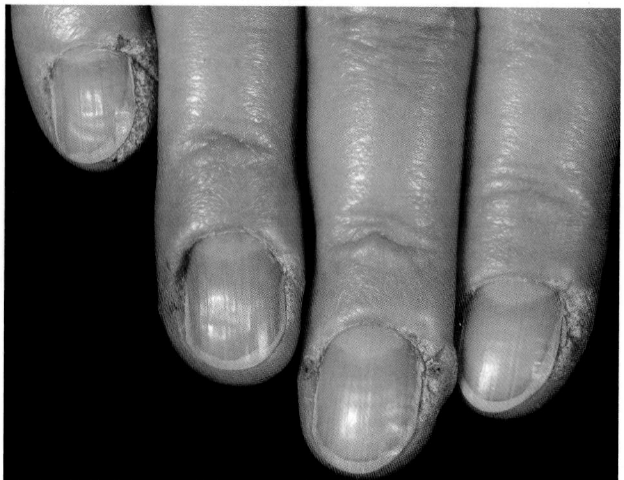

Figure 14.14 Periungal hyperkeratotic HPV warts.

in the environment at low temperatures for prolonged periods and therefore be contracted from contact with inanimate objects (changing room floors). The basal keratinocytes become infected, causing epidermal hyperplasia seen clinically as an exophytic warty lesion. Plantar warts (veruccae) form painful plaques (mosaic) containing black 'dots' (Figure 14.15) that represent thrombosed capillaries.

Cutaneous HPV lesions can undergo malignant transformation, particularly in individuals who are immunosuppressed by HIV or medication. If skin lesions suddenly increase in size or are painful then transformation to squamous cell carcinoma should be suspected. Acitretin is given to some transplant recipients to try to reduce the rate of cutaneous malignant transformation.

Treatment

Warts commonly occur in childhood and usually resolve spontaneously. There are however numerous treatment options available (indicating that not all warts respond to a particular treatment). Warts are generally slow to clear but studies show 70% will resolve following 4 months of salicylic acid applied once daily. Salicylic and lactic acids in various formulations can be

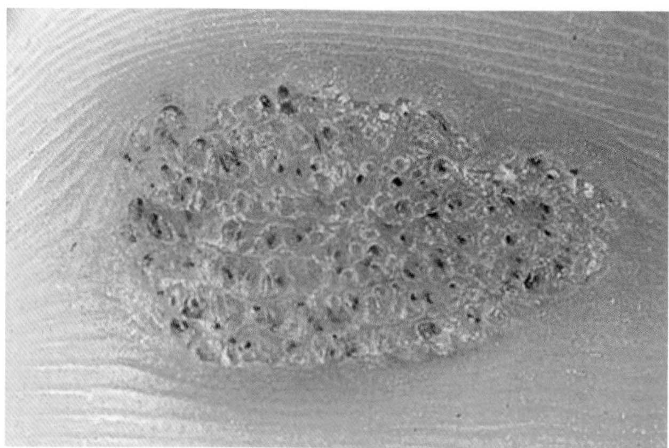

Figure 14.15 Plantar wart (verucca).

purchased over the counter and high percentages can be prescribed. Gels/ointments/paints/lotions should be applied daily after paring-down the wart surface.

Duct tape (used by builders) has been shown to be effective at treating HPV: 85% of warts resolved following 2 months of treatment with duct tape (which was cut to size, applied to the wart and renewed weekly).

For large/painful/recalcitrant warts other measures may be considered.

Liquid nitrogen is effective but has to be stored in special containers and replaced frequently. It can be applied with cotton wool or discharged from a special spray with a focused nozzle. Freezing is continued until a rim of frozen tissue forms around the wart, this is then repeated three times with thawing in-between cycles. Cryotherapy is accompanied by a burning sensation or pain and is not usually tolerated in young children. Subsequent pigment changes, blistering and even scarring may occur. Carbon dioxide is more readily available and can be transported in cylinders that produce solid carbon dioxide 'snow'. The temperature (about −64 °C) is not as low as that of liquid nitrogen (−196 °C).

Diathermy loop cautery under local anaesthetic is effective for perianal warts. Curettage and cautery for very large warts under local anaesthetic is often used to debulk the lesions prior to other measures.

Podophyllin derived from Mayapple is available in various formulations including ointment (Posalfilin®) for plantar warts (daily) and solution/cream (weekly) for genital warts (Warticon® and Condyline®). Podophyllin 15% paint should only be applied to warts by a trained practitioner as it can cause chemical burns. It should not be used on large numbers of warts simultaneously because of toxicity and must never be used in pregnancy.

Immune response modifier Imiquimod® 5% cream is licensed for the treatment of genital warts. It stimulates cytokine production at the site of application, which is carried out three times per week. Treatment should continue until the warts resolve or up to a maximum of 16 weeks. Local irritation and inflammation can be severe, especially on mucosal surfaces. Imiquimod 5% can also be used to treat cutaneous warts but daily application is usually required under occlusion to aid penetration and efficacy.

Immunotherapy with the contact sensitiser diphencyprone (DPC) can also be effective. Following sensitisation to DPC increasing concentrations are painted onto the warts to cause a local inflammatory response. At 6 months, 60% complete cure rates are reported in patients with previously highly recalcitrant warts.

Other treatments include carbon dioxide laser vaporisation, 5-fluorouracil, intralesional bleomycin and interferon alpha, oral cimetidine and oral isotretinoin.

Viral diseases with rashes

Many childhood viral illnesses have become less common because of increased availability of effective vaccines (Box 14.3). However, these vaccines are not universally available or accepted by parents, leading to regional outbreaks among susceptible populations. Approximately 880 000 deaths from measles occur worldwide each year. Recently, there has been a marked resurgence of measles in parts of the UK following a decline in take-up of MMR (measles/mumps/rubella) vaccinations. Measles is probably the best-known example of a viral exanthema – a widespread reactive cutaneous eruption that usually results from RNA viruses.

Box 14.3 **Viral diseases with rashes**

- Measles.
- Rubella.
- Infectious mononucleosis.
- Erythema infectiosum.
- Roseola infantum.
- Gianotti–Crosti syndrome.
- Hand, foot and mouth disease.
- Primary HIV infection.

Measles usually affects children under the age of 5 years and is highly contagious. The incubation period is 7–14 days. Prodromal symptoms include fever, malaise, upper respiratory symptoms, conjunctivitis and photophobia. Children are miserable and look unwell. Initially, Koplik's spots (white spots with surrounding erythema) (Figure 14.16) appear on the oral mucosa and then within 2 days a macular rash appears, initially behind the ears and on the face and trunk, and then on the limbs (Figure 14.17). Papules form and coalesce and may be haemorrhagic or vesicular, which fade to leave brown patches. Rarely encephalitis, otitis media and bronchopneumonia may complicate the infection. Reliable rapid diagnostic testing can be undertaken using oral fluid samples to detect measles virus RNA using real-time RT-PCR. Urine and serology tests are also available. There is no specific treatment for measles except supportive care; however, some studies have shown that vitamin A supplementation during the acute illness can reduce morbidity/mortality. Parents should be encouraged to get their children vaccinated with two doses of live-attenuated MMR.

Rubella affects children and young adults who may display prodromal fever, malaise and upper respiratory tract symptoms. The incubation period is 14–21 days. First signs of the disease

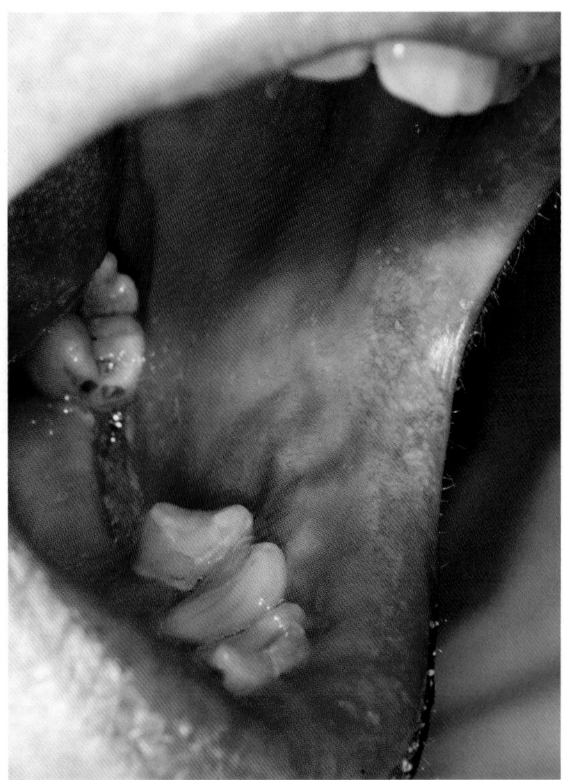

Figure 14.16 Koplick's spots in measles.

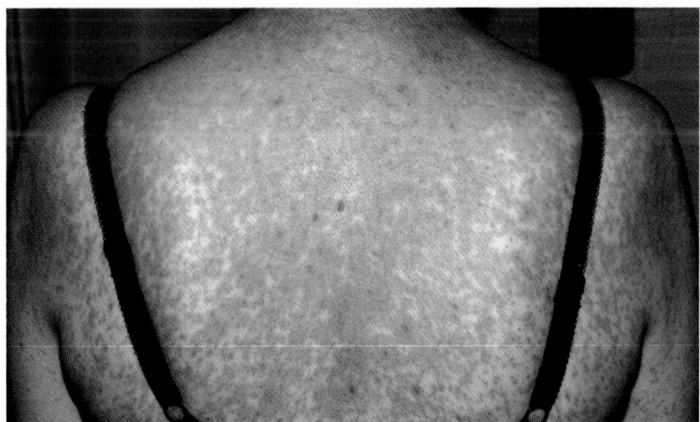

Figure 14.17 Measles rash.

include erythema of the soft palate and lymphadenopathy. Later, pink macules appear on the face, spreading to trunk and limbs over 1–2 days (Figure 14.18). The rash clears over 1–2 days (occasionally no rash develops). Infection during pregnancy can cause congenital defects. The risk is highest in the first trimester. The acute diagnosis is usually clinical with confirmation from convalescent serum antibody titres. Prevention through immunisation of school-aged girls is highly effective.

Erythema infectiosum (fifth disease) is caused by parvovirus B19, which mainly affects children aged 2–10 years. The incubation period is 5–20 days. The disease manifests as a prodrome of mild fever before the onset of a hot erythematous eruption on the cheeks – hence the 'slapped cheek syndrome'. Over 2–4 days

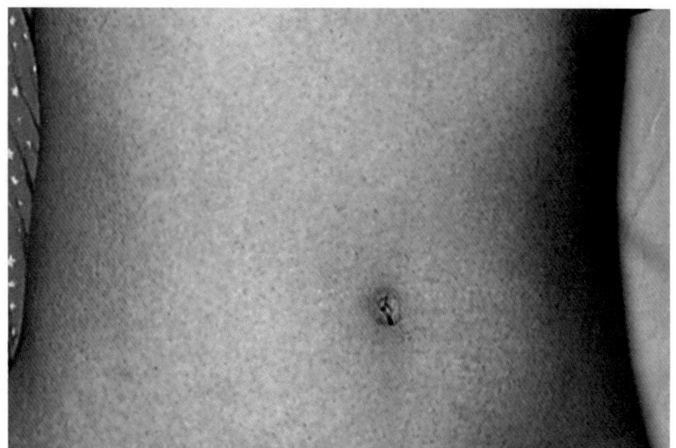

Figure 14.18 Rubella.

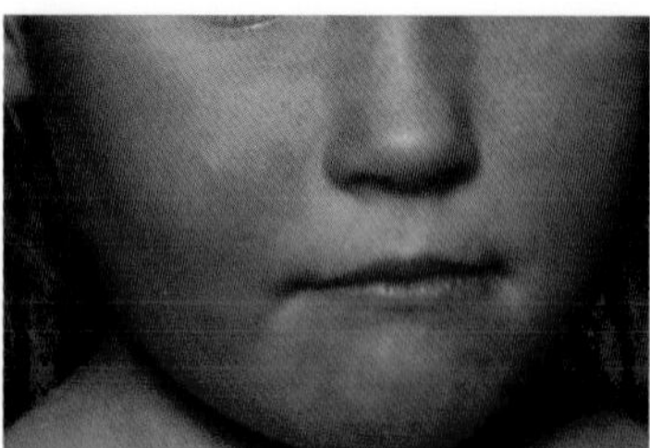

Figure 14.19 Erythema infectiosum.

a maculopapular eruption develops on the limbs and trunk (Figure 14.19), which can extend to the hands, feet and mucous membranes, and then fades over 1–2 weeks. The diagnosis can be confirmed by serology for parvovirus B19-specific IgM antibody. Complications include thrombocytopenia, arthropathy and foetal abnormalities if acquired in utero.

Roseola infantum (*sixth disease*) is caused by human herpesvirus type 6 (HHV6). This mainly affects infants below 2 years of age. The incubation period is 10–15 days. The onset of a rose-pink maculopapular rash appearing on the neck and trunk usually follows a few days of fever. The rash can spread to the limbs before clearing over 1–2 days. The diagnosis is made on clinical ground; however, HHV6 virus can be isolated from the blood or serology to detect antibody responses if necessary. Young infants may develop febrile convulsions. Care is supportive.

Gianotti–Crosti syndrome is the term given to a papular viral exanthem caused by infections due to Epstein–Barr virus (EBV) and hepatitis B. Children under the age of 14 years are most commonly affected. The incubation period is unknown; however, children generally present with malaise, lymphadenopathy and an acral eruption. Initially the rash consists of erythematous papules on the face, neck, limbs, buttocks, palms and soles (Figure 14.20). The rash is usually itchy and may become purpuric before it slowly settles over 2–6 weeks. Viral-specific serology can be requested. Rarely lymphadenopathy and hepatomegaly can persist for many months. The symptoms from the exanthem can be relieved with a topical steroid.

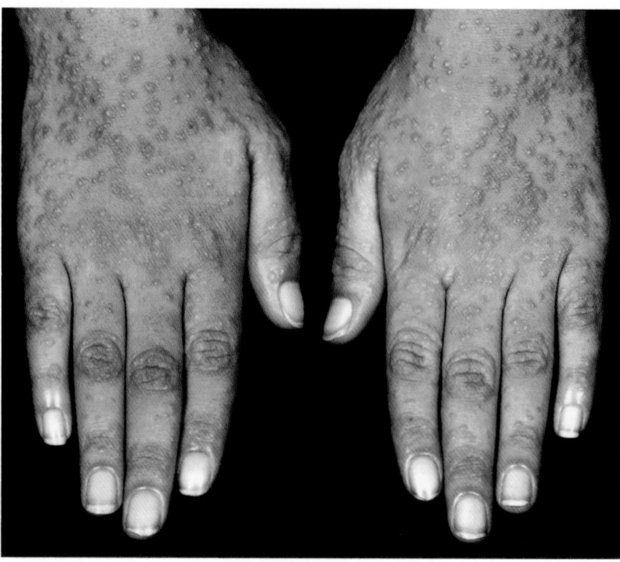

Figure 14.20 Gianotti–Crosti syndrome.

Hand, foot and mouth disease, as the name suggests, is an infection causing lesions on the hands/feet and in the mouth. It is most commonly associated with Coxsackievirus A and can affect children and adults. The virus is highly contagious with a short incubation period of 3–6 days. Young children in particular present with fever, headache and malaise alongside the rash. The characteristic rash consists of intense erythema surrounding yellow-grey vesicles 1–1.5 mm in diameter on palms/soles and lips (Figure 14.21). Rarely, a more generalised eruption develops.

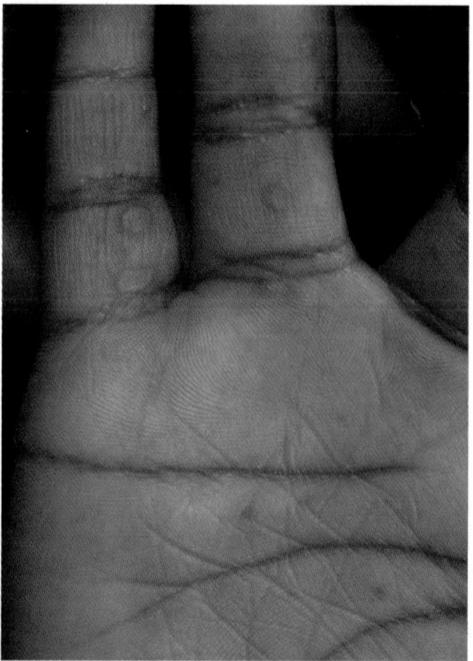

Figure 14.21 Hand, foot and mouth disease.

The rash and symptoms settle rapidly over 3–5 days. Coxsackie A (usually A16) virus can be rapidly isolated from lesions using viral swabs or be identified in the stools. Serology for viral-specific antibody can also be requested. Rarely, erythema multiforme can also occur.

Further reading

Biluk EJ. *Microbiology Cases Studies: Viral and Fungal Diseases of the Skin and Wounds*, Kindle Edition, 2011.

Straus EG and Strauss JH. *Viruses and Human Disease*, 2nd Edition, Academic Press, California, 2007.

CHAPTER 15

HIV and the Skin

Rachael Morris-Jones

Dermatology Department, Kings College Hospital, London, UK

OVERVIEW

- HIV infection leads to a progressive fall in the CD4 count with resultant immunosuppression and, if untreated, eventually AIDS.
- A widespread maculopapular rash occurs in 50% of patients during primary HIV infection.
- Cutaneous eruptions in the context of HIV are common, atypical and frequently severe.
- Common skin complaints associated with HIV include nodular prurigo, seborrhoeic dermatitis and pruritic papular eruption.
- Adverse drug eruptions are common in HIV patients, from mild toxic erythema to severe life-threatening toxic epidermal necrolysis.
- Skin conditions often improve as the immune system is restored with antiretroviral therapy.
- As the immune system reconstitutes there may be a brisk inflammatory response to high levels of antigen building up in chronic infections.

Introduction

The human immunodeficiency virus (HIV) is the cause of the acquired immune deficiency syndrome (AIDS). Worldwide, 34 million children and adults are currently living with HIV according to current WHO (World Health Organization) statistics (2013). 54% of those with HIV eligible for antiretroviral therapy have access to it. As yet there is no effective vaccine against HIV. Methods for reduced transmission of HIV include condoms, voluntary male circumcision, prevention of mother-to-child transmission, sterile injection equipment, screening blood products and pre-exposure prophylaxis for serodiscordant couples. Trials of pre-exposure prophylaxis with tenofovir disoproxil fumarate (TDF) 300 mg alone or with emtricitabine 200 mg have shown to reduce the risk of acquiring HIV by 60–90% depending on adherence.

HIV is an RNA retrovirus that replicates itself by reverse transcriptase to produce a DNA copy; this then becomes incorporated into the host DNA where further replication occurs. HIV persists in the body within the host's immune cells – the CD4 lymphocytes and monocytes – thereby directly weakening the host's immune system. Initially, the virus remains latent for an average of 10 years before causing profound immunosuppression. The extent to which an individual's immune system is affected by HIV is measured through the CD4 cell count and the HIV viral load. AIDS is defined as a CD4 count of less than 200 cells/μl, or HIV associated with any one of 26 (mainly opportunistic infections) conditions.

Patients with low CD4 counts who are profoundly immunosuppressed tend to have more frequent and more severe skin disorders. Common cutaneous diseases such as psoriasis, eczema, seborrhoeic dermatitis (SD) and acne tend to be more severe, have atypical features and are often resistant to conventional treatments. The spectrum of cutaneous manifestations in HIV has changed over the past decade because of the use of highly active anti-retroviral therapy (HAART). This treatment, however, is only available to 54% of individuals who need it and despite treatment 70% of patients still suffer from HIV-related skin problems with a high incidence of adverse drug rashes. In addition, patients taking HAART can develop problems when their immune system is reconstituted – the so-called immune reconstitution inflammatory syndrome (IRIS). In IRIS, the brisk inflammatory response relates to the immune system 'waking-up' to the presence of antigen previously unrecognised such as genital herpes simplex virus (HSV).

In general, HIV/AIDS should be considered in any patient with a florid or atypical inflammatory skin disease that is resistant to treatment or who has severe and extensive infection of the skin. Because of the atypical nature of cutaneous manifestations in HIV medical practitioners should have a low threshold for performing a skin biopsy for histology and culture (Box 15.1). Many modern heath

Box 15.1 **HIV and the skin**

- Skin disorders affect 80% of HIV patients.
- Fifty percent develop a rash during the primary HIV infection so-called 'seroconversion'.
- Severity of skin disorders usually increases with decreasing CD4 counts.
- Cutaneous presentations are frequently atypical.
- Consider taking a skin biopsy for histology and culture in any HIV patient with a rash.
- Management of skin diseases can be difficult; HAART is usually beneficial.
- Patients have a high risk of developing adverse drug reactions.

ABC of Dermatology, Sixth Edition. Edited by Rachael Morris-Jones.

care systems are introducing HIV screening for all patients newly registering at primary care facilities in the community or any patient who attends their local hospital. Diagnosing and treating those with HIV early on in the disease will result in less morbidity, less premature mortality and reduced onwards transmission and ultimately be cost-effective.

Stages of HIV

Primary HIV infection

Eighty percent of individuals have acute signs and symptoms associated with their primary HIV infection – the so-called 'seroconversion illness'. The incubation period is 2–6 weeks. Symptoms include fever, malaise, headache, nausea, vomiting and diarrhoea. Clinical signs include cervical lymphadenopathy, pharyngitis, weight loss and rash. The skin eruption associated with primary HIV infection is present in 50% of patients and consists of a maculopapular rash mainly on the face, neck and trunk lasting 2–3 weeks (Figure 15.1). Some patients develop a papulovesicular eruption or erosions in the mouth rather than a classic viral exanthem. During seroconversion abnormalities in the full blood count (FBC) may be seen (leukopenia, lymphopenia, thrombocytopenia, low haemoglobin) and diagnostically HIV RNA may be detected in the plasma.

Early stages

Within 1–2 months of the primary infection, 50% of patients will have detectable antibodies to HIV. The proportion of CD4 lymphocytes variably decreases and this is associated with an increased frequency and severity of skin disorders. Patients may experience worsening of premorbid skin complaints such as psoriasis or present *de novo* with sudden florid skin disease such as SD. Adverse drug reactions are more frequent and often severe.

Late-stage HIV infection

As the patient's immune system becomes increasingly suppressed and the CD4 count falls below 200 cells/μl he or she is classified as having AIDS. Patients with AIDS may present with severe widespread dermatoses including SD, crusted scabies, multidermatomal varicella zoster virus, Kaposi's sarcoma, widespread fungal/yeast infections, bacillary angiomatosis (BA) and eosinophilic folliculitis (EF). These conditions are described in more detail below.

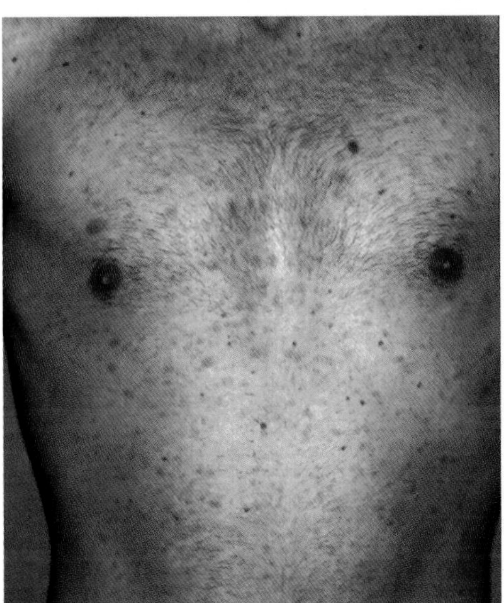

Figure 15.1 Primary HIV infection: seroconversion rash.

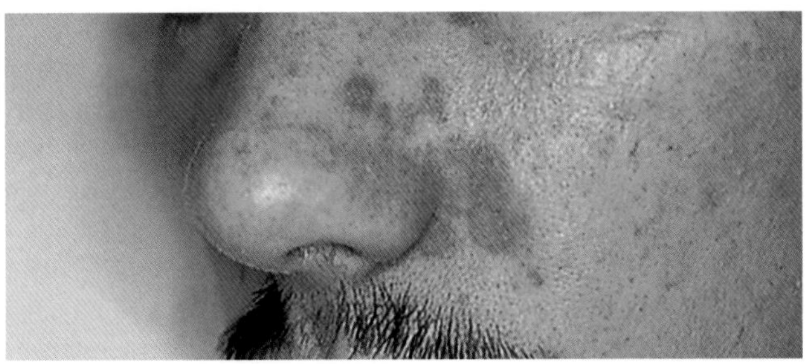

Figure 15.2 Seborrhoeic dermatitis.

Skin disorders in HIV

Seborrhoeic dermatitis

Fifty percent of HIV patients develop SD compared to 1–3% of the general population. SD may be one of the first indicators of HIV infection. It is interesting to note that as the immune system becomes increasingly suppressed by HIV, there is a higher incidence of allergic-type reactions. SD is an allergic contact dermatitis to the yeast *Malassezia furfur*, which is a normal skin commensal. SD classically affects the scalp, eyebrows, nasal creases, moustache and anterior chest. Adherent greasy scales cover underlying inflammatory eczema which may be very itchy (Figure 15.2). Management is aimed at reducing the numbers of yeast on the skin and suppressing the eczema. Ketoconazole shampoo can be used to wash the body and scalp once/twice weekly to reduce yeast carriage. Twice-daily topical steroids (±miconazole) can be used to control the dermatitis. In refractory cases systemic imidazoles such as itraconazole 200 mg daily for 1–2 weeks can be effective. However, if the patient's immune system reconstitutes with HAART, SD usually abates (Box 15.2).

Box 15.2 **Skin disorders in HIV/AIDS**

- Seborrhoeic eczema (severe)
- Psoriasis (severe)
- Fungal infections (extensive, recurrent)
- Bacterial infections
- Viral infections
- Kaposi's sarcoma (epidemic)
- Nodular prurigo
- Frequent adverse drug reactions (often severe)
- Oral hairy leukoplakia.

Psoriasis

It is estimated that 5% of HIV patients develop psoriasis and of those 50% suffer from psoriatic arthropathy. The pathophysiology of psoriasis is complex; however, there is a general consensus that it is a T-cell mediated autoimmune disease. The paradox in HIV is that immune dysregulation of T-cells goes hand in hand with severe, extensive and refractory psoriasis, indicating that there are likely to be other cells involved in the development of psoriasis such as Th17. A dermatology specialist is usually needed to manage patients with HIV and severe psoriasis. Conventional immunosuppressive treatments such as ciclosporin and methotrexate can be used with care. Drug interactions need to be considered with ciclosporin. PUVA (psoralen plus ultraviolet A) can be very useful at controlling extensive thick plaques, particularly in patients with pigmented skin.

Eosinophilic folliculitis

EF is an intensely pruritic condition of unknown aetiology that tends to occur when the CD4 count falls below 250 cells/μl. Speculation that the causative agent is *Demodex*, a commensal skin mite that lives in the perifollicular region, is based on responses to antiparasitic treatments including permethrin and ivermectin. Other studies suggest an autoimmune process with responses against the sebocytes/sebum. Clinically, patients present with multiple discrete, erythematous, perifollicular papules and pustules affecting the face and trunk (Figure 15.3) that can look like acne (but no comedones are seen). Differential diagnoses include *Staphylococcus* or *Pityrosporum* folliculitis and acne. Microbiological swabs are negative in EF. Peripheral eosinophilia and raised IgE may be noted. HAART therapy can help if the CD4 count rises above 250 cells/μl. UVB phototherapy can be very effective. Topical corticosteroids may reduce pruritus. Systemic indomethacin, minocycline and itraconazole have also been used.

Nodular prurigo

Non-specific pruritus is common in HIV patients, 30% developing itchy nodular lesions on the skin, called *nodular prurigo*. The cause is unknown. Classically, small red papules develop on the trunk and limbs, which itch intensely, and through scratching chronic nodules form (Figure 15.4). Nodular prurigo can be very aggravating and persistent. Relief from pruritus may be gained by regular applications of emollients. Potent topical steroids applied daily under occlusion of wraps or body suits may flatten lesions and relieve itching. UVB phototherapy and amitriptyline can also be used.

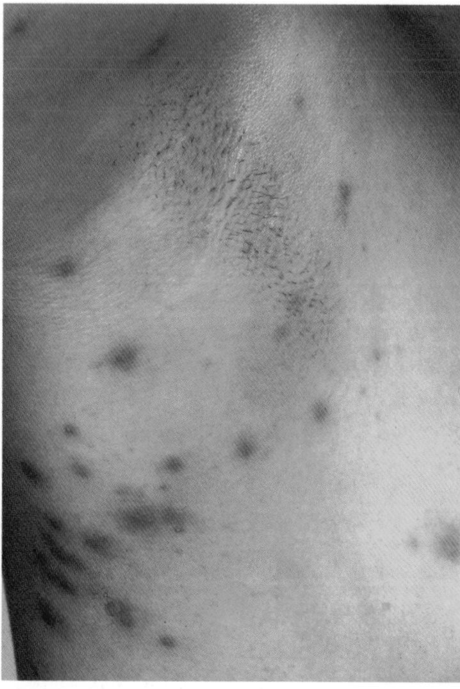

Figure 15.3 Eosinophilic folliculitis.

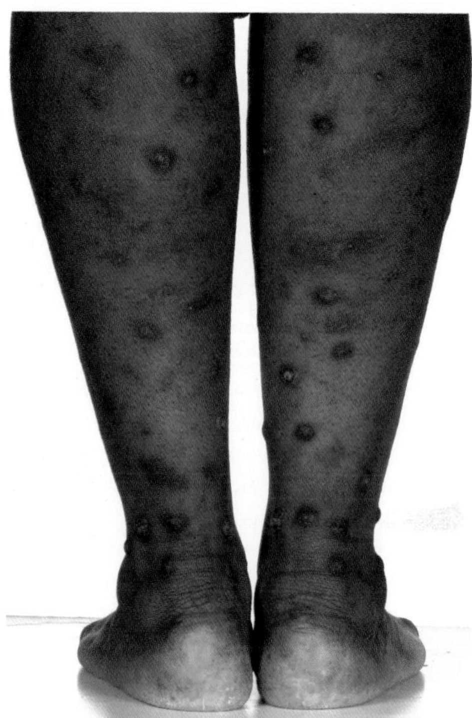

Figure 15.4 Nodular prurigo.

Infections

Fungal infections

Superficial dermatophyte and yeast infections are frequently more extensive in HIV patients with a higher incidence of dissemination systemically. Deep fungal infections that are not normally seen in healthy individuals occur in AIDS patients as opportunistic infections. *Cryptococcus neoformans* and *Histoplasma capsulatum* may cause inflammatory papular and necrotic lesions, particularly in the later stages of the disease.

Candidiasis is common and often associated with secondary bacterial infections. The oral mucosa can be extensively infected with *Candida albicans* that spreads to the pharynx and oesophagus. Clinically, there are extensive white plaques on a background of erythema. Candidiasis of the skin has a predilection for the flexures where classically there is confluent erythema with peripheral satellite lesions (Figure 15.5). Patients may complain of cutaneous discomfort and itching and oral ulceration and dysphagia (Figure 15.6). Women with HIV can develop severe vulvovaginitis caused by chronic candidiasis.

Bacterial infections

Impetigo caused by *Staphylococcus aureus* may be severe with large bullous lesions associated with strains producing exfoliative toxins

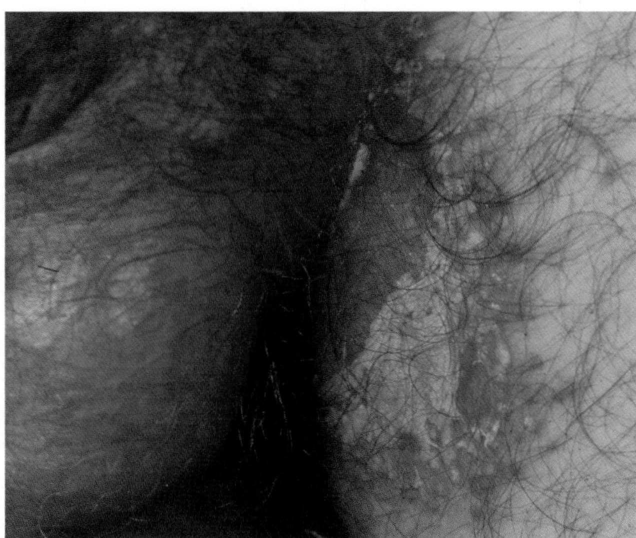

Figure 15.5 Flexural *Candida* infection.

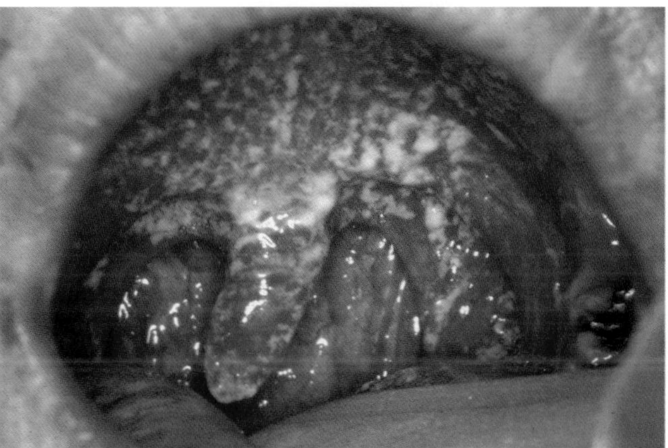

Figure 15.6 Pseudomembranous *Candida*.

A/B. Erythrasma (*Corynebacterium*) may be persistent and recurrent in the flexural areas and are often mistaken for a superficial fungal infection.

Bartonella henselae and Bartonella quintana infections can cause BA in AIDS patients, who present with multiple small haemangioma-like papules on the skin and mucous membranes. Skin lesions develop slowly over several weeks (Figure 15.7), and visceral organs may also be affected – most commonly, the liver. Differential diagnosis usually includes Kaposi's sarcoma. Blood cultures are usually diagnostic but the laboratory must be alerted to the possibility of *Bartonella* as blood cultures must be incubated for 3 weeks under specific conditions. Skin biopsy for histology is usually diagnostic. *Bartonella* are highly sensitive to macrolide antibiotics which are bacteriostatic and therefore an anti-angiogenic effect through down-regulation of endothelial cells has been postulated as the mechanism of action in BA. The treatment of choice is erythromycin 500 mg qds for up to 12 weeks. Azithromycin 500 mg on the first day and then 250 mg daily for 5 days is also highly effective.

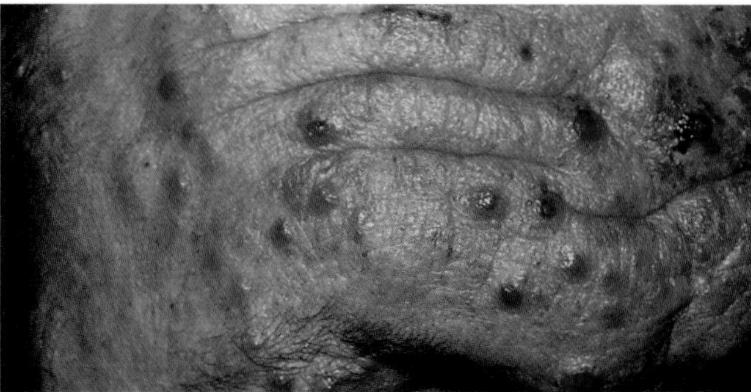

Figure 15.7 Bacillary angiomatosis.

Syphilis

Approximately 12 million new cases of syphilis infection are reported each year according to the WHO, with a notable resurgence in many parts of the world where the incidence was previously low. Between 20% and 70% of patients in the United States and Europe are co-infected with HIV and syphilis simultaneously. Syphilis is caused by the spiral bacterium (spirochaete) *Treponema pallidum*. Syphilis is the great mimicker of other diseases and in the context of HIV infection presentations may be atypical.

Classically, a painless genital ulcer develops 3–4 weeks after transmission via sexual intercourse. Secondary syphilis presents with a rash, fever, arthralgia and lymphadenopathy 4–8 weeks after the initial infection. The rash is usually asymptomatic and characteristically affects the trunk, palms and soles. Early lesions are usually annular erythematous macules that fade to a greyish brown (Figure 15.8). Serological testing for syphilis should be performed to confirm the diagnosis. Primary/secondary syphilis should be treated with a single dose of intramuscular benzathine penicillin 2.4 megaunits, or intramuscular procaine penicillin 600 000 units daily for 10 days. Latent syphilis requires prolonged treatment.

Mycobacteria may produce widespread cutaneous and systemic lesions. Varieties of mycobacteria that do not normally infect the skin may cause persistent necrotic papules or ulcers.

Viral infections

Herpesviruses

Herpesvirus types 1, 2 and 3 including herpes simplex (oral/genital) and herpes zoster infections may be unusually extensive, with large individual lesions in patients with HIV. Herpes zoster (shingles) classically spreads to involve adjacent dermatomes. Occasionally, persistent ulcerated lesions are seen with resultant squamous cell carcinoma, which can arise in any chronic ulcer. HSV infections may be particularly severe and recurrent such that patients require secondary long-term prophylaxis. In the context of HAART, an IRIS can occur in association with genital HSV with florid debilitating inflammatory reactions leading to extensive and persistent painful ulceration (Figure 15.9).

Epstein–Barr virus (*EBV*) is human herpesvirus type 4. Ninety percent of adults have evidence of past infection with EBV which remains latent in the body in B cells. In 30–50% of AIDS patients, EBV enters a replicative phase leading to oral hairy leukoplakia (OHL). OHL is characterised by overgrowth of epithelial plaques on

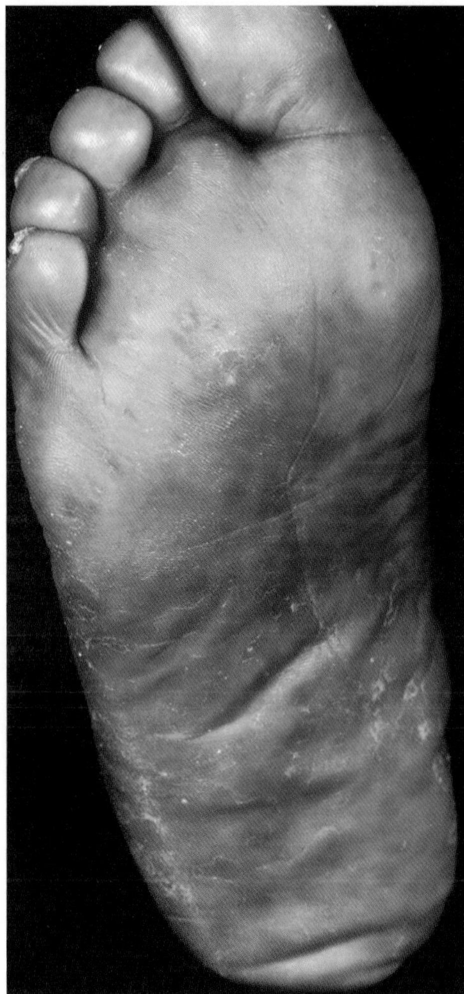

Figure 15.8 Secondary syphilis.

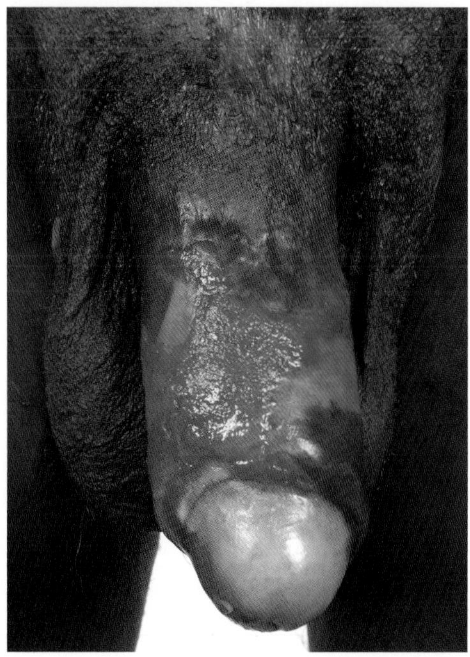

Figure 15.9 HSV (immune reconstitution inflammatory syndrome, IRIS).

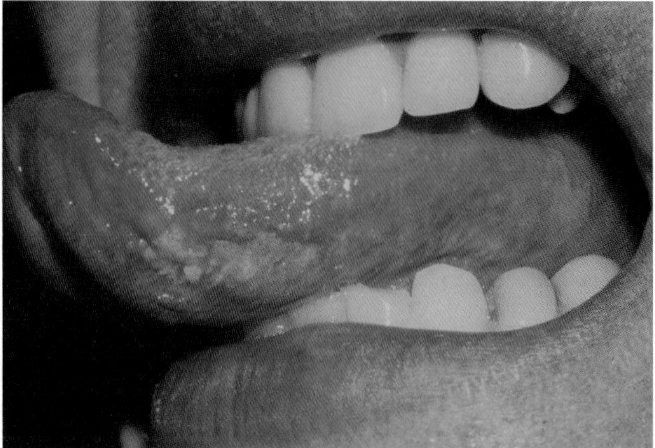

Figure 15.10 Oral hairy leukoplakia.

the sides of the tongue (Figure 15.10) with a verrucous grey/white surface. Biopsies from OHL show a lack of host Langerhans cells, which may account for the lack of immune response to the virus. Looking for OHL in the mouth can be a very quick and simple way of assessing potential immunosuppression in a previously undiagnosed individual in the clinic or field setting. OHL has also been reported in the context of haematological malignancy and after organ transplantation.

Kaposi's sarcoma (*KS*). Human herpesvirus type 8 is thought to be the causative agent in KS. In HIV patients lesions usually affect the face, oral cavity (Figure 15.11) and perineum. Early lesions may be erythematous-violaceous patches or papules which progress to firm nodules (Figure 15.12) or plaques with a purplish brown discolouration. Lesions may eventually ulcerate. KS koebnerises (occurs at sites of skin trauma) and secondary lymphoedema may occur, particularly in affected limbs. Histology from skin/mucosal lesions can be diagnostic. Patients traditionally had CD4 counts below 200 in order to present with KS; however, there are increasingly numbers of cases where patients present with CD4 counts between 300 and 400. Cutaneous therapy is directed at haemostasis, restoring function, improving the cosmetic appearance and debulking advanced disease. A variety of measures can be considered

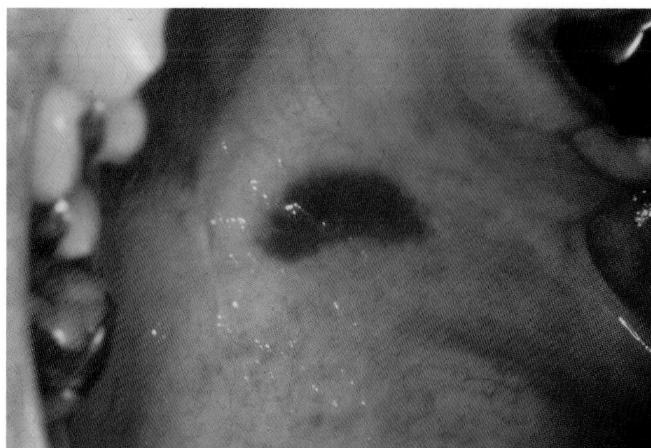

Figure 15.11 Kaposi's sarcoma on the hard palate.

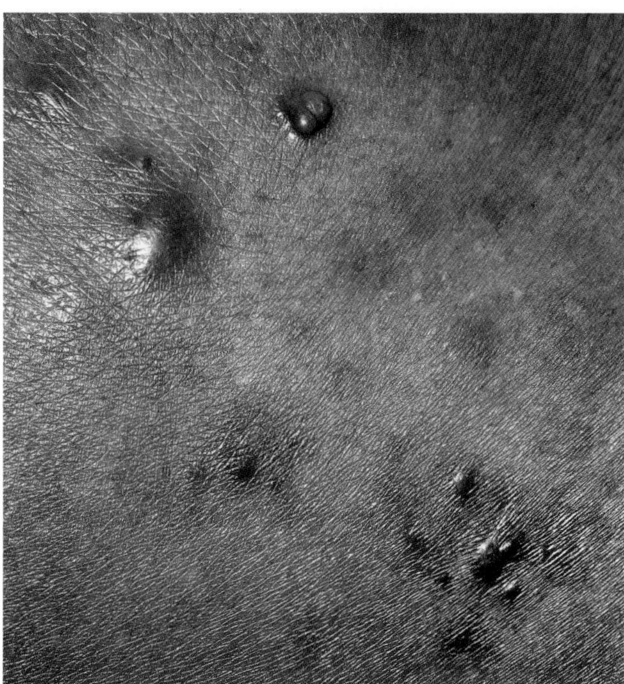

Figure 15.12 Kaposi's sarcoma nodules.

such as excision, radiotherapy, pulsed-dye laser and intralesional chemotherapy (vinblastine, vincristine and bleomycin).

Other viruses

Molluscum contagiosum infections are frequent in HIV patients. Individual lesions may be larger than usual (giant molluscum) and they may be extensive. Mollusca are readily identified as firm papules with an umbilicated centre (Figure 15.13). The differential diagnosis of large mollusca-like lesions in the context of HIV includes fungal infections due to *Cryptococcus* and histoplasmosis. If the diagnosis is in question then a skin biopsy for histology analysis can be very helpful.

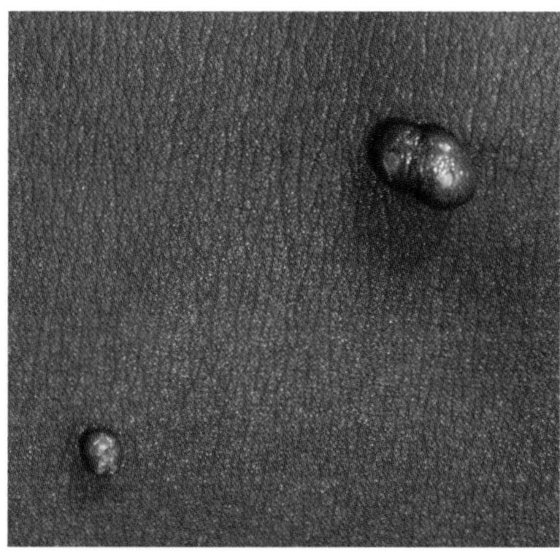

Figure 15.13 Molluscum contagiosum.

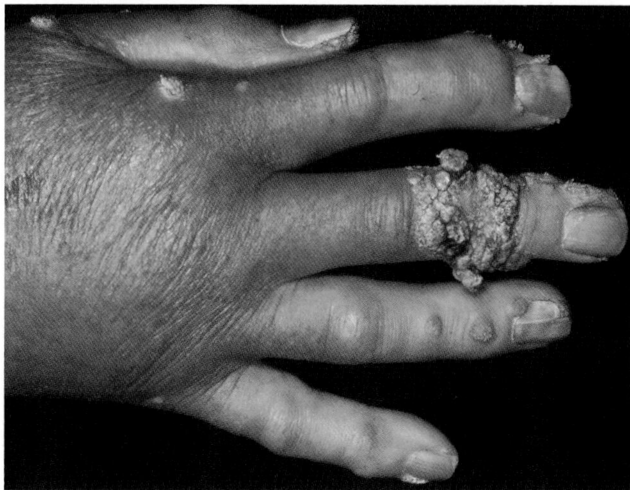

Figure 15.14 Human papillomavirus warts: extensive.

Human papillomavirus (*HPV*) warts may be numerous and large in HIV patients (Figure 15.14). Perianal and genital warts can be particularly troublesome and may be associated with intraepithelial neoplasia of the cervix and sometimes invasive perianal squamous cell carcinoma. With immune reconstitution HPV warts tend to resolve, but in the meantime, they may respond to wart therapies including salicylic acid, cryotherapy, imiquimod and diphencyprone therapy.

Infestations

Scabies in HIV patients may present with classic burrows on the fingers and genitals or as widespread crusted scabies which is highly contagious (Figure 15.15). Patients present with hyperkeratotic papules and plaques with relatively little inflammation (helping to distinguish it from psoriasis). Itching may be mild or intractable. Microscopic examination of the crusts is a simple rapid diagnostic test. Topical treatment with 5% permethrin (two applications 7 days apart) may be effective, but ivermectin 200 μg/kg as a single dose (or repeated after 7 days) may be needed in refractory/crusted and recurrent infestations.

Drug rashes

HIV patients frequently take multiple medications, many of which have a reputation for causing drug rashes (sulphonamides and antibiotics). Nonetheless, the frequency of drug rashes in HIV patients is extremely high (10 times higher than in the general population), especially at CD4 counts below 200 cells/μl. This is partially explained by the fact that HIV itself affects the metabolism of many drugs. The majority of drug rashes occur within 7–20 days after starting the offending drug, and take the form of toxic erythema (maculopapular eruption), which is usually mild and resolves when the medication is stopped.

However, severe life-threatening drug reactions such as toxic epidermal necrolysis (TEN) are 1000 times more common in HIV-positive individuals. In HIV patients, TEN has been reported

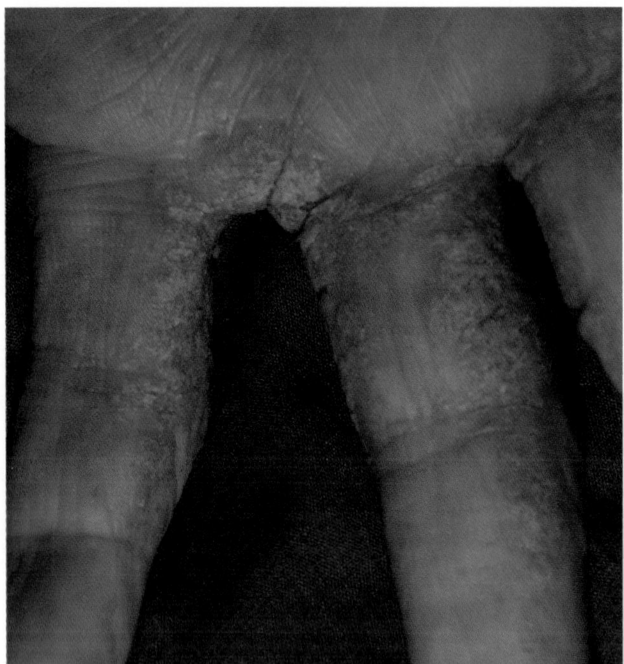

Figure 15.15 Crusted scabies on the hand.

in association with nevirapine, abacavir and co-trimoxazole. Clinically, patients present with rapid, widespread (>30% of skin surface area), painful, full-thickness skin necrosis, which is associated with a 25–30% risk of mortality (Figure 15.16).

Other drug rashes in HIV patients include pigmentation of nails/tongue/skin (zidovudine and clofazimine), hyperpigmentation of the palms and soles (emtricitabine) mucosal ulceration (zalcitabine, foscarnet and saquinavir), rash and pruritus (abacavir and raltegravir), alopecia and ingrowing nails (indinavir), diffuse erythema (abacavir), phototoxic rashes (St John's wort), injection site reactions (enfuvirtide) Stevens–Johnson syndrome (co-trimoxazole and dapsone) and TEN.

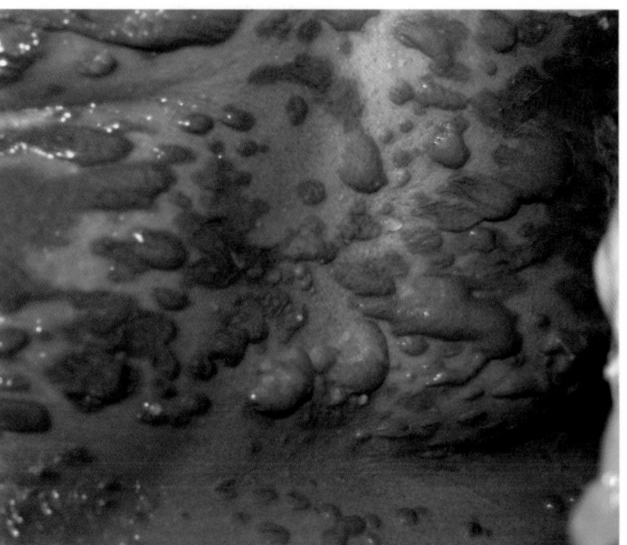

Figure 15.16 Toxic epidermal necrolysis.

Further reading

Adler MW et al. *ABC of HIV and AIDS*, 6th Edition, Wiley-Blackwell, Oxford, 2012

www.ashm.org.au.

CHAPTER 16

Fungal Infections

Rachael Morris-Jones

Dermatology Department, Kings College Hospital, London, UK

OVERVIEW

- Fungi can cause infections of the skin, hair, nails and orogenital tract.
- Fungal infections are more common in hot climates and in immunosuppressed individuals.
- A diagnosis of fungal infection is usually made clinically; however, it may be confirmed by culture of skin scrapings/scalp brushings.
- Tinea capitis usually needs to be treated with systemic antifungals.
- Onychomycosis (fungal infection of the nails) affects mainly adults and may be chronic.
- *Candida* (yeast) causes lesions in the mucous membranes and flexures where it should be differentiated from psoriasis, seborrhoeic dermatitis and contact dermatitis.
- Deep fungal infections may occur in diabetics, neutropenic, debilitated patients and the immunosuppressed.

Introduction

One million species of fungi are currently recognised, of which 300 are pathogenic to humans and of these over three-quarters primarily infect the skin and subcutaneous tissues. Superficial fungal pathogens are the fourth commonest cause of any human disease worldwide. Historically, superficial fungal infections have caused minimal disease in temperate climates, with the most severe outbreaks occurring in the tropics and subtropics. The use of potent immunosuppressant and antimicrobial drugs has increased the incidence of fungal infective episodes in temperate climates. Currently, there is emerging resistance to antifungal medications and to date no human fungal vaccine exists.

Some fungi live on the skin as part of the normal skin flora while others come into contact with the skin through the environment and animals. Superficial fungal infections attack the epidermis, mucosa, nails and hair, and are divided into two groups: moulds (e.g. dermatophytes) and yeasts (e.g. *Candida*).

ABC of Dermatology, Sixth Edition. Edited by Rachael Morris-Jones.

Yeast that comprise part of the normal skin flora can become pathogenic because of a change in the host's immune system. This allows the yeast to disseminate throughout the body, causing serious life-threatening disease. Conversely, mycoses that originate as systemic infections can become deposited in the skin via haematogenous spread.

Investigations

Diagnosis of fungal infections can be made by taking skin scrapings, nail clippings, scalp brushings and skin biopsies for mycological analyses (Box 16.1). A moistened bacterial swab taken from the affected skin and inoculated into standard fungal media can be a useful additional test. Expert mycologists who perform fungal microscopy may be able to make an immediate diagnosis through recognition of characteristic fungal features. Macroscopic patterns of fungal growth from cultures may also lead to species diagnoses; however, fungi are usually slow to grow. Modern fungal diagnostics are moving towards the use of rapid PCR tests and ELISA, which can rapidly process numerous specimens simultaneously. Some mycology reference laboratories may also be able to provide a sensitivity profile to antifungal drugs from any fungal strain isolated.

Box 16.1 **Principles of diagnosis**

- Consider a fungal infection in any patient with itchy, dry, scaly lesions (usual distribution is asymmetrical).
- Skin samples are taken by scraping the edge of the lesion with a blunt blade held at right angles to the skin and collected onto a piece of dark paper
- Nail clippings should be taken from the nail including subungal debris.
- Scalp brushings should be taken from the scalp (a travel toothbrush can be used).
- Laboratories will report initially on direct microscopy but culture results take 2–4 weeks.
- Lesions to which steroids have been applied are often quite clinically atypical because the normal inflammatory response is suppressed – *tinea incognito*.
- Wood's light (ultraviolet light) can reveal *Microsporum* infections of hair, as they produce a green-blue fluorescence.

General features of fungi in the skin

Superficial dermatophyte infections are named according to the body site affected: tinea capitis (scalp), tinea corporis (body), tinea cruris (groin) and tinea pedis (feet). Fungal infections invariably cause itching; the skin may be dry and scaly or in flexural areas wet maceration can result.

Zoophilic (animal) fungi generally produce a more intense inflammatory response with deeper indurated lesions (Figure 16.1) than fungal infections due to anthropophilic (human) species. Some lesions have a prominent scaling margin with apparent clearing in the centre, leading to annular or ring-shaped lesions – hence the term 'ringworm'.

Children below the age of puberty are susceptible to scalp ringworm, termed tinea capitis. In many inner city areas the most common fungus isolated is caused by a human species *Trichophyton tonsurans*, but fungi from animals (cattle, dogs, and cats) may also occur. Infection from dogs and cats with a zoophilic fungus (*Microsporum canis*) to which humans have little immunity can occur at any age (Figure 16.2). *Adults* typically are more commonly affected by tinea pedis. Tinea cruris in the groin is seen mainly in men, and fungal nail infections (onychomycosis) are particularly common in the elderly and debilitated.

Scalp and face

Tinea capitis (scalp ringworm) mainly affects pre-adolescent children. The main fungal pathogens isolated include *Trichophyton, Microsporum* and *Epidermophyton*. The most commonly isolated fungus in urban settings is *T. tonsurans*; it penetrates the hair shaft (endothrix fungus) and is characterised by single or multiple patches of alopecia, often minimal scaling and occasionally inflammation. *T. tonsurans* must be treated with systemic antifungal therapy to clear the endothrix infection.

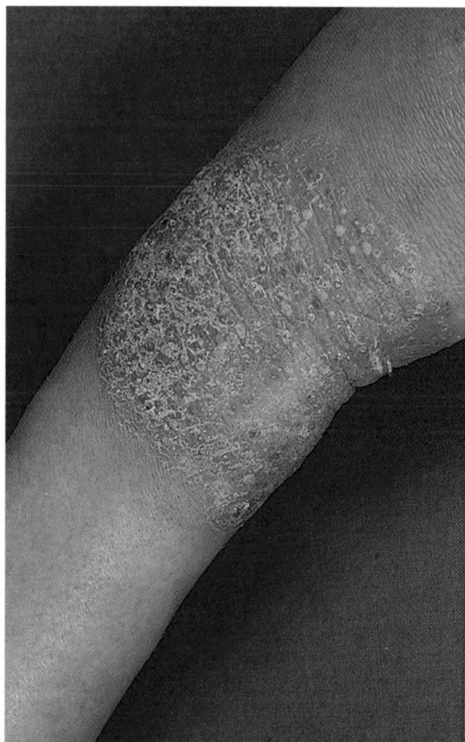

Figure 16.1 Animal ringworm.

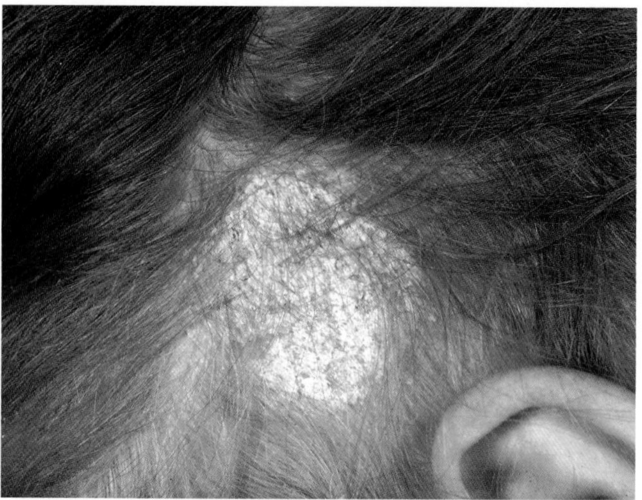

Figure 16.2 Tinea capitis: *Microsporum*.

Clinically, features are highly variable: diffuse scaling, grey patches, black dots (broken-off hairs), multiple pustules, patchy alopecia (Figure 16.3), extensive alopecia with inflammation (Figure 16.4) kerion formation and occipital lymphadenopathy. A *kerion* is an inflamed, boggy, pustular lesion on the scalp (Figure 16.5) that occurs when there is a brisk inflammatory response. This settles with systemic antifungal treatment and does not require surgical drainage. The clinical differential diagnosis of tinea capitis includes scalp eczema/psoriasis, folliculitis, alopecia areata and seborrhoeic dermatitis.

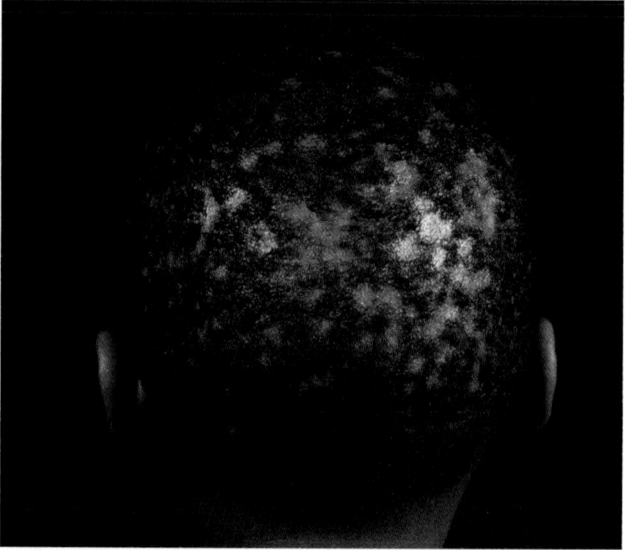

Figure 16.3 Patchy alopecia in tinea capitis caused by *Trichyophyton tonsurans*.

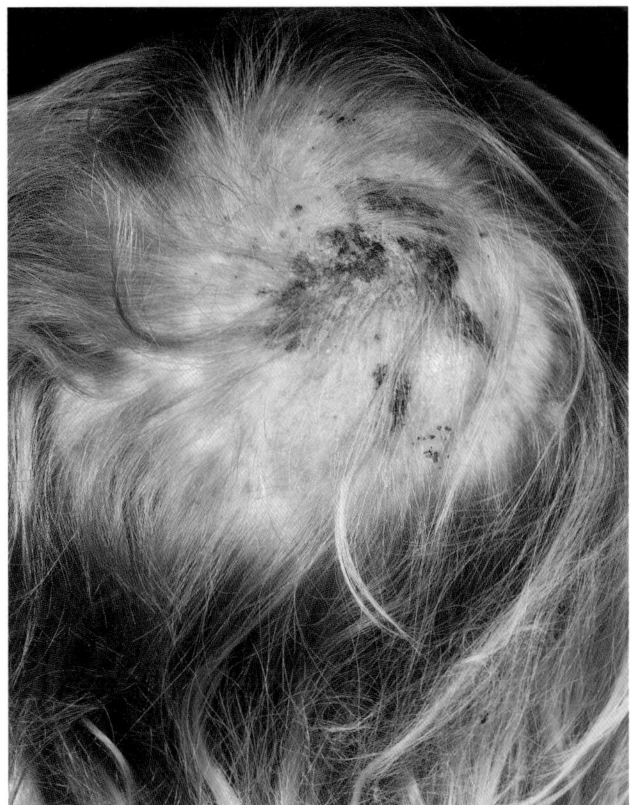

Figure 16.4 Extensive alopecia and inflammation caused by *T. tonsurans* infection.

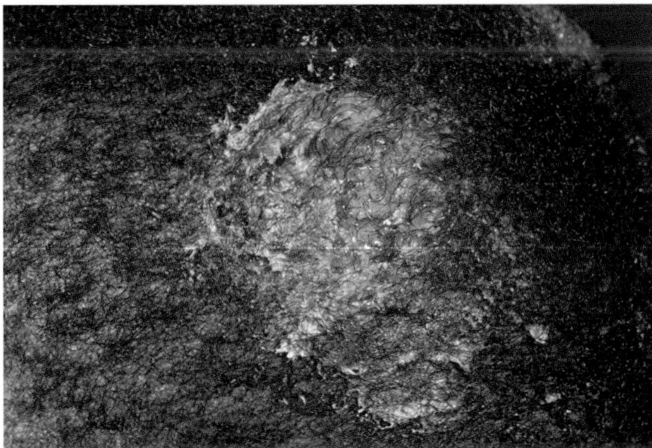

Figure 16.5 Kerion in *T. tonsurans* tinea capitis.

Scalp brushings should be taken to isolate the fungal pathogens from index cases and close family contacts. Parents may have tinea corporis on the shoulder/neck area where their child's infected head has come to rest.

Topical antifungals are unable to penetrate the hair shaft sufficiently to eradicate endothrix infections and therefore systemic antifungal agents are required for rapid clinical and mycological cure. Oral griseofulvin (10 mg/kg if over 1 month of age; occasionally 20 mg/kg is required) is the current FDA-approved treatment. It is effective for the treatment of *Microsporum* infections when given for 8–10 weeks but may cause gastrointestinal side effects. However, many dermatologists are using oral terbinafine as first-line therapy as it has a comparable safety profile and greater efficacy against *T. tonsurans* and is half the cost. Terbinafine is given daily for 1 month (dosage according to weight: <20 kg, 62.5 mg; 20–40 kg, 125 mg; >40 kg, 250 mg daily). Ideally, repeat scalp brushings should be taken after treatment to ensure mycological as well as clinical cure. Occasionally, a papular/pustular widespread cutaneous eruption appears after the commencement of systemic antifungal treatment – this is a so-called 'id reaction' (Figure 16.6) which is an immunological response and not an adverse drug reaction.

Tinea incognito is the term used for the indistinct appearance of a superficial fungal infection on the skin caused by use of topical/systemic steroids. Therefore, because the typical clinical features of the fungal infection (raised scaly margin with inflammation) are lost, the diagnosis becomes more difficult (Figure 16.7).

Figure 16.6 'Id reaction' after commencing oral treatment for tinea capitis.

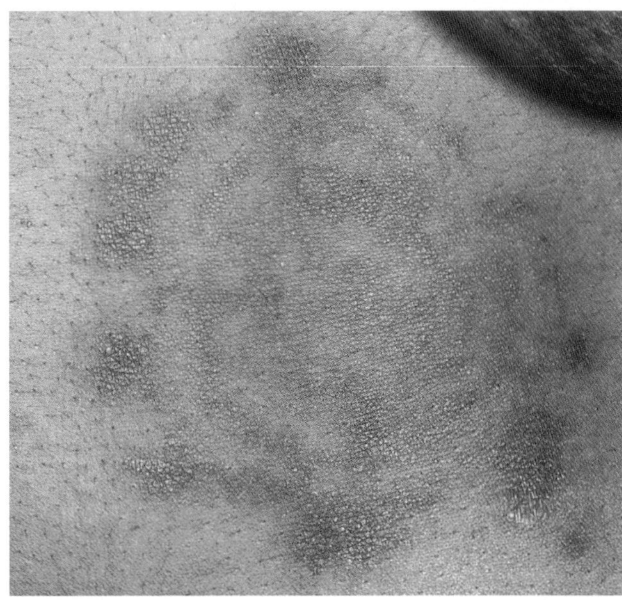

Figure 16.7 Tinea incognito.

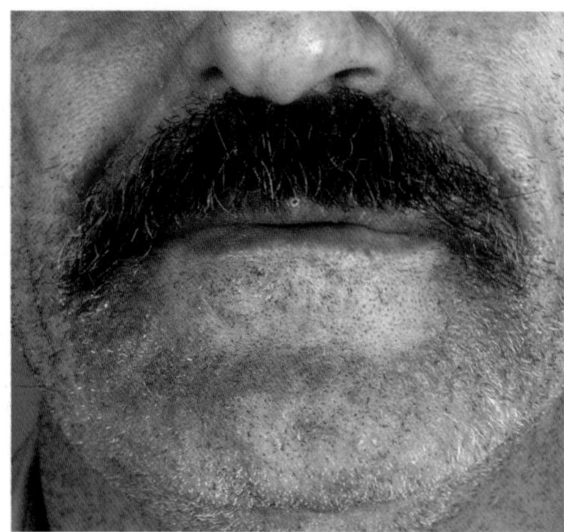

Figure 16.8 Seborrhoeic dermatitis.

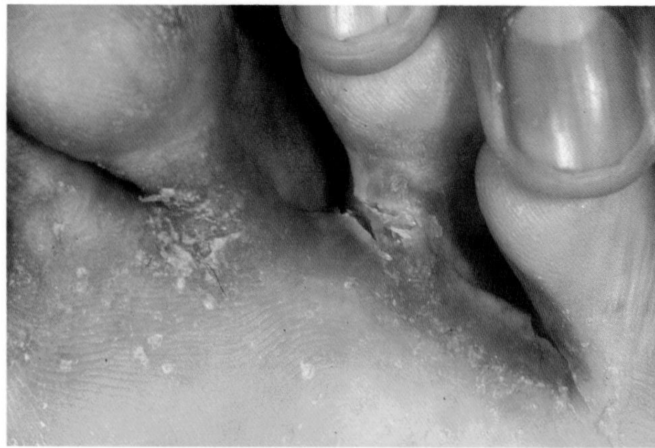

Figure 16.10 Toeweb tinea pedis.

The groin, hands, and face are sites where this is most likely to occur. Management is to stop the steroids and treat with topical antifungal agents.

Seborrhoeic dermatitis (SD) is an allergic contact dermatitis due to the yeast *Malassezia furfur* which is part of the normal skin flora; therefore, the condition is usually chronic. SD most frequently affects the hair-bearing skin (scalp, eyebrows, moustache and anterior chest) and nasal creases (Figure 16.8). There is marked scaling with associated eczema and adherent greasy scales. SD may be very itchy. The differential diagnosis of SD includes atopic eczema/psoriasis. It should be explained to patients that the problem will always tend to recur following treatment, which is aimed at reducing the numbers of yeast on the skin and controlling the eczema. Ketoconazole shampoo can be used to wash the body and scalp once weekly to reduce yeast numbers. Twice-daily topical steroids (± miconazole) can be used to treat the eczema. In refractory cases, systemic imidazoles such as itraconazole can be effective.

Feet (and hands)

Tinea pedis or athlete's foot is a common disease mainly affecting adults. It is easily acquired in public swimming pools or showers, and industrial workers appear to be particularly predisposed to this infection. Tinea pedis is very itchy and can affect any part of the foot (Figure 16.9) but frequently occurs between the toes (especially the fourth toe web) where the skin becomes macerated (Figure 16.10). Across the plantar and dorsal aspects of the feet there is usually a dry, scaling rash occasionally with vesicles at the active margins. The hands may be similarly affected. The condition needs to be differentiated from psoriasis and eczema (particularly pompholyx) and therefore scrapings for mycology can be helpful. Terbinafine 1% cream twice daily for 2–4 weeks is usually effective but recurrent infections may occur.

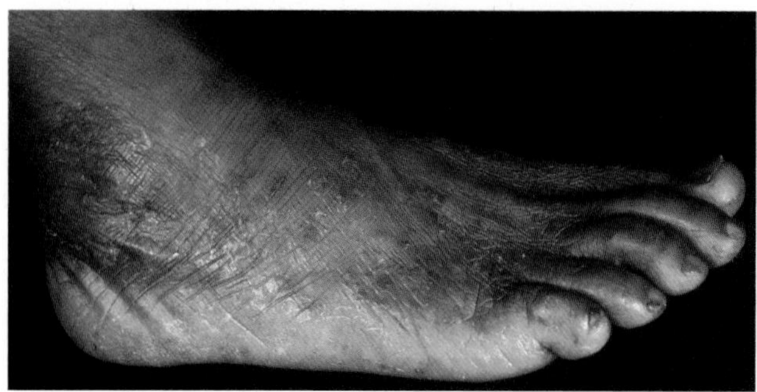

Figure 16.9 Tinea pedis.

Trunk

Tinea corporis also causes pruritus. Lesions tend to be erythematous with a well-defined scaly edge (Figure 16.11). In the groin, tinea cruris (Figure 16.12) is usually symmetrical dry scaling and may spread to the upper inner thighs. Conversely, intense erythema and satellite lesions suggest a *Candida* yeast infection. The differential diagnosis includes erythrasma due to *Corynebacterium minutissimum* (which may require a systemic erythromycin/tetracycline), psoriasis, mycosis fungoides and eczema. Terbinafine 1% cream is the most effective topical treatment for tinea corporis/cruris; other agents include miconazole, clotrimazole, ketoconazole and econazole for 2–4 weeks. If systemic therapy is required, itraconazole (100 mg daily) or terbinafine (250 mg daily) for 2 weeks is usually effective.

If systemic antifungals are not available, then simple measures such as antiseptic paints – Neutral Red or Castellan's paint – can be used. Whitfield's ointment (benzoic acid ointment) is easily prepared and is reasonably effective for superficial fungal infections.

Pityriasis versicolor affects the upper back, neck, chest and arms. It usually becomes apparent when the skin is exposed to the sun as these areas fail to tan. Well-defined macular lesions of variable colour (hence the name 'versicolor') from darker brown (Figure 16.13) to pale tan coloured fine scale (Figure 16.14) appear. The differential diagnosis includes seborrhoeic dermatitis, pityriasis rosea, guttate psoriasis and vitiligo. In skin scrapings, the causative organism *M. furfur* can be readily identified. Topical selenium sulphide (Selsun®) and topical ketoconazole 2% cream applied once daily for 2 weeks reportedly cures between 70 and 80% of patients, but one-third relapse. Systemic treatment with ketoconazole (200 mg once daily for 2 weeks), fluconazole (300 mg once

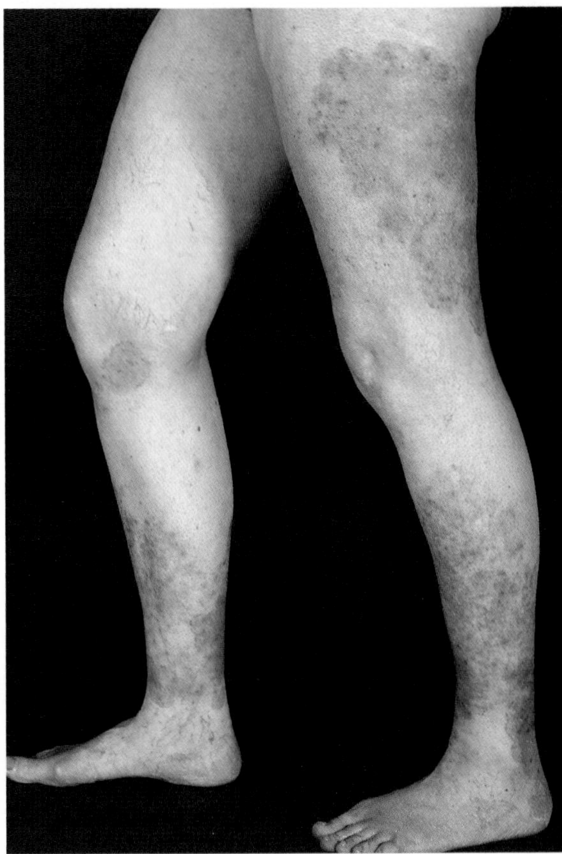

Figure 16.11 Tinea corporis.

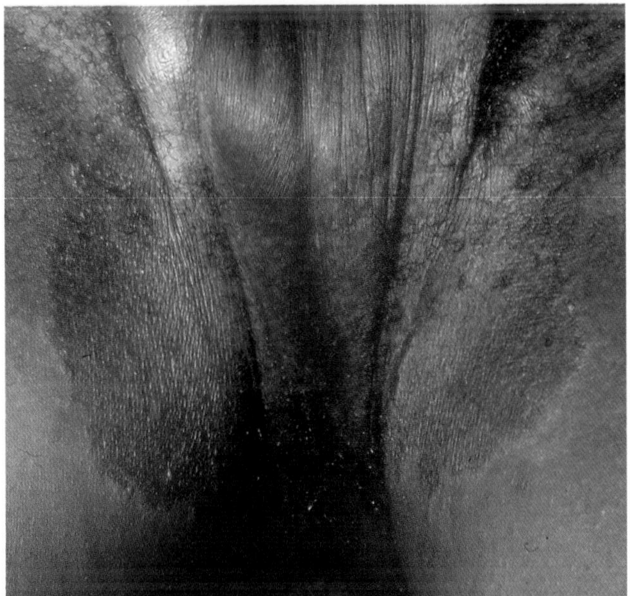

Figure 16.12 Tinea cruris.

weekly for 2 weeks) or itraconazole (200 mg once daily for 7 days) gives comparable results. The pale areas left behind after treatment will only repigment once the patient is re-exposed to sunlight.

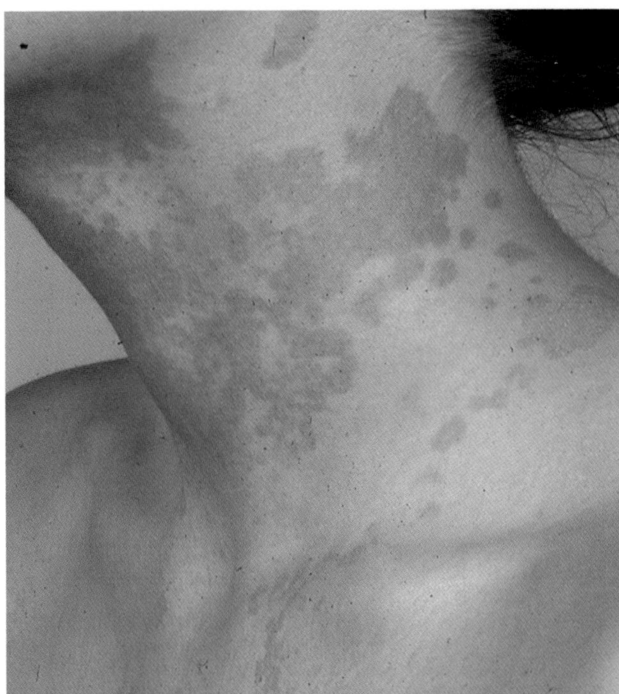

Figure 16.13 Pityriasis versicolor with hyperpigmented scaling.

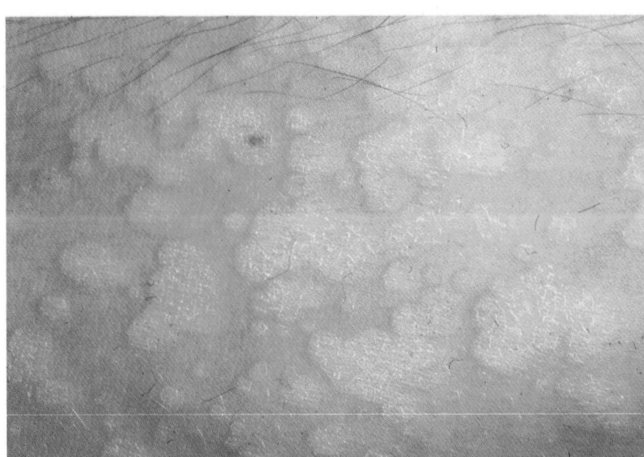

Figure 16.14 Pityriasis versicolor with hypopigmented scaling.

Nails

Onychomycosis affects mainly adult toenails and is usually caused by dermatophytes. Nail plates become thickened, brittle and white to yellow/brown (Figure 16.15). The distal nail plate is usually affected initially with spread proximally to involve the nail fold. In psoriasis of the nail, the changes occur proximally and tend to be symmetrical and are associated with pitting and other evidence of psoriasis elsewhere. Lichen planus may also cause nail dystrophy but this is usually manifested by vertical ridging and nicks in the nails (see Chapter 20). Onychomycosis may be caused by yeast infection such as *Candida albicans* (Figure 16.16).

Topical treatment should be considered for a single nail or very mild distal nail-plate onychomycosis. Agents available include amorolfine and ciclopirox olamine 8% nail lacquer solutions, sodium pyrithione, bifonazole/urea, imidazoles and allylamines.

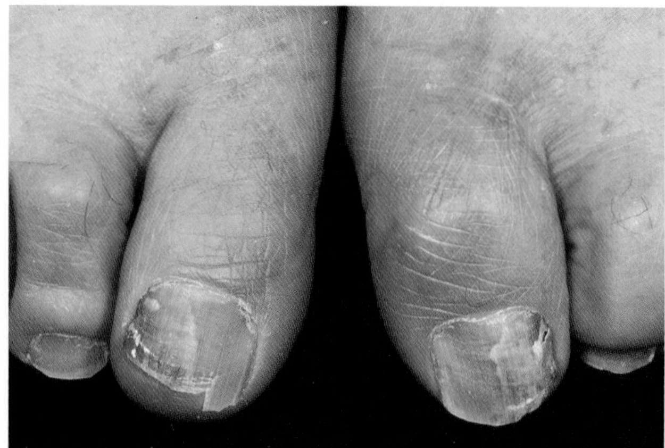

Figure 16.15 Onychomycosis caused by *Trichophyton rubrum*.

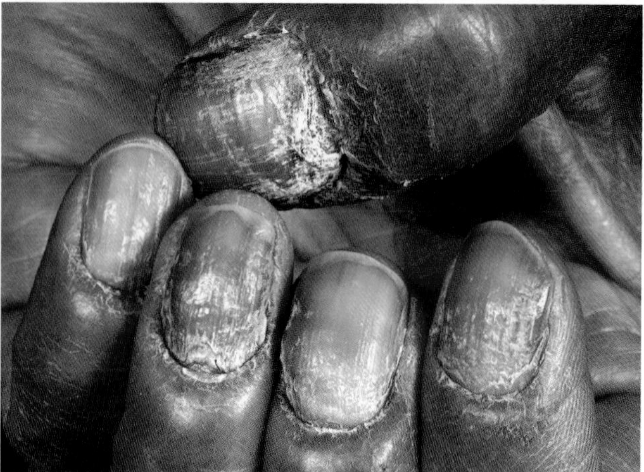

Figure 16.16 Candida onychomycosis.

Diseased nail plates may be 'dissolved' using 40% urea preparations (Canespro®) applied carefully to the nail plate, occluded with clingfilm left on overnight and then scrapped off before repeating each night for about 2 weeks. This helps to physically remove the infected nail without the need for medications or surgery. As the nail plates regrow, a topical antifungal such as amorolfine should be used twice weekly to prevent re-infection. Systemic therapy with terbinafine 250 mg daily for 16 weeks (toenails) or 8 weeks (fingernails) is usually considered first line. Terbinafine continues to be effective for many months after stopping the drug, and the abnormal nails should be seen to 'grow-out' with time. Pulsed itraconazole (200 mg twice daily for 1 week per month, for a total of 4 months) is also highly effective. Care should be taken to avoid drug interactions with itraconazole.

Chronic paronychia occurs around the nails of individuals involved in 'wet-work' who repeatedly put their hands in water (such as child carers, chefs, doctors, dentists, nurses and hairdressers). Other predisposing factors include diabetes, poor peripheral circulation, removal of the cuticle and artificial nails. There is erythema and swelling of the nail fold, often on one side with brownish discolouration of the nail. Pus may be exuded. There is usually a mixed infection including *C. albicans* and bacteria.

Pushing back the cuticles should be avoided. This is commonly a long-term condition, lasting for years. The hands should be kept as dry as possible, an azole lotion applied regularly around the nail fold, and in acute flares a course of erythromycin prescribed. Oral itraconazole (1 week per months for 3 months) or fluconazole (one dose per week for 3 months) can be used to treat severe infections.

Yeast infections

Candida infection may occur in the flexures of infants, elderly or immobilised patients, especially under the breasts and abdominal skin folds. This should be differentiated from (a) psoriasis, which does not usually itch; (b) seborrhoeic dermatitis, a common cause of a flexural rash in infants; and (c) contact dermatitis/discoid eczema. *Candida* intertrigo is symmetrical and 'satellite' pustules or papules outside the outer rim of the rash are typical (Figure 16.17). Yeast, including *C. albicans*, may be found in the mouth (Figure 16.18) and

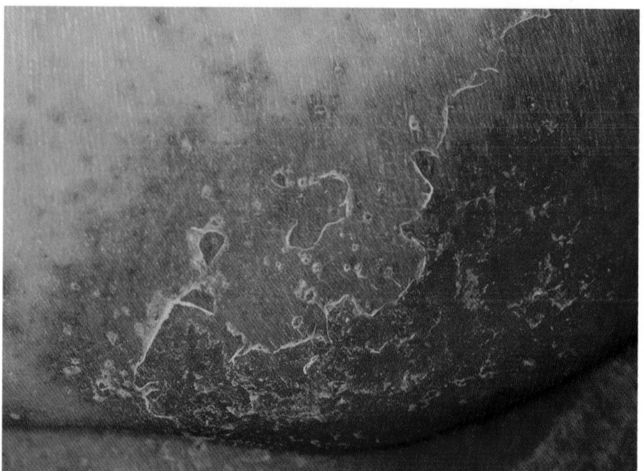

Figure 16.17 Candida infection in the groin.

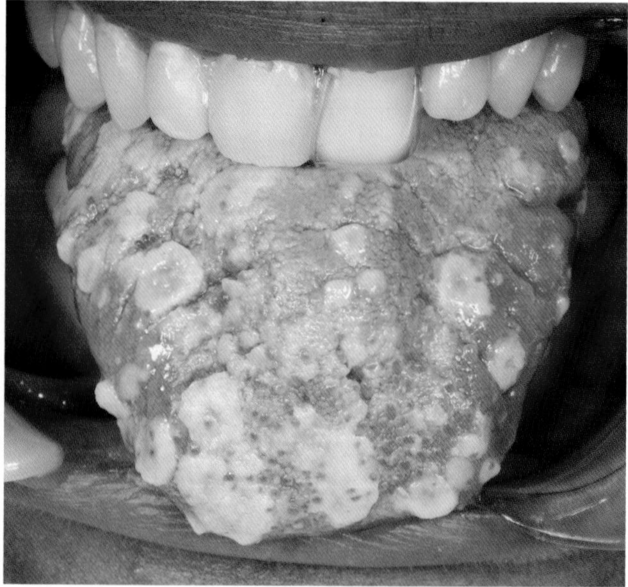

Figure 16.18 *Candida albicans* stomatitis.

vagina of healthy individuals. Clinical lesions in the mouth – white buccal plaques or erythema – may develop. Predisposing factors include general debility, impaired immunity (including HIV), diabetes mellitus, endocrine disorders and corticosteroid treatment. Vaginal candidosis or thrush is a common (occasionally recurrent) infection of healthy young women, leading to itching, soreness and a mild discharge.

The majority of superficial *Candida* infections can be treated using topical antifungals including clotrimazole, miconazole and nystatin in various formulations including pastilles, lozenges, oral gel, mouthwashes, pessaries, creams and lotions. Many patients find systemic treatments more convenient such as fluconazole 150 mg as a single dose or itraconazole 200 mg twice for 1 day. Some drugs interact with azole drugs, the main ones being terfenadine, astemizole, digoxin, midazolam, cyclosporin, tacrolimus and anticoagulants.

Deep fungal infections

Fungal infections of the deeper tissues are rare in healthy individuals and usually only affect those who have underlying medical problems or are immunocompromised by illness or medication. However, implantation of fungi into the skin through trauma may precipitate a chronic deep localised infection in otherwise healthy individuals. Fungal infections that involve the deeper skin tissues include histoplasmosis, cryptococcosis, sporotrichosis, *Fusarium* spp. (Figure 16.19) and *Penicillium marneffei.* In HIV patients, papules resembling molluscum contagiosum may be the earliest feature of deep fungal infections with *P. marneffei* and histoplasmosis. In the immunocompromised, neutopenic and diabetic ketoacidosis patients, severe life threatening infections may result from mucormycosis species such as Rhizopus (found in moldy bread). These fungi usually infect the facial sinus and may spread to the brain. Initially, symptoms can mimic sinusitis (nasal stuffiness) followed by facial swelling and black pus followed ultimately by necrotic tissue.

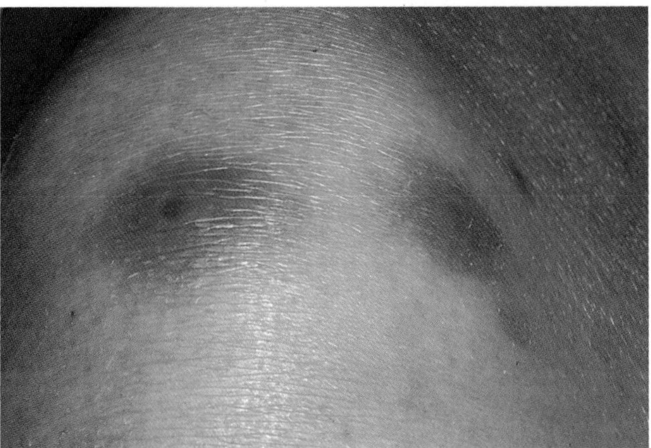

Figure 16.19 Fusarium infection in a bone marrow recipient.

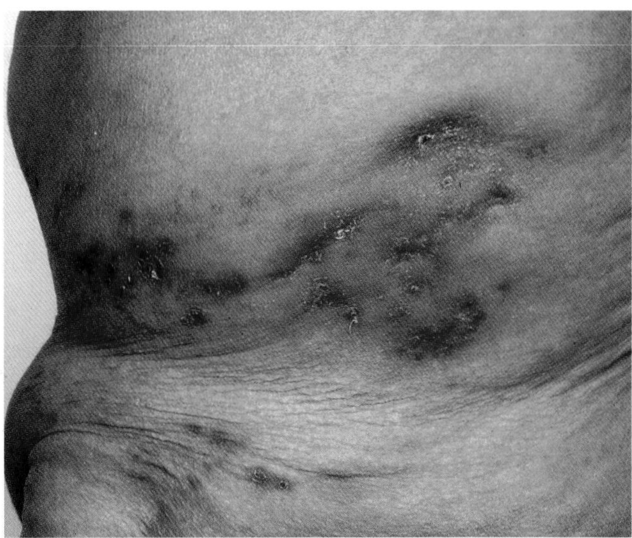

Figure 16.20 Deep fungal infection.

In tropical countries, deep fungal infections are more common. These are described in Chapter 18. They should be considered in any patient from a tropical country with chronic indurated and ulcerating lesions (Figure 16.20).

Systemic antifungal drugs

Severe or disseminated cutaneous fungal infections may require prolonged treatment with a systemic antifungal drug. Oral preparations available include terbinafine, which can be used to treat widespread dermatophyte infections (scalp, nails, skin) and sporotrichosis. Itraconazole is effective against candidiasis, seborrhoeic dermatitis, pityriasis versicolor, aspergillosis, histoplasmosis and blastomycosis. Griseofulvin is mainly used to treat tinea capitis but may also be used to treat tinea corporis. Voriconazole is effective against invasive candidiasis and aspergillosis. Recent evidence suggests that it is also beneficial in treating *Fusarium* infections. Voriconazole is available as an oral preparation and is therefore useful for outpatient management. Posaconazole is used as prophylaxis against invasive fungal infections post bone marrow transplantation, for severe *Candida* infections, chromoblastomycosis and zygomycosis. Liposomal amphotericin B is often used empirically to treat presumed fungal infections, disseminated Candida, aspergillosis, Cryptococcus and histoplasmosis. Caspofungin may be used as empirical therapy in febrile neutropenic patients and for the management of disseminated aspergillosis and candidaemia.

Further reading

Goering et al. *MIM's Medical Microbiology*, 5th edition, Saunders, 2012.

Richardson MD and Johnson EM. *Pocket Guide to Fungal Infection*. 2nd Edition, Wiley-Blackwell, 2006.

CHAPTER 17

Insect Bites and Infestations

Rachael Morris-Jones

Dermatology Department, Kings College Hospital, London, UK

OVERVIEW

- Bites can cause a local skin reaction and/or systemic disease in humans through the transmission of parasites, bacteria or viruses.
- Biting insects (including mosquitoes, midges, bedbugs, fleas, sandflies, mites, ticks and lice) cause erythematous pruritic lesions on exposed skin, usually in groups/clusters.
- A generalised anaphylactic reaction to an insect sting can be life threatening. Patients known to be at risk should carry a preloaded syringe of adrenaline to use when reactions occur.
- Worldwide, scabies is the most common infestation. Female mites burrow through the skin, resulting in intense itching.
- Other infestations include lice (which may transmit trench fever and typhus). Pubic lice may be associated with other sexually transmitted diseases.
- Cutaneous larva migrans occurs when larvae from the dog/cat hookworm penetrate human skin, causing a superficial creeping eruption.

Insect bites and stings

When insects bite, they inject their saliva into the skin and ingest blood, which usually causes localised areas of discomfort and itching (Figure 17.1), which may be clustered or in a linear distribution (Figure 17.2). Stinging insects inject venom through the sting that causes a more severe local reaction. More serious effects are due to (a) anaphylactic reactions from the bite/sting or (b) the introduction of infectious diseases.

Most cases of bites from fleas, midges and mosquitoes are readily recognised (Box 17.1) and cause few symptoms apart from discomfort/itching. Occasionally, an allergic reaction confuses the picture, such as large bullae (Figure 17.3). Persuading patients that their recurrent itchy spots are due to flea bites can be difficult and they may reject the suggestion (Box 17.2). Some patients develop a persistent insect bite reaction which lasts for many months (Figure 17.4).

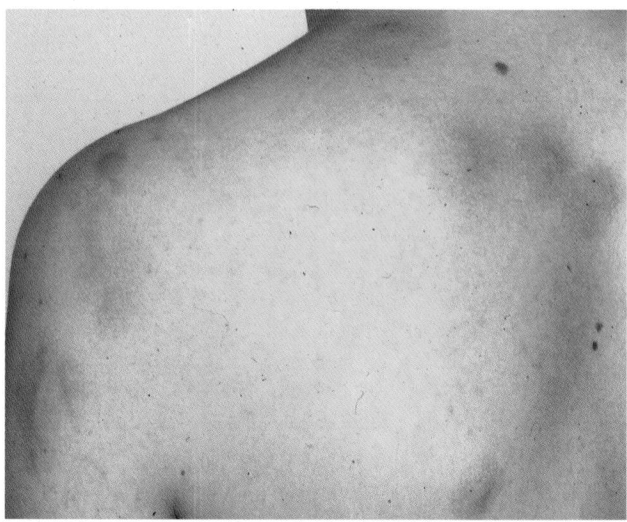

Figure 17.1 Papular and inflammatory insect bite reactions.

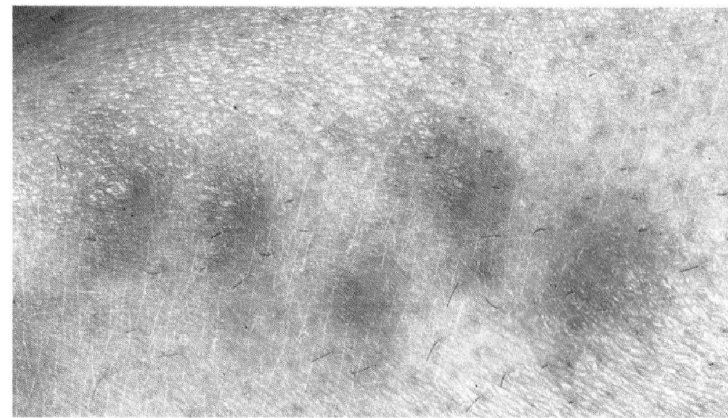

Figure 17.2 Linearity of insect bite reactions.

Box 17.1 **Clinical features of bites**

- Exposed skin sites, especially lower limbs
- Clustering or linear groups of lesions
- Papules, nodules, urticated lesions
- Blisters or ulceration
- Excoriations with secondary bacterial infection.

ABC of Dermatology, Sixth Edition. Edited by Rachael Morris-Jones.

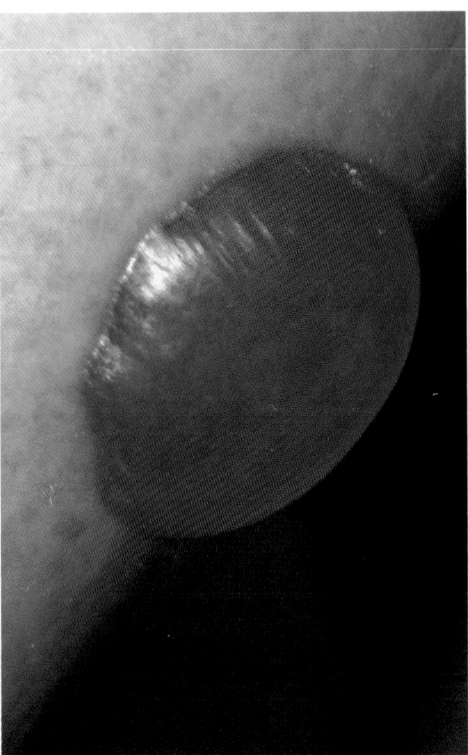

Figure 17.3 Bulla bite reaction.

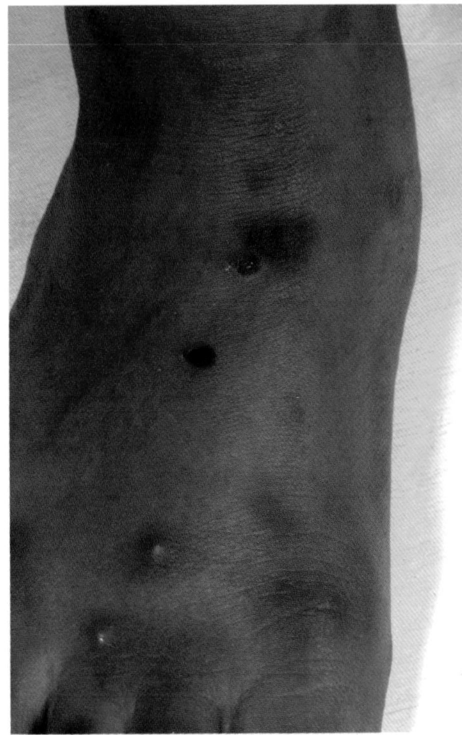

Figure 17.4 Persistent insect bite reaction.

Box 17.2 **Risk factors for bites**

- Outdoor activities
- Travel
- Poor-quality accommodation
- Contact with animals
- Recent death of a family pet.

Delusions of parasitosis

Patients are convinced they have an infestation with parasites when they do not; the term *pseudoparasitic dysesthesia* may helpfully be used with patients. Those affected often bring samples in jars of 'insects' (Figure 17.5). Examination shows these to be pickings of keratin, cotton or thread. Sympathy and tact should help reassure the patient and help build confidence; derision and disbelief will tend to trigger seeking a second opinion elsewhere. Two thirds of patients have the unshakable belief that they are infested with parasite. Application of topical creams and bandaging may help heal the affected excoriated skin; however, antipsychotic drugs are usually required to treat the psychosis and should be prescribed in conjunction with advice from a psychiatrist. Drugs such as risperidone can be of benefit but care must be taken because of potential side effects, particularly if the patient has epilepsy or cardiovascular disease. More recently, aripiprazole (15 mg for 8 weeks and then 7.5 mg/day) has been shown to be effective. Antidepressants including citalopram have also shown benefit especially in those with concomitant depression.

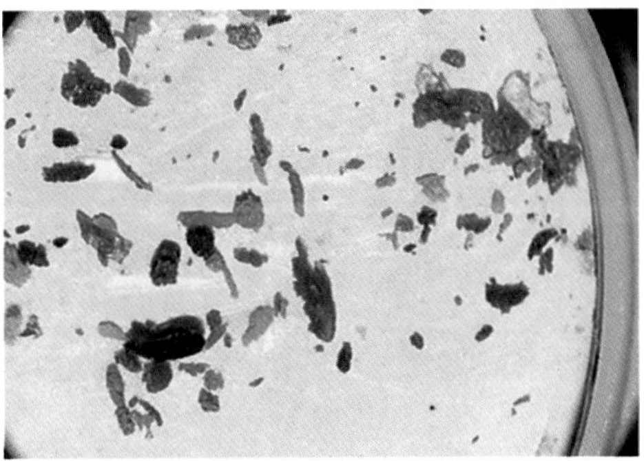

Figure 17.5 Parasitophobia specimens.

Allergic reaction to bites

Commonly, insect bite reactions cause local irritation, and rarely (often to stings rather than bites) a generalised anaphylactic reaction may occur. For localised allergic reactions oral antihistamines and topical steroids are effective and for more generalised reactions oral antihistamine, intramuscular (IM) adrenaline (injected into the lateral thigh) and systemic steroids may be required. In those identified as having severe reactions to stings they should be given a self-injectable epinephrine pen to use in subsequent severe reactions.

Management of bite reactions

- Over-the-counter preparations can be used in the majority of cases, such as bite-soothing spray, lidocaine and hydrocortisone ointment.

- Antihistamine creams (crotamiton and doxepin) or tablets (cetirizine and desloratadine) can help reduce itching.
- If blisters are present they can be deflated with a sterile needle.
- Topical steroids such as Betnovate ointment twice daily can be applied to reduce inflammation, swelling and itching.
- If bite reactions are secondarily infected, topical or oral antibiotics may be needed. Topical fucidin ointment or Fucibet cream (a combination steroid and antibiotic) can be used twice daily. Flucloxacillin usually covers secondary staphylococcal infections (erythromycin in penicillin-sensitive patients).
- In very severe cases, a short course of oral prednisolone may be needed (30 mg daily for 5 days).

Prevention of bites

Keep the skin covered with clothing (especially dark colours), wear insect repellent (WHO recommends Icaridin (Autan®, chemical KBR 3023) and DEET (*N,N*-diethyl-meta-toluamide)) and sleeping under bed nets off the ground.

Insect bites transmitting parasites

The identity of the biting insect can be important information if a parasitic infection is suspected. Insects that bite humans include mosquitoes, midges, bed bugs, fleas, sand flies, mites, ticks and lice. Each insect has its own specific distribution, preferred location, seasonal activity and preferred skin sites. All these factors can help pinpoint the offending insect (see Table 17.1). It may therefore be significant to know where the patient has been and his or her activities. Travel to tropical areas raises the possibility of parasite infection, while Lyme disease may occur from walking in endemic areas. Handling grain at harvest time may lead to harvest mite (*Pyemotes* spp.) bites.

Lyme disease

Tick and mosquito bites can lead to infection with *Borrelia burgdorferi*, causing arthropathy, fever and a distinctive rash (erythema chronicum migrans) (Figures 17.6 and 17.7). The bite may not be recalled by the patient. The tick needs to stay on the skin for many hours to take the blood meal and transmit the disease. If the patient is unwell and has visited an area where Lyme disease is endemic (parts of the United States and Europe) or gives a history of a tick bite, then check serology for *B. burgdorferi*. Do not wait for the results, however, but treat with doxycycline 100 mg twice daily for 10–30 days. Children under 8 years and pregnant or breastfeeding women can be given amoxicillin or azithromycin.

Table 17.1 Skin lesions associated with insect bites.

Rash morphology	Differential diagnosis	Vectors (organisms)
Maculopapular	Human typhus Rocky mountain spotted fever Scrub typhus Relapsing fever	Human louse (*Rickettsia*) Ticks (*Rickettsia*) Mites (*Rickettsia*) Lice/ticks (*Borrelia recurrentis*)
Vesicular	Rickettsial pox	Mouse/louse (*Rickettsia*)
Annular	Lyme disease	Tick/blackfly (*B. burgdorferi*)
Nodules (pruritic)	Onchocerciasis	Blackfly (*Filaria, Onchocerca volvulus*)
Nodules (ulcerating)	Leishmaniasis	Sand fly (*Leishmania*)
Necrotic lesions	Tick typhus	Ticks (*Rickettsia*)
Facial flushing	Yellow fever/dengue	*Aedes* mosquito (*Arbovirus*)

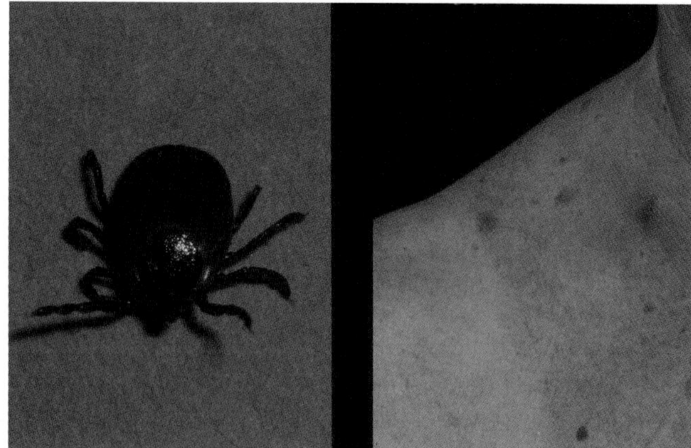

Figure 17.6 Tick bite reaction.

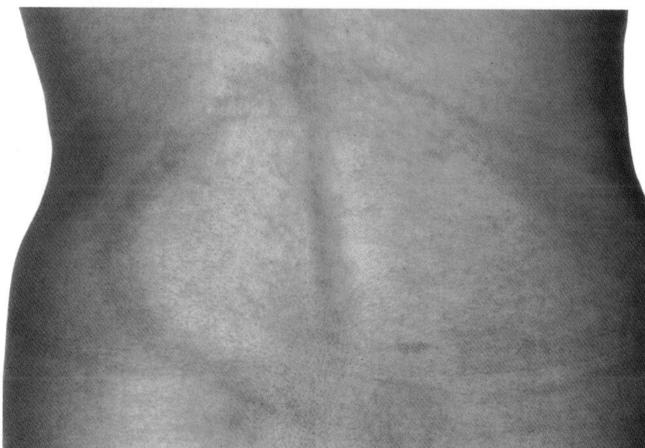

Figure 17.7 Erythema chronicum migrans in Lyme disease.

Spider bites

Bites from spiders found in the tropics and subtropics can be quite severe (Figure 17.8). The bite of the brown recluse spider (found in parts of the United States) can become necrotic resembling pyoderma gangrenosum (i.e. a necrotic ulcerated lesion). Some spiders inject venomous neurotoxins that may be fatal – for example, bites from the 'black widow' (*Latrodectus mactans*), 'fiddleback' (*Loxosceles veclusa*) and *Atrax* species found in Australia. European spiders may cause a painful bite reaction, but they are not venomous. However, with increasing transportation of fresh produce from topical/subtropical countries, there are incidents of venomous spiders arriving by ship in consignments of fruit to non-endemic areas.

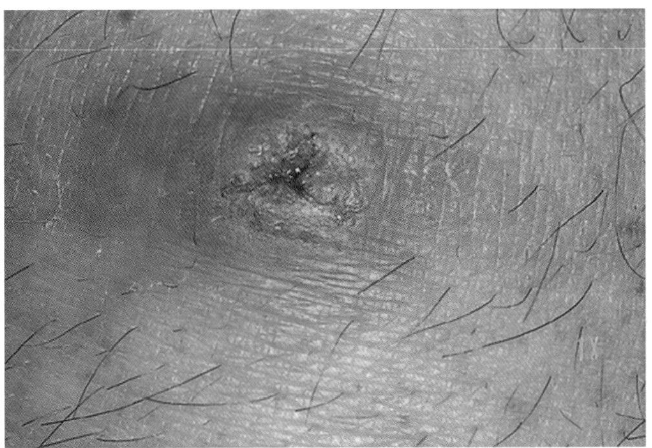

Figure 17.8 Spider bite (Nigeria).

Wasp and bee stings

The Hymenoptera are a large order of insects, which inject venom through the sting apparatus. Both bee and wasp venom contains histamine, mast cell-degranulating peptide, phospholipase A2 and hyaluronidase. Local reactions are usually insignificant but generalised systemic reactions with massive respiratory tract oedema can be fatal.

Treatment

Mild local reactions can be treated with oral antihistamines. If anaphylaxis occurs then an epinephrine autoinjection can be given (currently available in two fixed doses: 0.15 and 0.30 mg) immediately if available. In the emergency room, epinephrine is given IM (1:1000 adrenaline, 500 μg in 0.5 ml IM given in the lateral thigh to children >12 years and adults, children 6–12 years 300 μg IM, children <6 years 150 μg IM), repeated every 5 min if necessary. Consider giving additional IV fluids, chlorpheniramine (chlorphenamine) and hydrocortisone. IV adrenaline should only be given by experienced specialists. Desensitisation with venom extract carried out in a specialised unit is effective in those sensitive to bee venom.

Infestations

Scabies (*Sarcoptes scabiei*)

The most common infestation worldwide is scabies, which causes intense itching that characteristically keeps those affected awake at night. The female mite burrows into the epidermis and lays eggs which hatch into larvae within a few days. See Box 17.3.

Transmission occurs because of close personal contact (at least 15 min of skin-to-skin contact) with an infected individual. The first symptoms of itching occur 2 weeks later when the immune system reacts to the proteins in the mites, eggs and faeces in the skin. Most infestations in immunocompetent individuals carry 10 adult mites, but in crusted scabies mite numbers will be in the hundreds because of failure of the host's immune system.

Box 17.3 **Scabies – points to note**

- There may be very few burrows, though the patient has widespread itching.
- The distribution of the infestation is characteristically the fingers, wrists, nipples, abdomen, genitalia, buttocks and ankles.
- Close personal contact is required for infestation to occur – for example, within a family, through infants in playgroups, and through regular nursing of elderly patients.
- Itching may persist even after all mites have been eliminated; itching papules on the scrotum and penis are particularly persistent.

Diagnosis

Scabies infestations may be difficult to diagnose because of the wide variation in clinical presentations. However, key points in the history include several individuals in the same household/institution/classroom/ward being affected simultaneously by a rash that is intensely itchy at night. Clinically, burrows can be seen, especially in the finger-web spaces and on the genitals. Burrows are linear palpable ridges on the skin with a black speck indicating the position of the mite (Figure 17.9), which can be teased out of its

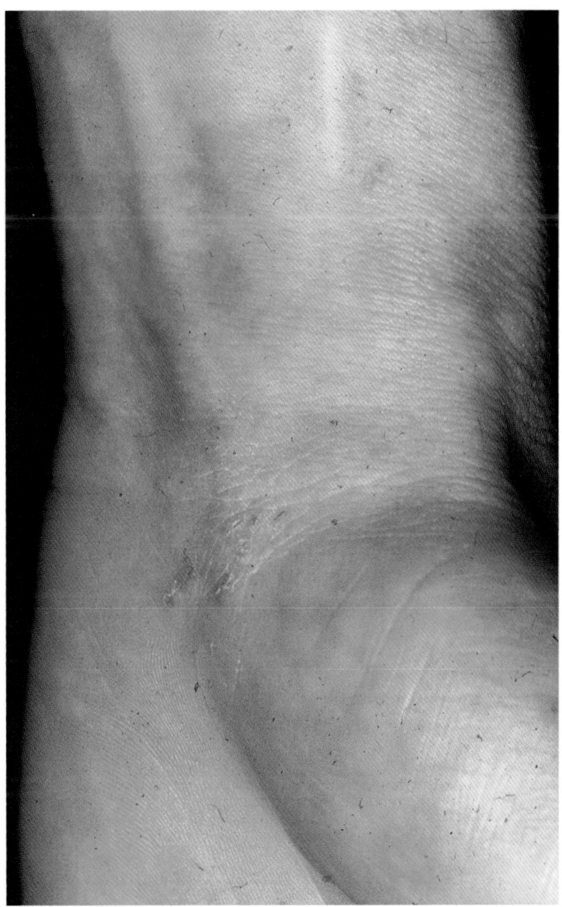

Figure 17.9 Scabies burrows.

burrow using a sterile needle and mounted onto a microscope slide. Patients often have a widespread papular rash, which is due to a reaction to the infestation, with multiple excoriation marks which can become secondarily infected with staphylococcus.

Scabies in children

Babies and young children infested with scabies characteristically present with erythematous cutaneous papules and nodules in the axillae and on the soles of the feet (Figures 17.10 and 17.11). It is not unusual for the lesions to blister. Classic burrows are rarely seen in this age group.

Crusted scabies

Crusted scabies can look similar to dry scaly skin rashes such as psoriasis and eczema, and consequently can be misdiagnosed. Patients are usually immunosuppressed or elderly and do not complain of itching, as their immune cells are not reacting against the mite proteins. Consequently, mite numbers are usually in the hundreds. Clinically patients have a crusted fine scaling on the skin, which is superficial with very little erythema (unlike psoriasis and eczema) (Figure 17.12). If the diagnosis is missed then numerous close contacts such as nurses and carers develop classic scabies and small outbreaks can occur.

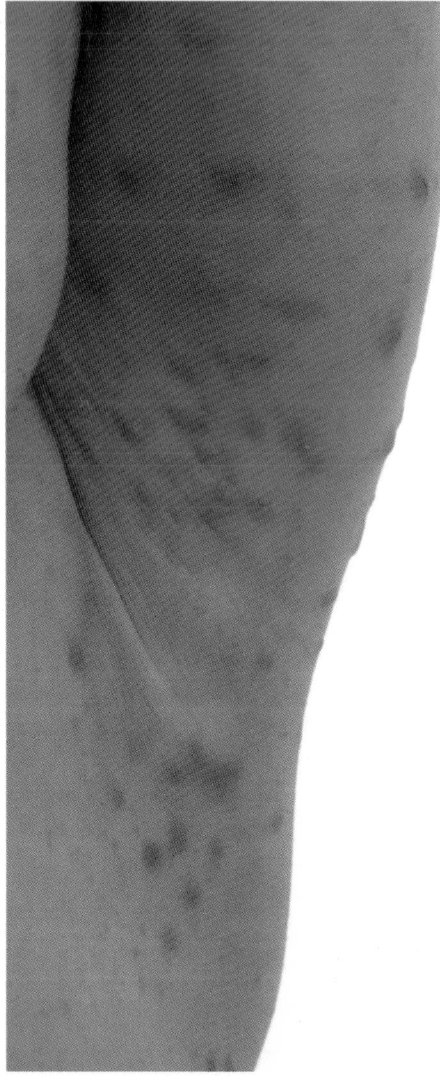

Figure 17.10 Scabies nodules in a child.

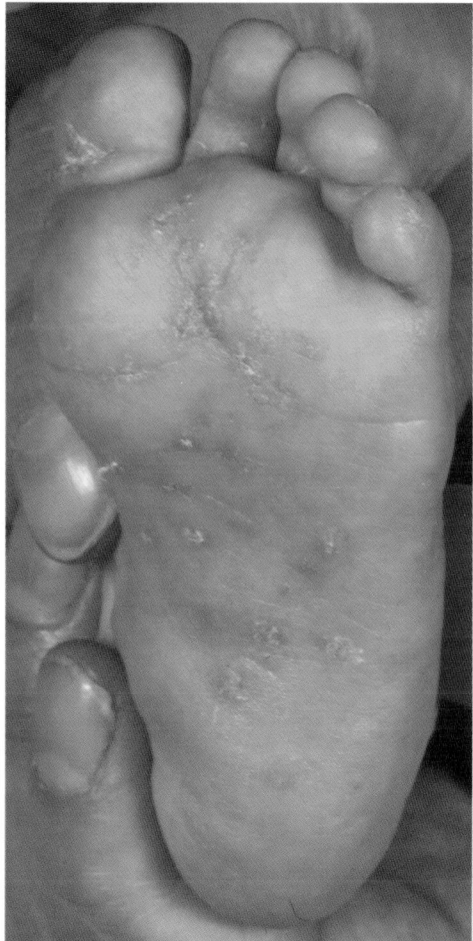

Figure 17.11 Scabies on sole of an infant.

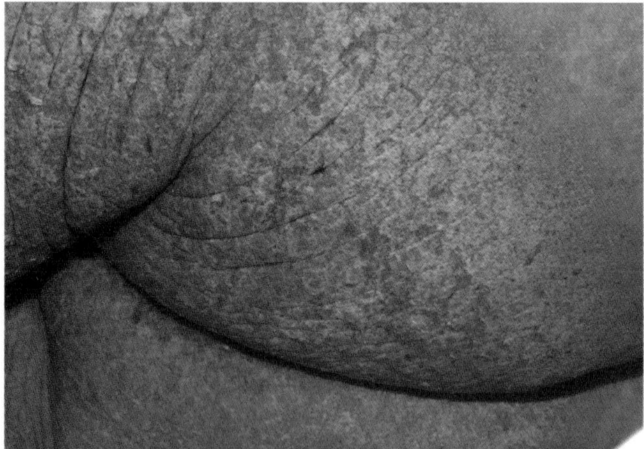

Figure 17.12 Crusted scabies on buttocks.

Management

A full explanation of how to use topical therapy is essential if infestations are to be successfully managed. The most common cause of treatment failure is incorrect use of insecticides. Patients should be told that they and all their close personal contacts need to be treated at the same time, the lotions should be applied from the neck downwards (although the head and neck of babies should also be treated), the treatment left on overnight, and then repeated after 7 days. They should pay particular attention to the web spaces and genital areas. They should reapply the lotion after washing their hands (Box 17.4).

Towels, bedding and underwear should be washed. Patients should be warned that the skin itching will take 6–8 weeks to subside. Persistent itching often leads patients to conclude that the mites are still active and they subsequently treat themselves repeatedly, leading to an irritant dermatitis. The itching resolves when the mites, eggs and faeces have been removed from the skin by the host's immune cells.

Box 17.4 **Management of scabies**

- First-line treatment for scabies is 5% permethrin cream left on overnight, two applications 7 days apart. Adults apply from neck downwards; babies/infants apply to all the skin.
- Second line is 0.5% malathion lotion left on overnight (applied as above).
- Ivermectin 200 μg/kg, two doses 7 days apart (named-patient basis), can be given to immunocompromised patients and those with crusted scabies (avoid in patients <15 kg and in pregnancy).
- If you suspect genuine resistance (i.e. the treatment has been carried out according to your instructions), then switch to a different class of insecticide.
- Pruritus can be alleviated with menthol in aqueous cream, crotamiton or doxepin. In severe cases, a topical steroid can be applied twice daily to settle persistent nodular skin reactions.
- If permethrin and malathion are not available, then 10% sulphur in yellow soft paraffin is effective and safe; 25% benzyl benzoate emulsion may also be used.

Lice

Head lice

Head lice have infested humans for thousands of years. They have a worldwide distribution and can affect anyone. Children are the most common hosts. The exact prevalence is difficult to estimate with 0.1–66% of schoolchildren shown to be infected in different areas of rural Africa and 11% in Australia.

Lice are transmitted by head-to-head contact, and on combs, brushes and hats. Girls are more commonly affected than boys; this is thought to be due to their close contact with others during play. Mild itching may be the only symptom of head lice. Careful inspection of the hair close to the scalp may reveal adult lice and nits (white empty egg cases) in infested individuals (Figure 17.13). Patients may develop an itchy irritant looking dermatitis on their upper back and neck area (Figure 17.14). Fine-toothed combs can aid detection.

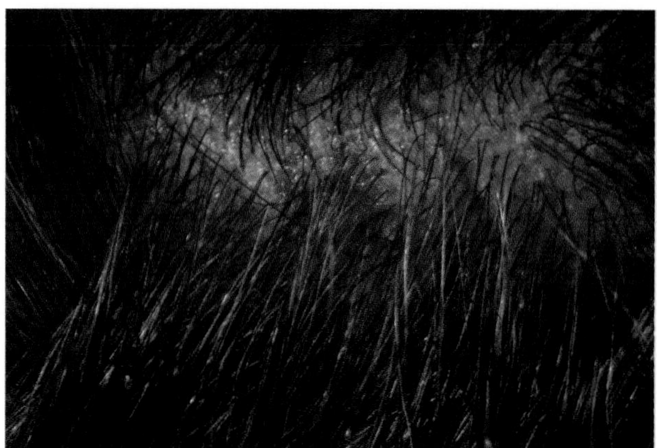

Figure 17.13 Head lice.

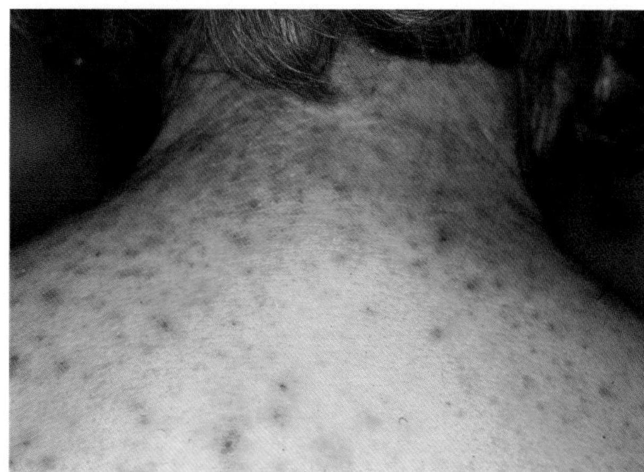

Figure 17.14 Pediculosis (head lice) causing an irritant rash on the posterior neck and upper back.

Management

- Only treat individuals with live lice visible on the scalp. Fine-toothed nit-combs can be used to comb out lice and eggs over a basin ('bug-busting'). An application of hair conditioner usually allows the comb to pass more easily through the hair. Wet combing alone (30 min every 3 days for 2 weeks) has been shown to be inferior to insecticides, but in highly motivated families it can be very successful.
- First-line treatment is permethrin 1–5% crème rinse applied to dry hair and left on overnight. This should be repeated after 7 days.
- Alternative agents include phenothrin 0.5% or malathion 0.5% (applied as above).
- Combinations of insecticides and bug-busting can be used.

Body lice

Body lice are the vectors of several human pathogens including *Bartonella quintana* (agent of trench fever, bacillary angiomatosis and endocarditis) and *Rickettsia prowazekii* (agent of typhus). Body lice tend to affect individuals from poorer economic backgrounds and those sleeping rough. The lice live in the host's clothes and bite the skin. Close inspection, especially of the clothing seams, reveals the adults and eggs. Infested individuals have a widespread papular eruption with excoriations. If the patient has a fever or constitutional symptoms then the possibility of louse-borne systemic infection should be raised.

Management

- Wash clothing in hot water, 'tumble-dry' or place infested clothes in a sealed plastic bag for 2 weeks to kill adults and eggs.
- Treat the skin reactions with a moderately potent topical steroid, plus topical antibiotic if secondarily infected with bacteria.
- Take blood for culture and serology if louse-borne systemic disease is suspected. Refer to cardiologists if endocarditis is suspected.

Pubic lice

These lice prefer the sparser hair-bearing sites on the skin such as the pubic, axillary and eyelash areas (Figure 17.15). The so-called crab lice are slow moving and are spread by close personal contact. Check the patient for other sexually transmitted diseases.

Management

- Use topical permethrin 5% cream or 0.5% malathion to the skin from the neck downwards, left on overnight, repeated after 7 days.

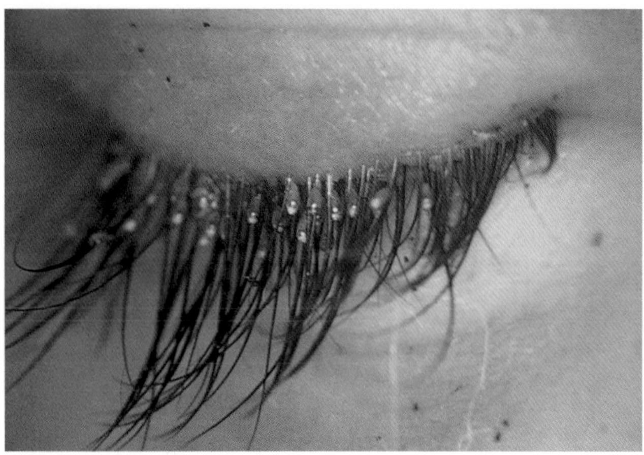

Figure 17.15 Pubic lice on eyelashes.

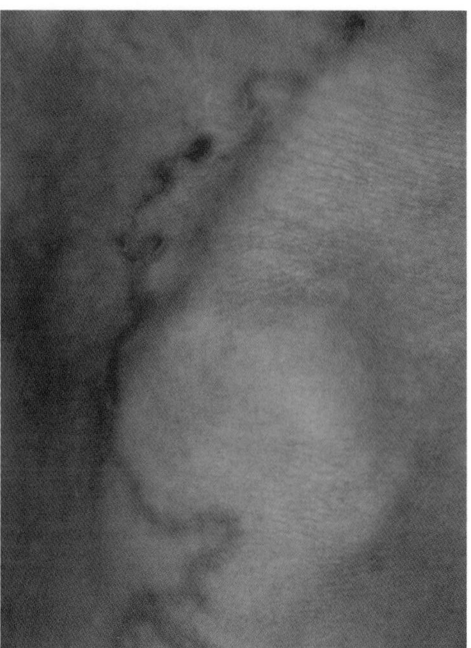

Figure 17.16 Cutaneous larva migrans.

- If the eyelashes are involved use petrolatum only, as insecticides can damage the eyes.

Cutaneous larva migrans

Larvae from nematodes such as the dog/cat hookworm (*Ancylostoma caninum*) and *Strongyloides* parasites accidentally penetrate human skin and then wander aimlessly, unable to invade the deeper tissue causing a superficial creeping eruption (Figure 17.16). In their animal host, the larvae eventually make their way to the gut to complete their lifecycle. Treat the patient with albendazole 400 mg daily for 3 days or ivermectin as a single dose of 200 mg/100 kg body weight.

Further Reading

www.dermnet.com.
www.phmeg.org.uk.

CHAPTER 18

Tropical Dermatology

Rachael Morris-Jones

Dermatology Department, Kings College Hospital, London, UK

OVERVIEW

- The majority of tropical diseases are due to infections and infestations, a large proportion involving the skin.
- Hot humid conditions in the tropics and frequent lack of effective health care mean skin diseases are common and recurrent.
- Pyogenic bacteria commonly involve the skin, causing impetigo and erysipelas.
- The intensity and type of immune response to tropical diseases such as leprosy and leishmaniasis determine the clinical manifestations.
- Cutaneous fungal infections can be very florid, persistent and recurrent.
- In deep fungal infections, there is chronic inflammation in the subcutaneous tissues. These include chromoblastomycosis, mycetoma, blastomycosis and histoplasmosis.
- The most common infestations affecting the skin are scabies and lice. Others include tungiasis, myiasis, onchocerciasis, loiasis (*Loa loa*) and dracunculiasis.

Introduction

Tropical dermatology is a diverse topic covering a multitude of different skin diseases many of which are infections and infestations. This chapter concentrates on tropical diseases involving the skin (bacterial, viral, protozoan, helminth and arthropod related). Health workers in the tropics and subtropics may be familiar with many of the cutaneous presentations in the local population. However, due to the relative ease of world travel more visitors who are immunologically naïve may present locally with atypical features or florid disease. In addition, when these individuals return home they can present to their family medical practitioner who may be unfamiliar with tropical skin diseases.

Hot humid conditions in the tropics and subtropics provide an ideal environment for the proliferation of many organisms. Up to 50% of the local population is estimated to be affected by a skin disease in the tropics, the majority being infections or infestations such as impetigo, tinea and scabies. Many of these conditions are amenable to treatment. However, the hot humid conditions, overcrowding, poverty and the lack of resources mean that skin diseases are common and frequently recurrent. Local simple therapies can be very effective and may be administered by those with only minimal training. Health care infrastructure in the tropics is improving although many areas still suffer from lack of basic medicines and trained healthcare personnel.

Many tropical dermatoses have distinctive clinical features. Skin changes may result from the presence of the organisms, ova or larvae or a reaction in the skin to disease at a distant site.

Bacterial infections

Individuals living and travelling in the tropics are prone to *Staphylococcus aureus* infections on the skin in the form of impetigo (see Chapter 13). Bacterial infections may arise secondary to minor trauma or may be superimposed on any other skin disease. Clinical features include erythema, exudates, vesicles/bullae and crusting. Impetigo is highly contagious and many family members may be infected.

Deeper infections mainly caused by *Streptococcus* result in erysipelas or cellulitis, which may be accompanied by systemic symptoms. The face and limbs are most frequently affected. Deep infections may occur following minor trauma or impaired barrier function due to pre-existing skin diseases such as tinea, scabies, atopic or irritant dermatitis.

The skin changes are characterised by marked erythema and tissue swelling. The patient may have systemic symptoms such as fever, rigors and malaise. Individuals who do not have immediate access to antiseptics or antibiotics may develop severe skin changes and ultimately bacteraemia.

Leprosy

Leprosy is caused by *Mycobacterium leprae*, which results in a chronic granulomatous infection of the skin and peripheral nerves. Leprosy is endemic in Africa, south-east Asia, the Indian subcontinent and South America. Aerosols from the nasal mucosa are thought to be the mode of transmission between humans, but animal reservoirs do exist (nine-banded armadillo, chimpanzees and some monkeys). The incubation period is highly variable (6 months to 40 years) with a mean of 4–6 years.

ABC of Dermatology, Sixth Edition. Edited by Rachael Morris-Jones.

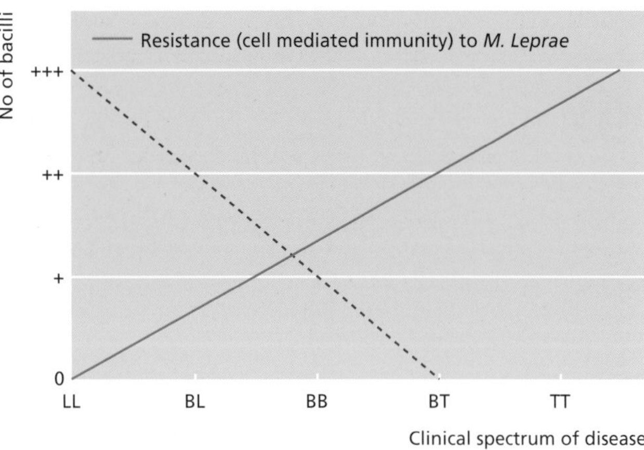

Figure 18.1 Spectrum of clinical disease in leprosy. BB, mid-borderline leprosy; BL, borderline lepromatous leprosy; BT, borderline tuberculoid leprosy; LL, lepromatous leprosy; TT, tuberculoid leprosy.

There is a spectrum of clinical disease (Figure 18.1) depending on the patient's cell-mediated immunity to *M. leprae*. Patients whose immune systems respond poorly have clinical disease characterised by numerous skin lesions with numerous mycobacteria (multibacillary). Patients whose immune systems are responding well to the infection have very few mycobacteria present (paucibacillary) in isolated skin lesions. These two ends of the spectrum are referred to as *tuberculoid leprosy* (good immune response) and *lepromatous leprosy* (*LL*) (poor immune response). Clinical intermediates exist and these are termed *borderline* cases (Figures 18.2–18.5).

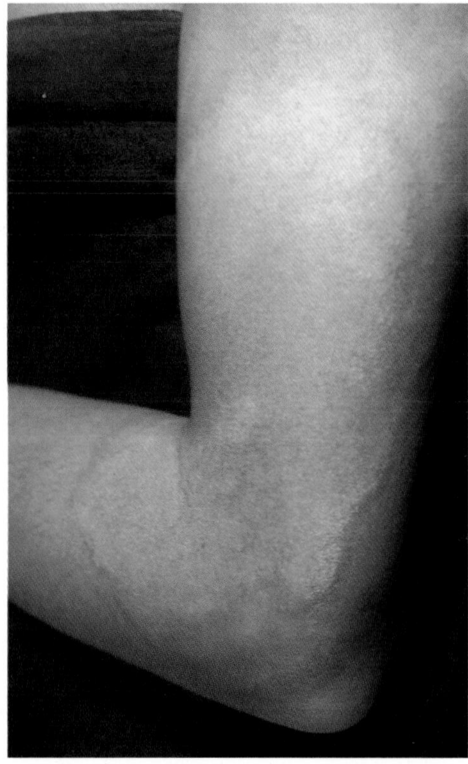

Figure 18.2 Tuberculoid leprosy: hypopigmented patches.

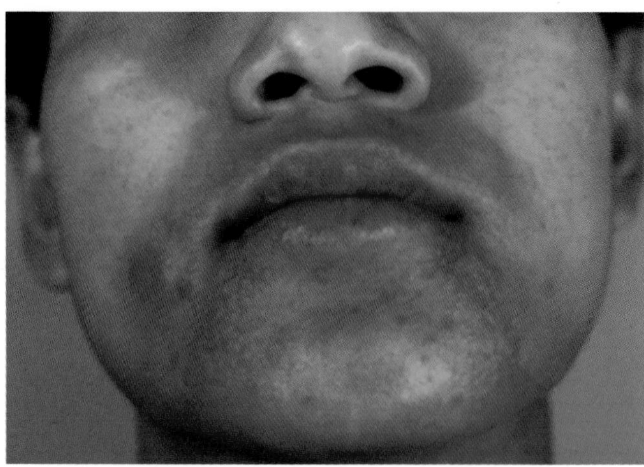

Figure 18.3 Tuberculoid leprosy.

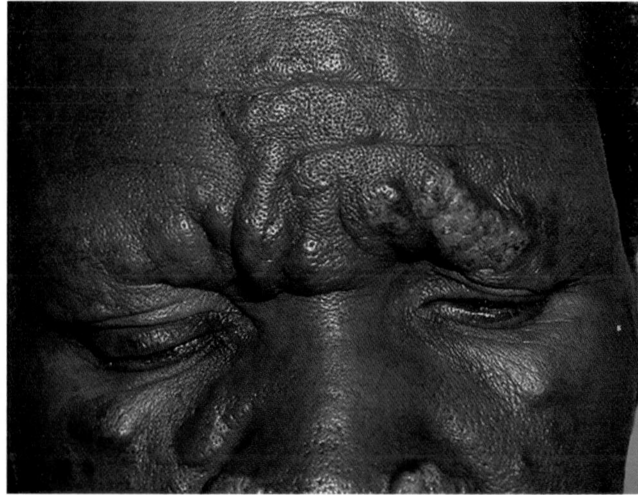

Figure 18.4 Lepromatous leprosy.

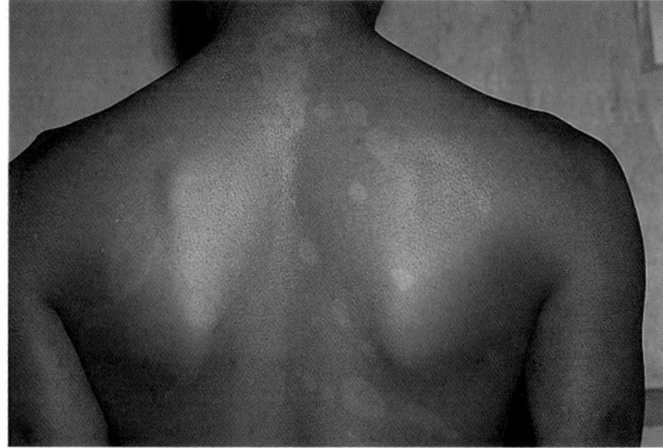

Figure 18.5 Borderline leprosy.

Diagnosis

Typical clinical findings are as follows.

- In tuberculoid leprosy (TT) there is a single anaesthetic patch or plaque with a raised border.
- In LL, there are widespread symmetrical shiny papules, nodules and plaques which are not anaesthetic.
- In borderline leprosy (BT, BB, BL), there are varying numbers of lesions, few in BT and numerous in BL. They may be widespread but are asymmetrical. BB is mid-borderline leprosy.
- Palpably enlarged cutaneous nerves (great auricular nerve in the neck, the superficial branch of the radial nerve at the wrist, the ulnar nerve at the elbow, the lateral popliteal nerve at the knee and the sural nerve on the lower leg).
- Glove and stocking sensory loss leads to secondary changes through trauma such as blisters, erosions and ulcers (neuropathic) on anaesthetic fingers/toes.
- Deformity due to invasion of the peripheral nerves with leprosy bacilli, a leprosy reaction or recurrent trauma to anaesthetic limbs.

Slit skin smears measure the numbers of bacilli in the skin (bacterial index, BI – see Box 18.1) and the percentage of these that are living (morphological index, MI).

Box 18.1 **Bacterial index (BI)**

0 No bacilli seen
1+ 1–10 bacilli in 100 oil immersion fields
2+ 1–10 bacilli in 10 oil immersion fields
3+ 1–10 bacilli in 1 oil immersion field
4+ 10–100 bacilli in an average oil immersion field
5+ 100–1000 bacilli in an average oil immersion field
6+ >1000 bacilli in an average oil immersion field

Treatment

Paucibacillary leprosy (BI of 0 or 1+):

- rifampicin 600 mg once a month
- dapsone 100 mg daily
- for 6 months.

Multibacillary leprosy (BI of 2+ or more):

- rifampicin 600 mg once a month
- clofazimine 300 mg once a month
- clofazimine 50 mg/day
- dapsone 100 mg/day
- for 12 months.

An estimated 20–40% of patients with leprosy develop immunologically mediated reactions (most common in borderline leprosy cases) that can permanently damage nerve function. These so called 'reversal reactions' can be type 1 (T1R delayed hypersensitivity) or type 2 (T2R immune complex mediated). Type 1 reactions are characterised by marked inflammation and oedema in skin lesions, acral oedema and acute neuritis manifested by nerve pain/sudden onset of loss of sensation/function. Urgent treatment with 40–60 mg oral prednisolone daily should be given and then tapering doses over 3–6 months, in addition to the anti-lepromatous therapy. Type 2 reactions resemble erythema nodosum but are generally more widespread and the erythematous nodules may be superficial as well as deep, and may ulcerate. Neuritis may accompany the erythema nodosum leprosum, systemic upset (fever, malaise), photophobia and iritis and so on. Patients should be treated promptly with aspirin and oral prednisolone.

Cutaneous leishmaniasis

Leishmaniasis affects approximately 12 million people worldwide and is found in over 80 countries (in the 'Old World' in Africa, Asia and Europe and in the 'New World' in Central and South America). Leishmaniasis is caused by *Leishmania* protozoan parasites transmitted by the bite of the female sandfly (usually at night). Rarely in humans transmission via blood transfusion, congenital passage and sexual intercourse have been reported. Animal reservoirs include dogs, rodents, foxes and jackals. Clinically, leishmaniasis is classified into cutaneous, mucocutaneous and visceral, depending on the parasite's ability to proliferate at a particular temperature. Therefore, the amastigote parasites may remain in the skin or be carried by macrophages to internal organs. There are many different species of *Leishmania* parasites, each restricted to a particular geographical region (Box 18.2).

Box 18.2 **Cutaneous leishmaniasis**

New World (Americas)

Leishmania tropica mexicana, *Leishmania amazonensis*, *Leishmania brasiliensis* (cutaneous + mucocutaneous)

Old World

L. tropica, *Leishmania major*, *Leishmania aethiopica* (mucocutaneous), *Leishmania infantum* (cutaneous + visceral)

Cutaneous lesions usually on exposed skin sites develop within weeks of the sandfly bite. Children are more frequently affected than adults. Several family members may be affected simultaneously, often bitten by the same sandfly. Painless erythematous papules leading to nodules and eventually ulceration can classically be seen. The clinical presentation varies according to the host's nutritional state, their immunity and the *Leishmania* species involved. Spontaneous resolution may occur after 2–10 months, but latent reactivation after several years in an area of minor skin trauma means leishmaniasis can be an unpredictable disease.

Mucosal involvement may occur in isolation or concurrently with cutaneous lesions, and in some cases there may be a delay of up to 20 years between the appearance of cutaneous and mucosal lesions. Mucosal lesions may be painful and can lead to nasal obstruction, congestion, tissue destruction and bleeding.

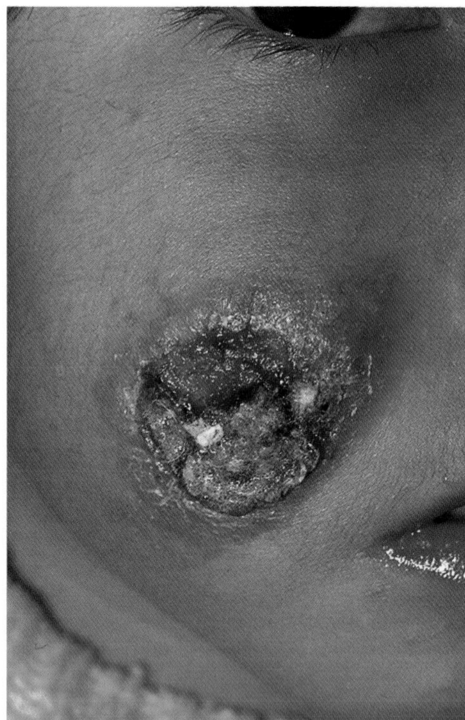

Figure 18.6 Acute leishmaniasis.

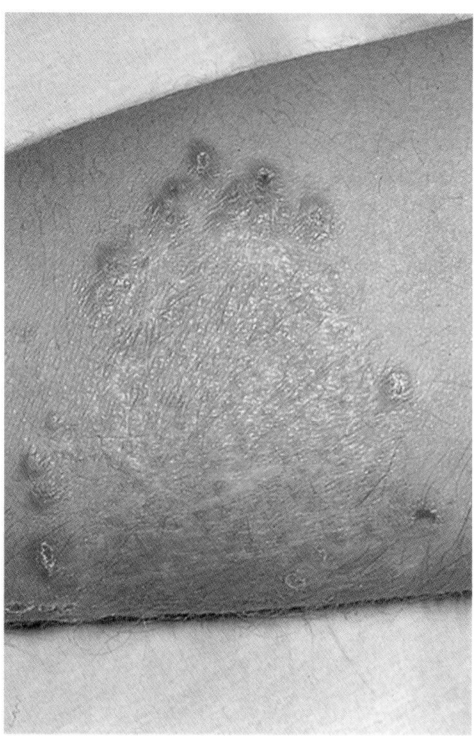

Figure 18.7 Chronic leishmaniasis.

Acute leishmaniasis

A red nodule similar to a boil ('Delhi boil', 'Balkan sore') occurs at the site of the bite. The nodules enlarge and may ulcerate (moist and exudative or dry and crusted) (Figure 18.6). Lesions usually heal spontaneously after approximately 1 year, leaving a pale cribriform scar.

Chronic leishmaniasis

In a patient with good cell-mediated immunity, after the acute leishmaniasis has healed, new granulomas appear at the edge of the scar; these do not heal spontaneously (Figure 18.7).

Diffuse cutaneous leishmaniasis

This is leishmaniasis in a patient with no immunity to the organism (equivalent to LL). Extensive skin nodules occur with numerous organisms (Figure 18.8).

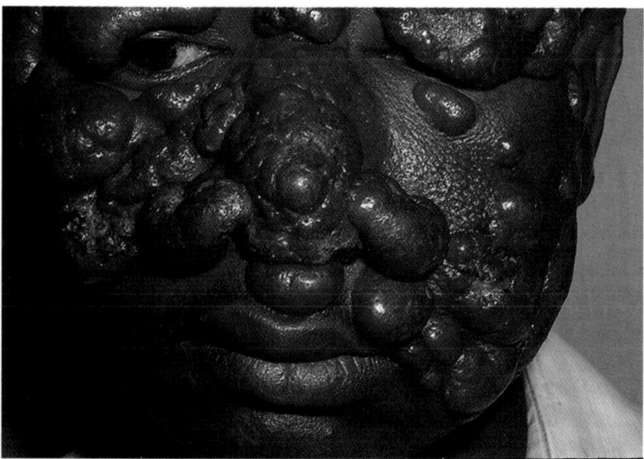

Figure 18.8 Diffuse cutaneous leishmaniasis.

Diagnosis

Diagnosis is usually made from a history of travel to an endemic area and clinical appearances of the lesions. Skin biopsy stained with Giemsa will demonstrate the parasites in over 50% of cases, and modern polymerase chain reaction (PCR) techniques can be useful in determining the species responsible which can help guide management.

Leishmaniasis skin testing is used in some countries where killed parasites are injected into the dermis and the reaction measured at 48 h. This is, however, not positive in acute infections and in endemic areas is often positive in over 70% of the population. If visceral leishmaniasis is suspected then serology testing with an indirect fluorescent antibody test (IFAT)/Western blot or ELISA can be highly specific and sensitive.

Treatment

A proportion of cutaneous lesions will heal spontaneously or resolve following simple treatments such as cryotherapy, heat treatment or surgery.

Pentavalent antimonials sodium stibogluconate (Pentostam) or meglumine antimoniate are the main therapeutic agents used to treat cutaneous leishmaniasis in most countries. Intralesional stibogluconate can be injected into the affected skin (1–3 ml injected around the active edge of the lesion – repeated fortnightly over approximately 6–8 weeks is highly effective) or local applications of paromomycin can be effective for isolated cutaneous lesions. Systemic stibogluconate i.v./i.m. (200 mg test dose followed by 20 mg/kg daily) should be used until healing occurs (usually 2–3 weeks, although some experts consider four treatments sufficient).

Amphotericin B deoxycholate and liposomal amphotericin B (AmBisome) 0.5–3 mg/kg given on alternate days have been shown to be highly effective but must be administered intravenously and can be expensive. An alternative agent is pentamidine 2–4 mg/kg on alternate days (maximum 15 doses). Miltefosine is the first highly effective oral preparation for the treatment of leishmaniasis. A 28-day treatment course leads to 90% cure rates. It is currently used in India, Colombia and Germany, and although it is generally well tolerated it is teratogenic. There is some evidence that itraconazole and ketoconazole can be effective for treating leishmaniasis.

Superficial fungal infections

The warm moist conditions in the tropics and subtropics are ideal for the survival and proliferation of fungal species in the environment and on the skin. Cutaneous fungal infections can be very florid, persistent and recurrent (Figure 18.9). There are also many fungal infections that are specifically found in the tropics. These include tinea imbricata, tinea nigra, piedra and favus (Table 18.1).

Superficial dermatophyte fungal infections (see Chapter 16) generally present with itching. Lesions often expand slowly from a small focus on the skin to form rings or annular lesions, where the edge is active and there is central clearing. The margins are usually palpable and the lesions scaly.

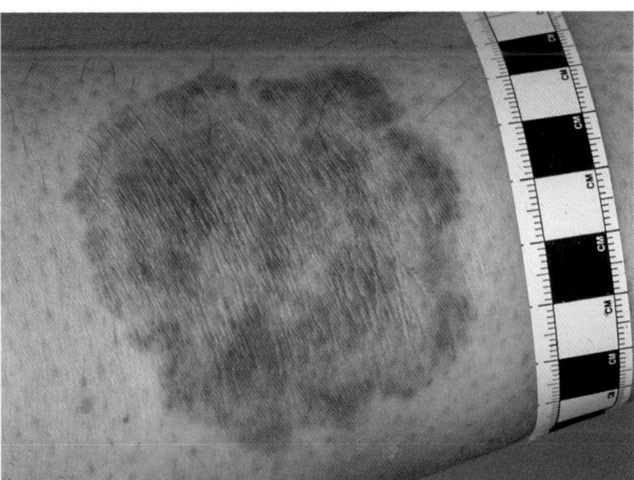

Figure 18.9 Superficial fungal infection.

Table 18.1 Tropical fungal infections of the skin.

Superficial cutaneous infection	Black/white piedra, tinea nigra, *Malassezia* yeast
Cutaneous infection	Tinea, *Trichophyton*, *Scytalidium*, *Candida*
Subcutaneous infection	Sporotrichosis, chromoblastomycosis, mycetoma
Systemic infection with cutaneous signs	*Fusarium*, *Penicillium marneffei*, *Histoplasma*, lobomycosis, blastomycosis

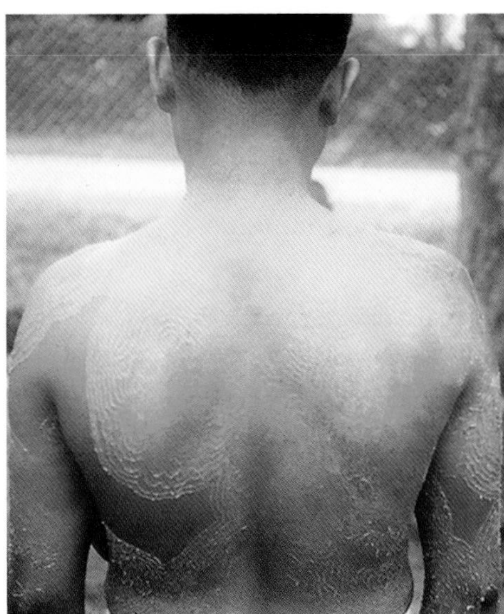

Figure 18.10 Tinea imbricata.

Tinea imbricata due to *Trichophyton concentricum* is characterised by superficial concentric scaling rings spreading across the trunk (Figure 18.10). The condition is frequently chronic and relapsing. It occurs mainly in Central/South America and Asia. Topical Whitfield's ointment may be effective or oral griseofulvin or terbinafine.

Tinea nigra caused by *Cladosporium werneckii* occurs in the tropical areas of America, Asia and Australia. The pigmented fungus invades the stratum corneum usually through contact with contaminated soil, vegetation or sewage. Hyperpigmented brown or black macules are seen most commonly on the palms and soles. Treatment with keratolytic agents (salicylic acid preparations and topical retinoids) can be effective due to the very superficial nature of the infection. Topical antifungals such as terbinafine, miconazole, ketoconazole and clotrimazole are also effective.

Piedra is a fungal infection of the hair producing hard nodular lesions on the hair shaft. The lesions may be black (due to *Piedraia hortae*) or white (due to *Trichosporon beigelii*). The nodules consist of clumps of fungal hyphae that can be difficult to remove from the hair shaft when the fungus is pigmented. Hair removal has traditionally been used to clear infections. Salicylic acid, formaldehyde preparations and antifungal creams are also effective. Re-infection rates are high.

Favus is most commonly seen in North/South Africa, Brasil, Pakistan and the Middle East and rarely in Europe (Poland). Favus is caused by an endothrix fungus – *Trichophyton schoenleinii* – which causes a thick yellow crust (honeycomb appearance) usually on the scalp, but nails and glabrous skin may also be affected. The confluent areas of yellow adherent crusts are frequently secondarily infected with bacteria and have an unpleasant odour. Erythematous areas of scarring occur that must be differentiated from lichen planus and other causes of scarring alopecia.

Prolonged systemic treatment with griseofulvin, terbinafine or itraconazole is usually effective.

Deep fungal infections

In these conditions, there is chronic inflammation in the subcutaneous tissues leading to granulomatous and necrotic nodules.

Mycetoma (Madura foot)

This is a chronic granulomatous infection of the dermis and subcutaneous fat caused by various species of fungus (eumycetoma) or bacteria (actinomycetoma). Endemic areas include Asia, Africa and South America. Mycetoma most commonly occurs on the foot of an agricultural worker but any skin site can be affected. Traumatic implantation is thought to be the mode of transmission of the organism into the subcutis. Patients most commonly present with a swollen foot and multiple discharging sinuses (Figure 18.11). The infective 'grains' can be seen as tiny dark or pale bodies within the discharging purulent exudate. These can be teased out with a sterile needle and identified by microscopy and culture. Many fungal species (*Acremonium*, *Fusarium*, *Aspergillus*, *Madurella*, *Exophilia*) and actinomycetes bacteria (*Nocardia*, *Actinomadura*, *Streptomyces*) have been implicated in the aetiology of mycetoma. Identification of the organism is important as this guides treatment.

Diagnosis

- Examination of the discharging grains (colour will give a clue as to the cause).
- Culture of the grains to identify the causative fungus or bacterium.
- If no grains can be found, a skin biopsy may be needed.
- Radiological imaging may demonstrate bone involvement.

Treatment

Fungal mycetoma

A combination of medical and surgical treatment is frequently recommended for these difficult infections.

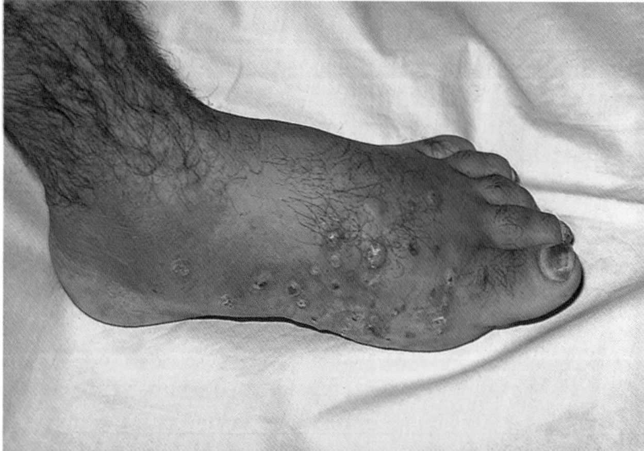

Figure 18.11 Madura foot.

- Surgical excision of affected tissue if disease is limited. Amputation if extensive.
- Ketoconazole (200–400 mg daily) or itraconazole (200 mg twice daily) for at least 12 months. In addition, the newer agent posaconazole 800 mg daily for up to 34 months has been shown to be highly effective.

Bacterial mycetoma

Two drugs may be used for a synergistic effect.

- Sulfamethoxazole/trimethoprim mixture 960 mg twice daily (for up to 2 years).
- Other agents include dapsone, streptomycin, rifampicin, amikacin and imipenem.

Chromoblastomycosis

This is a chronic granulomatous condition that mainly affects the legs. Chromoblastomycosis results from traumatic implantation of a variety of parasitic fungi including *Fonsecaea*, *Cladosporium* and *Philalophora* into the skin. The disease is characterised by large spreading verrucous nodules or plaques from the site of implantation (Figure 18.12). In some cases, the whole of the lower leg can be affected, with blockage of lymphatic ducts leading to an elephantiasis-type appearance.

Diagnosis is usually straightforward with typical fungal Medlar (thick walled sclerotic) bodies being visualised on microscopy from a scraping or skin biopsy. Treatment has been extremely difficult in the past; cryosurgery has been used with some success as has itraconazole 200 mg twice daily. However, recent reports of cure rates around 80% with posaconazole 800 mg daily are highly encouraging. Healing usually occurs with depressed pale scarring. In refractory cases surgery may be required.

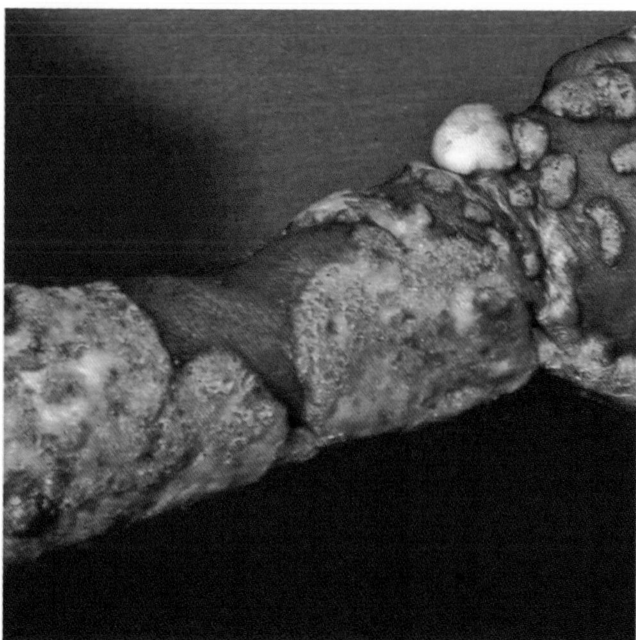

Figure 18.12 Chromoblastomycosis.

Blastomycosis

The spores of the fungus *Paracoccidioides brasiliensis* are most commonly inhaled leading to respiratory infection; however, skin lesions occur in 20% of patients leading to single or multiple cutaneous nodules. Skin lesions most commonly affect the face/neck and extremities and appear as violaceous papules/nodules that expand and may ulcerate, with studded pustules around the edge of the lesions. The differential diagnosis of the skin lesions includes tuberculosis and other mycoses such as sporotrichosis, chromoblastomycosis and coccidiomycosis. Blastomycosis most commonly occurs in Central and South America. In suspected cases, patients should be investigated with a chest X-ray, sputum culture, bronchoscopy, skin biopsy (Periodic acid Schiff (PAS) stain) and serological tests if available. Treatment options include itraconazole 200 mg three times a day for 3 days and then twice daily for 6 months, or liposomal amphotericin B 3–5 mg/kg/day for 2 weeks initially before switching to oral itraconazole.

Histoplasmosis

Histoplasma capsulatum is the fungal organism responsible for histoplasmosis. Two forms of the fungi exist: *H. capsulatum var. capsulatum* and *H. capsulatum var. duboisii*. The former mainly in North/Central America and Eastern Asia, causes respiratory disease, and the latter skin and bone disease in West Africa. In endemic areas up to 80% of the local population has been infected; however, the majority of infections are asymptomatic with spontaneous resolution. Disseminated disease can occur in immunocompromised individuals, the elderly and young children. The cutaneous form leads to nodules and ulcers at the site of traumatic implantation that can progress to deeper tissues leading to bony involvement. The disease is usually treated with itraconazole 100–400 mg daily for 3 months or amphotericin B (Figure 18.13).

Infestations

Tungiasis

Invasion of the skin by sand fleas (*Tunga penetrans*) causes tungiasis in tropical areas of Africa, America and India. Pregnant female fleas (measuring 1 mm across) burrow into the plantar skin, especially under the toes and toe nails (Figure 18.14). A marked inflammatory reaction occurs at the skin site, leading to encapsulation of the parasite. Clinically, lesions can appear white with a black central dot – not dissimilar to a plantar wart. Dermoscopy can help visualise the central plugged opening of the flea's burrow. The release of flea eggs through the central opening may be seen if one is lucky.

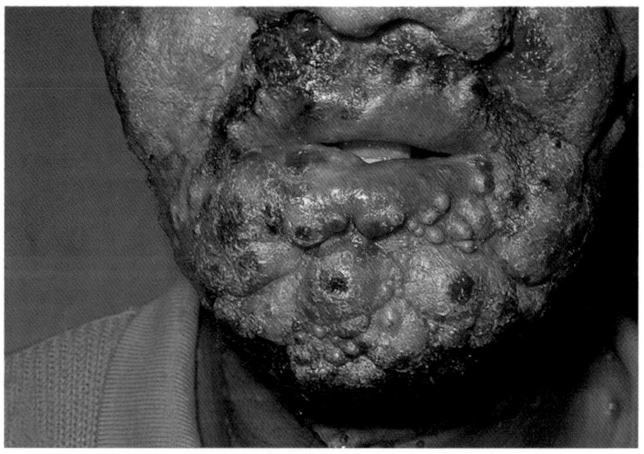

Figure 18.13 Histoplasmosis in HIV infection.

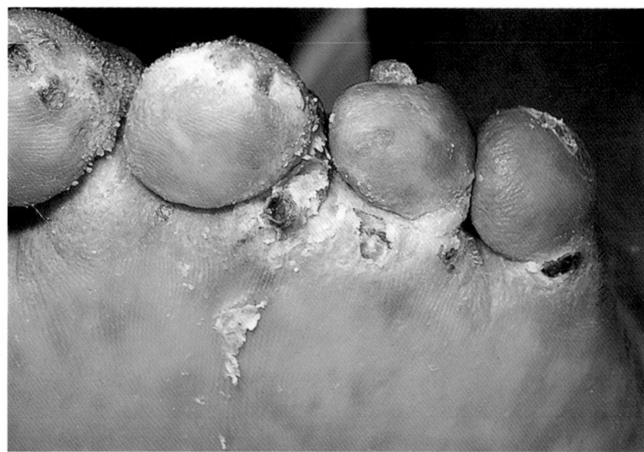

Figure 18.14 Tungiasis.

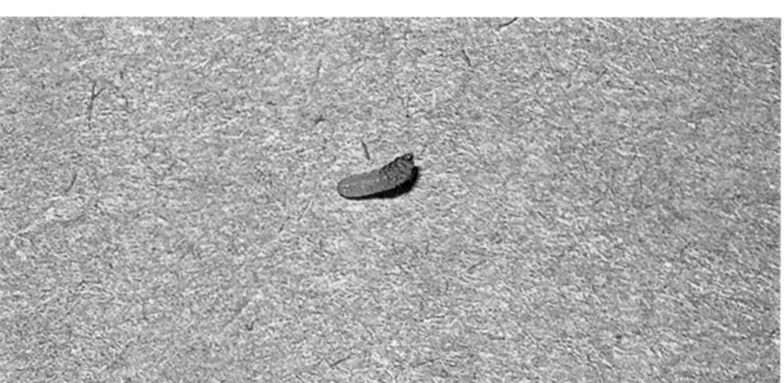

Figure 18.15 Myiasis: larva.

The disease can usually be prevented by wearing shoes and keeping skin exposure to a minimum. (Vaseline with 10% kerosene applied daily can prevent the tunga flea from penetrating.)

Removal of the flea is both diagnostic and therapeutic. The flea can be winkled out with a pin or sterile needle (most individuals in endemic areas perform this themselves). If the fleas are very extensive, soak the feet in kerosene or treat with a single dose of ivermectin 200 μg/kg body weight.

Subcutaneous myiasis

Invasion of the skin by the larvae of the tumbu (mango) fly (*Cordylobia anthropophaga*) in sub-Saharan Africa causes myiasis. The fly lays her eggs on dry soil or clothes laid out to dry; these hatch out 2 days later and the larvae can survive up to 2 weeks waiting for an opportunity to invade a new host animal. When the clothes are worn the larvae burrow into the skin, causing a red painful or itchy papule/nodule, predominantly on the trunk, buttocks and thighs (Figure 18.15).

Other flies that cause myiasis:

- *Dermatobia hominis* – tropical Bot fly, in Mexico, Central and South America, with tender nodules developing on the scalp, legs,

forearms and face. The bot fly lays her eggs on the abdomen of a blood-sucking insect (usually a mosquito) and when that insect subsequently takes a blood meal the eggs hatch and penetrate the skin through the bite site or broken skin. Larvae are able to 'grab' onto hair while the mosquito is feeding leading to a high proportion of myiasis infestations affecting the scalp skin.
- *Aucheronia* sp. – Congo floor maggot, in Central and southern Africa; bites of the larvae cause intense irritation.
- *Callitroga* sp. in Central America causing inflamed lesions with necrosis.

Preventative measures include ironing clothes before wearing them to kill the eggs. Treatment of skin lesions with an application of petroleum jelly or grease (applied in a thick layer – left in place for 30–60 min under an occlusive dressing) causes the larvae either to suffocate or crawl out of the skin.

Filariasis

Thread-like helminths ('filum' from the Latin: thread) cause an infestation in humans when transmitted by insect vectors such as mosquitoes. There are many different species of filarial worms that live in the lymphatics and connective tissue. The basic life cycle starts in humans when the fertilised eggs develop into microfilariae. These are taken up by insect vectors (intermediate hosts) in which further development occurs; the mature stages are then inoculated back into humans when the insects bite.

Three diseases are caused by filarial worms.

- Lymphatic filariasis due to *Wuchereria bancrofti*, which liberate microfilariae into the bloodstream.
- Onchocerciasis due to *Onchocera volvulus*. The microfilariae are liberated into the skin and subcutaneous tissues.
- Loiasis due to *L. loa*, in which microfilariae are found in the blood.

Lymphatic filariasis affects 120 million people in 73 countries (34% in sub-Saharan Africa). The adult worms can live for up to 4–6 years in the lymphatic vessels leading to dilatation, tortuosity and malfunction. Lymphoedema results in the draining tissues, usually the legs, genitalia and breasts (Figure 18.16). Individuals may be asymptomatic for long periods with adult worms producing thousands of microfilariae each day. These are picked up by mosquitoes when they take a blood meal and are passed on to the next host when they feed again.

The diagnosis can be confirmed by examining a thick blood smear taken at midnight. More convenient detection of filarial antigens can be done at any time and takes just 5 min to complete. Fingerprick blood is placed on an immunochromatographic filariasis card to detect circulating *W. bancrofti* antigens. PCR techniques are highly sensitive and can detect one microfilaria in 1 ml of blood.

Treatment

In endemic areas, the whole community should be treated with a single dose of two of the following three drugs once a year for 4–6 years:

- Ivermectin 400 μg/kg body weight
- diethylcarbamazine (DEC) 6 mg/kg body weight
- albendazole 600 mg.

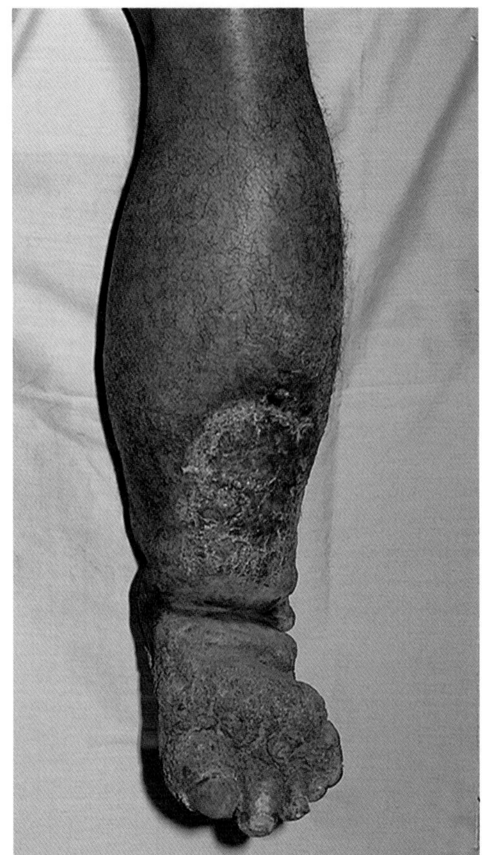

Figure 18.16 Lymphoedema of the legs in filariasis.

The chronic lymphoedema can be improved by keeping the legs moving and raising the legs when sitting, and secondary bacterial infection can be prevented by regular washing and moisturising of the skin.

Podoconiosis is a non-filariasis cause of lymphoedema of the lower legs in people exposed to red volcanic soil high in silicates. Endemic areas include the highlands of Ethiopia, parts of India and Central America. The aetiology is thought to be a combination of genetic predisposition and chronic exposure to particular soil types of bare skin of the feet. The most commonly affected are those working the land who do not wear shoes. The resultant inflammation in the skin causes damage to the lymphatics, which lead to a 'mossy' appearance of the foot with papules, nodules, swelling and marked lymphoedema which may be uni- or bilateral. Treatment includes washing the feet, compression and getting patients into shoes (those made initially need to be custom made to fit the enlarged feet). Prevention through education and getting local populations to wear shoes should help reduce the incidence of this neglected tropical disease.

Onchocerciasis

Onchocerciasis (river blindness) occurs in Africa south of the Sahara and in Central America. It is due to *O. volvulus* transmitted by the bite of blackflies *Simulium damnosum* which breed by fast-flowing rivers. The inoculation of microfilariae by the bite of

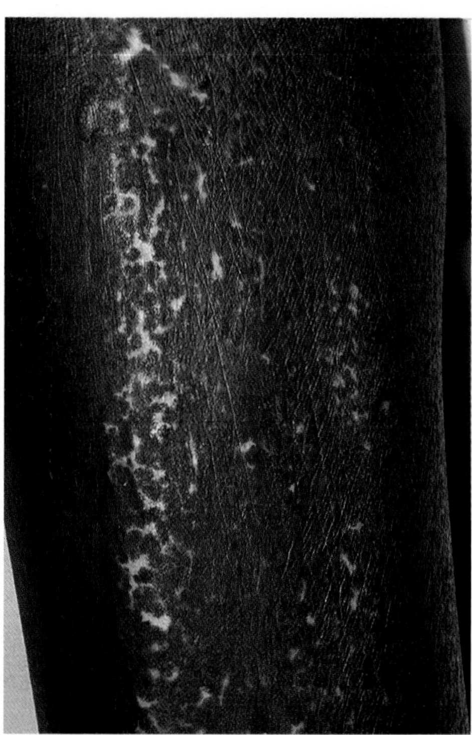

Figure 18.17 'Leopard skin' in onchocerciasis.

a blackfly causes intense local inflammation and is followed by an incubation period of 1–2 years. The adult worms live in nodules around the hips and in themselves cause no harm. However, they produce thousands of microfilariae each day which travel to the skin and eyes. In the skin, they produce a very itchy rash which looks similar to lichenified eczema. On the lower legs, there is often spotty depigmentation (Figure 18.17). Involvement of the eyes causes blindness.

Risk factors for being infected

- Living, working or playing near fast-flowing rivers.
- Not wearing enough clothes so that the skin is exposed to insect bites.
- The construction of dams leading to less breeding of blackflies within the dam itself but increased breeding in the dam spillways.

Diagnosis

The microfilariae can be demonstrated by skin snips or slit-lamp examination of the eyes. Skin snips are usually taken from six sites (iliac crests, scapulae and calf bilaterally). Very superficial samples of skin (without drawing blood) are taken and placed in saline; within an hour the microfilariae can be seen on microscopy. Removal of a skin nodule can reveal the adult worms. PCR to show parasite DNA and ELISA tests are now available in some countries.

Treatment

Spray the breeding areas with insecticides. An annual dose of ivermectin (400 μg/kg for 4–6 years) should be taken by all those living in endemic areas to prevent the release of microfilariae from the adult worms. In addition, Doxycycline 100 mg daily for 6 weeks helps kill the adult worms or sterilise the females by killing the symbiotic bacteria Wolbachia in their gut, leading to lower worm burdens.

Loiasis (*Loa loa*)

Loiasis occurs in the rain forests of Central and West Africa. It is transmitted by mango flies, deer and horseflies. The adult worms live in the subcutaneous tissues where they can be seen in the skin and under the conjunctivae. The microfilariae are only found in the blood. Hypersensitivity to the worms shows itself as swelling of the skin, particularly of the wrists and ankles (Calabar swellings), which are itchy and erythematous.

Diagnosis

- Thick blood film to look for microfilariae (sample taken between 10 AM and 2 PM).
- Adult worms can be identified by soft-tissue ultrasound examination.
- Immunoassay for antigen detection may be the most reliable test.

Treatment

- A single dose of ivermectin 400 μg/kg body weight or a 3-week course of albendazole 400 mg/kg body weight/twice daily.
- Diethylcarbamazine (DEC) should be avoided as this can cause death as a result of a reaction to toxins from the rapid destruction of the microfilariae.

Dracunculiasis

Dracunculus medinensis or 'Guinea worm' is a nematode that infests the connective tissue of humans. It is acquired from drinking fresh water containing the intermediate host, a copepod (*Cyclops*) that contains the parasitic larvae. From the gastrointestinal tract, the female mature nematode migrates to the subcutaneous tissue, usually of the lower leg. Papules develop at the skin site containing the female worm and numerous microfilariae which are released on contact with water. Treatment consists of very carefully extracting the worm by winding it onto a stick (a few centimetres per day) over several weeks (adults can be 1 m long). Symptomatic treatment of secondary infection and allergic reactions is also required. If the adult worm dies in the extremity it may become encased in calcium, causing chronic pain and leg swelling.

To prevent exposure to the larvae, water should be filtered or boiled before drinking. Swimming in fresh water in endemic areas should be avoided, in order to break the life cycle.

Further Reading

Lucchina LC, Wilson M et al. *Colour Atlas of Travel Dermatology*, Blackwell Publishing, Oxford, 2006.

Tyring SK, Lupi O and Hengge UR. *Tropical Dermatology*, Churchill Livingstone, Oxford, 2005.

CHAPTER 19

Hair and Scalp

Kapil Bhargava and David Fenton

St. John's Institute of Dermatology, Guy's and St. Thomas' Hospitals, London, UK

OVERVIEW

- Hair grows in a cyclic manner.
- Hair loss or alopecia may be scarring or non-scarring, resulting in permanent loss of hair follicles. It may be generalised or localised, with or without inflammation.
- Androgenetic alopecia is the most common cause of hair loss and affects men and women. Topical, oral and surgical therapies can provide benefit.
- Common types of non-scarring alopecia include androgenetic alopecia, alopecia areata, telogen effluvium and tinea capitis.
- Scarring alopecia is less common and maybe divided into lymphocytic and neutrophilic disorders.
- Hair treatments and styling can result in scarring alopecia.
- Excess or diminished growth of hair may indicate underlying disease.

Introduction

Human hair plays a significant role in the self-image of individuals and the image they present to the world. Healthy hair conveys a sense of well-being, vitality and youthfulness and as such it cannot be overestimated how devastating diseases affecting this vital organ can be. Excess hair growth in females, particularly in prominent sites such as the face, is not only an embarrassment but may indicate underlying systemic disease.

Hair cycle

Hair is a modified type of keratin and is produced by the hair matrix, which is equivalent to the epidermis. Three types of hair occur in humans.

1. Lanugo hair covers the foetus in utero and is normally shed before birth. This is long and silken.
2. Vellus hair covers the whole body (sparing the palms and soles only) and is short, fine and non-pigmented.
3. Terminal hair is limited to the eyebrows, lashes and scalp until puberty; following puberty secondary terminal hair develops in the axillae, pubic region and on the central chest in men in response to androgens. It is coarser than vellus hair and tends to be darker and longer.

The hair follicle is unique among epidermal structures in that it grows in cycles (Figure 19.1). There are three phases.

1. Anagen – the active growth phase, which typically lasts 1000 days depending on predetermined genetic factors (as opposed to body hair which lasts from 1 to 6 months).
2. Catagen – the short growth arrest phase, of approximately 10 days.

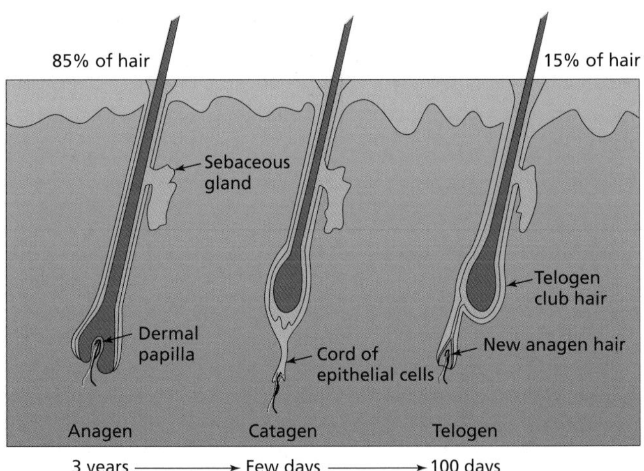

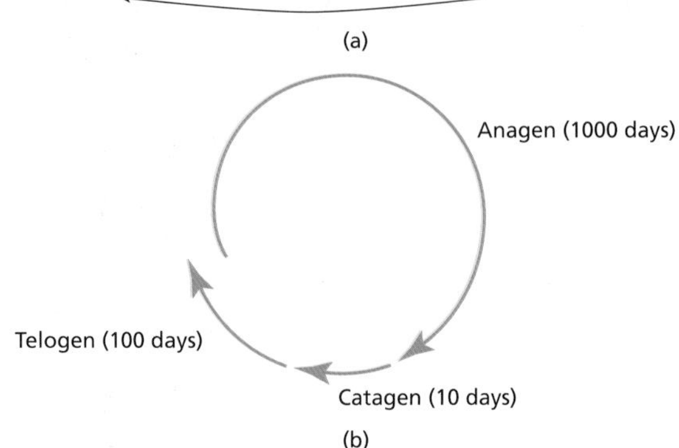

Figure 19.1 (a) Diagrammatic cross-section of hair at various growth phases. (b) Hair growth cycle.

ABC of Dermatology, Sixth Edition. Edited by Rachael Morris-Jones.

3 Telogen – the resting phase, lasting approximately 100 days irrespective of location.

The ratio of anagen to telogen hairs is 9:1 reflecting the fact that only a few hairs at a time are in catagen phase. On average, 100 hairs are shed per day although seasonal variation does occur.

Hair loss

Hair loss or alopecia can be divided into scarring and non-scarring types depending on the underlying pathological process, and these can then be further categorised according to distribution, either diffuse or localised.

Non-scarring alopecias

Androgenetic alopecia

Androgenetic alopecia (AGA) is synonymous with male-pattern baldness and is the most prevalent form of hair loss, affecting about 50% of Caucasian males to some extent by the age of 50. It also affects a significant number of women and is synonymous with female pattern hair loss (FPHL) (Figure 19.2). It is an androgen-dependent trait, requiring a genetic predisposition, and becomes more prevalent with advancing age. It causes hair loss over the temples (fronto-temporal recession) or vertex in men and may progress to leave a horse-shoe distribution of hair over the ears and occipital scalp. Women experience thinning over the central scalp, often presenting with a widening of their parting. In contrast to men, there is usually preservation of the frontal margin. Over time, the follicles become smaller, producing shorter and finer hairs.

The more potent androgen, dihydrotestosterone (DHT), formed by the action of 5α-reductase on testosterone is the main driver of hair loss, particularly in men. Circulating levels of androgens are often within the normal range in both sexes, however. In some premenopausal women, there may be other signs of androgenisation suggesting gonadal (e.g. polycystic ovarian syndrome) or rarely adrenal disorders and elevated circulating androgens maybe present. The diagnosis particularly in men is straightforward; however, chronic telogen effluvium and rarely diffuse alopecia areata (AA) may be considered.

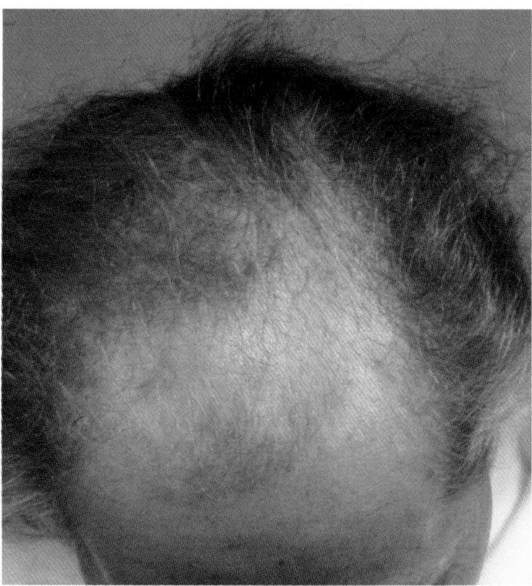

Figure 19.2 Female androgenetic alopecia.

There is currently no cure for AGA and few treatments have been shown to be effective. Two drugs which are currently licensed to promote hair growth in men with AGA are oral finasteride and topical minoxidil. Minoxidil provides improvement in around 60% of men after use for at least 3–6 months. Benefit may be sustained from continued use, but is lost on cessation. Finasteride is a 5α-reductase inhibitor and reduces circulating DHT levels. Daily dosing with 1 mg orally may slow hair loss and improve growth. There is a small increased incidence of sexual dysfunction, for example, impotence in men.

Minoxidil also provides benefit in FPHL. Combined oral contraceptives may increase sex-hormone-binding globulin (SHBG) levels, leading to a reduction in free testosterone. Anti-androgens such as spironolactone, flutamide and cyproterone acetate are most useful in women with hyperandrogenism, although each requires monitoring for side effects, some of which are significant. Finasteride and dutasteride may also be beneficial; however, the dose of finasteride required maybe higher than in men.

Hair transplantation is an option where medical therapy fails. It is only possible if there is an adequate donor area, which in AGA is usually the occiput or the sides of the scalp. For follicular unit hair transplantation (FUT), hair follicles are harvested by excising a strip of skin, and individual follicular units, each consisting of 1–4 hairs, are dissected out and implanted into the bald areas. Consideration should be made of future areas of loss pre-operatively, and any progressive pathology should be treated or accounted for.

Alopecia areata

AA is an organ-specific autoimmune disease, which leads to non-scarring alopecia. It affects 0.15% of the population and can affect any hair-bearing part of the body. Extensive involvement may lead to total scalp hair loss (alopecia totalis), total body hair loss (alopecia universalis) or localised hair loss along the scalp margin (ophiasis).

AA typically presents with smooth round or oval patches of non-scarring hair loss on the scalp (Figure 19.3). Exclamation mark hairs, when present, are diagnostic of AA. These characteristic hairs break at their distal point as they taper and lose pigment proximally, giving them the appearance of an exclamation mark and occur at the periphery of patches of alopecia (Figure 19.4). Nail abnormalities, predominantly pitting or roughening, may occur in association with this condition (Figure 19.5). Other organ-specific autoimmune disorders such as vitiligo and thyroiditis are occasionally associated with AA. Investigation of associated diseases is usually indicated if symptomatic.

The age of onset is usually in the first two decades. The course of AA is difficult to predict. Poor prognostic markers include

- childhood onset of disease
- atopy
- ophiasis (band of alopecia in occipital region)
- nail dystrophy
- family history of other autoimmune disorders
- presence of autoantibodies.

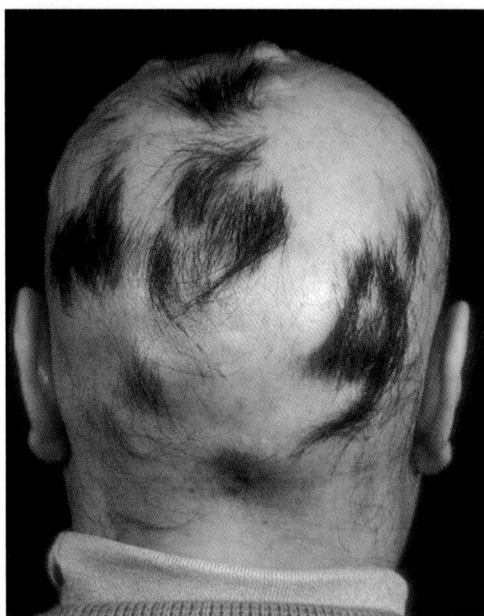

Figure 19.3 Alopecia areata.

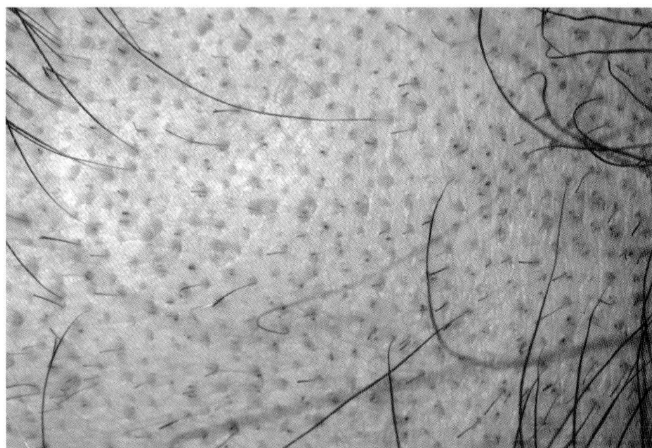

Figure 19.4 Exclamation mark hairs.

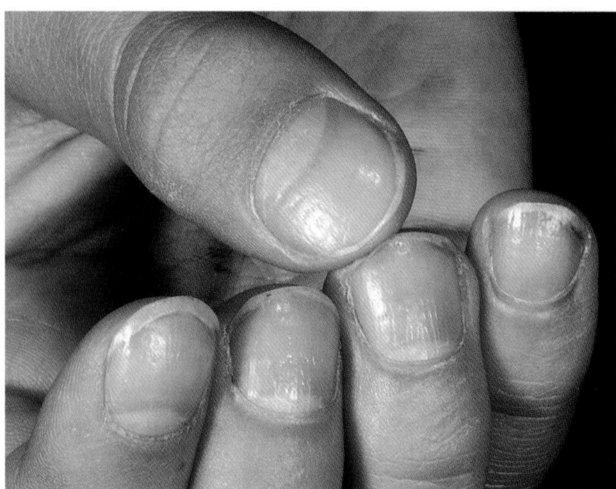

Figure 19.5 Nail pitting associated with alopecia areata.

Trichotillomania, traction alopecia, telogen effluvium, AGA and tinea capitis should all be excluded by clinical examination, appropriate mycology and skin biopsy where there is diagnostic difficulty. In AA, the hair follicle is not injured and maintains the potential to regrow hair should the disease go into remission. There is, however, no cure for AA and no universally proven treatment to stimulate hair regrowth and sustain remission. It is unclear if any of the treatment options available alter the course of the disease. Treatment is therefore guided by the extent of the disease and the age of the person being treated.

Current treatments include the following.

Topical/intralesional corticosteroids. Potent topical corticosteroids can be used on the scalp for 2–3 months on localised patches of alopecia. Intradermal injection of triamcinolone diluted with local anaesthetic can be used. This may stimulate localised regrowth of hair. Unfortunately, it often falls again and there is a risk of causing atrophy. Topical steroid lotion can be used but results are variable.

Systemic immunosuppression. This includes short-term systemic corticosteroids and oral psoralens with exposure to ultraviolet light A (PUVA).

Contact sensitisation using either irritants (dithranol or retinoids) or allergens (diphencyprone).

Topical minoxidil (also used in combination with corticosteroids).

Platelet rich plasma injected into the affected scalp areas.

Other non-scarring alopecias

Telogen effluvium

In the normal scalp, each hair follicle passes through the growth cycle independently, or asynchronously. However, following a number of stimuli the majority of hair follicles may enter the resting phase (telogen) at the same time (synchronously) resulting in diffuse shedding approximately 2 months after the triggering event, often described as the hair 'falling out by the roots'. This is usually an acute self-limiting phenomenon, usually resolving within 6 months; however, chronic telogen effluvium may occur (Table 19.1).

Post-febrile alopecia refers to hair loss as a result of high fever. It has been reported in a wide range of infectious diseases (including glandular fever, influenza, malaria and brucellosis) and inflammatory bowel disease.

Dietary factors such as iron deficiency and hypoproteinaemia may play a role in diffuse alopecia and may be accompanied by nail dystrophy.

The assessment of a patient with suspected telogen effluvium should include investigations based on the history and physical examination. Thyroid function, ferritin, vitamin B12, folate and zinc

Table 19.1 Causes of telogen effluvium.

Hormonal (e.g. pregnancy and post-partum)
Nutritional (e.g. iron deficiency)
Acute weight changes
Drugs (e.g. β-blockers, anti-coagulants, retinoids, immunisation)
Systemic disease (e.g. chronic inflammatory diseases, malignancy)
Stress (e.g. pyrexia, major surgery or trauma)

levels may be considered. Iron replacement should be implemented to achieve serum ferritin of 70 μg/l. Ultimately the condition will resolve once the precipitating factor has been removed and reassurance is all that is required.

Tinea capitis

Tinea capitis (see Chapter 16) is a fungal infection, which causes patchy usually non-scarring hair loss associated with short broken-off hairs, scaling and erythema of the underlying skin (Figure 19.6). It occurs almost exclusively in children. The most common fungi causing disease in urban areas are *Trichophyton tonsurans* (spread from human to human by direct contact) and *Microsporum canis* (caught from kittens or puppies). The diagnosis can be confirmed by taking hair pluckings and performing microscopy to look for spores inside the hair shaft; culture identifies the underlying organism. Scalp brushings can be taken and the bristles directly inoculated into the culture medium. Tinea capitis due to *M. canis* fluoresces green under Wood's light.

Kerion formation (Figure 19.7) is an inflamed, boggy, pustular lesion on the scalp that may result from tinea infections (cattle ringworm in rural areas and human *T. tonsurans* in urban areas). This swelling will resolve with systemic antifungal treatment and should not be surgically drained.

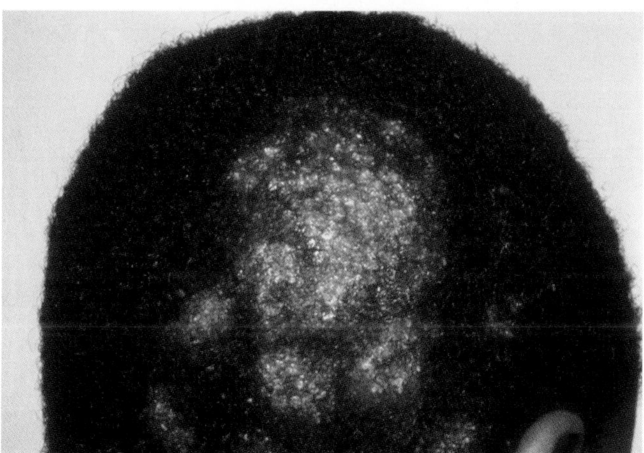

Figure 19.6 Tinea capitis.

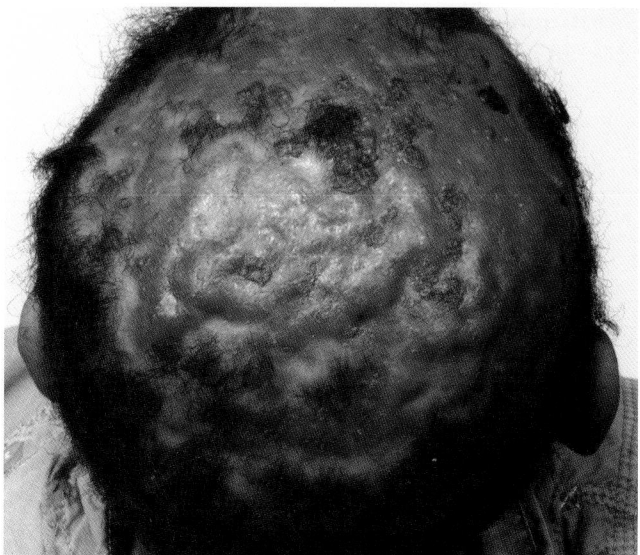

Figure 19.7 Kerion.

Oral griseofulvin or terbinafine is given daily for 4–6 weeks. Secondary bacterial infection should be treated with appropriate antibiotics (usually flucloxacillin to cover for *Staphylococcus aureus*). If infection is due to *M. canis*, it is also important to treat the affected pet.

Scarring alopecia

Scarring alopecias are characterised by permanent hair loss due to replacement of hair follicles by scar tissue. Scarring alopecia may be primary or secondary, depending on whether the hair follicle acts as the primary target or is damaged incidentally by non-follicular events. Permanent alopecia may also occur in conditions not traditionally considered as scarring processes such as in traction alopecia or trichotillomania in which follicular drop-out may occur.

Primary causes

These are best considered according to the underlying pathological process, and skin biopsy can be very helpful in establishing a diagnosis.

Lymphocytic disorders

Discoid lupus erythematosus and lichen planopilaris are both causes of scarring alopecia associated with a lymphocytic inflammatory infiltrate histologically. Both conditions present initially in a localised manner and may be associated with cutaneous findings, which may be diagnostic of the underlying disease. Scarring alopecia is associated with scaling, erythema and the presence of follicular plugging (Figure 19.8) with lupus affecting the scalp. Lichen planopilaris is characterised clinically by perifollicular erythema, follicular spines and scarring (Figure 19.9). Frontal fibrosing alopecia is an increasingly prevalent variant, which affects predominantly postmenopausal women. There is commonly symmetric frontotemporal recession with associated complete or partial alopecia of the eyebrows.

Skin biopsy with direct immunofluorescence is helpful in confirming the underlying diagnosis in those patients where there is doubt about the diagnosis. Treatment options include topical or systemic corticosteroids, oral antimalarials, retinoids or immunosuppressants.

Pseudopelade of Brocq is the label given to patients with a non-inflammatory scarring alopecia (Figure 19.10) in the absence of any other underlying pathology on biopsy. It may represent end-stage lichen planopilaris.

Central centrifugal cicatricial alopecia (CCCA) is seen in black women. It commonly presents with asymptomatic loss in the mid scalp or vertex and progressively enlarges centrifugally. It is thought to result from common practices of hot comb, chemical relaxant or pomade use; however, a definite causal link has not been established. The condition tends to progress despite cessation of these practices. Traction alopecia is a non-inflammatory scarring alopecia usually presenting with frontal or temporal hair loss. Hair styling

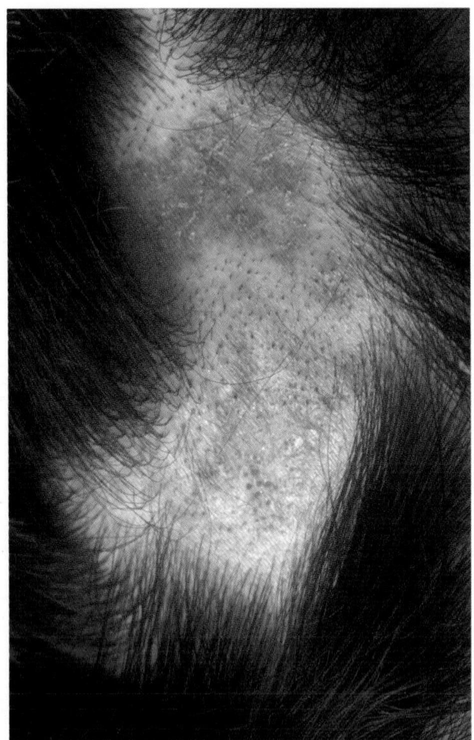

Figure 19.8 Discoid lupus erythematosus.

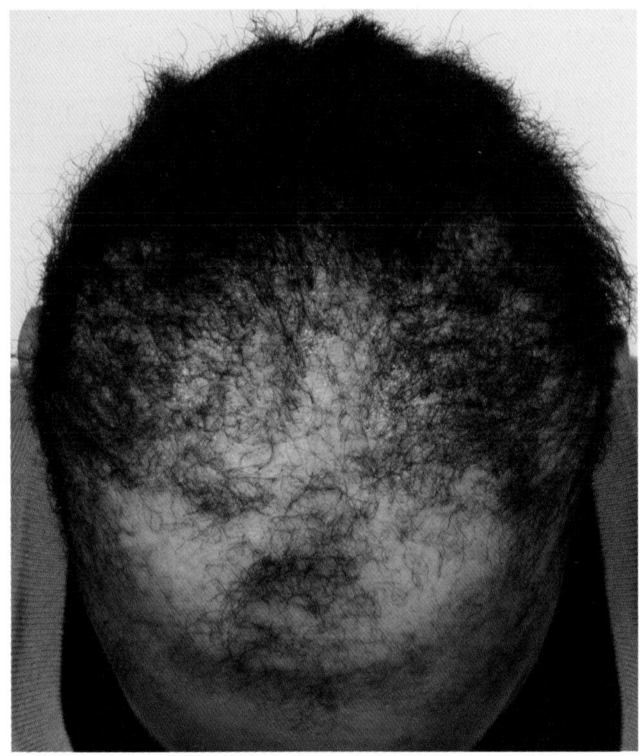

Figure 19.9 Lichen planopilaris.

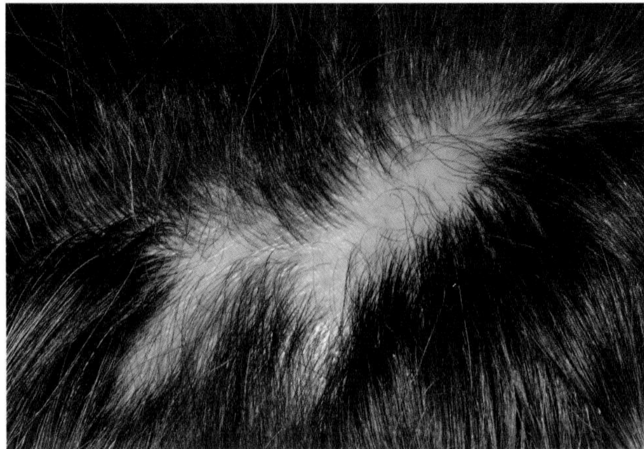

Figure 19.10 Pseudopelade of Brocq.

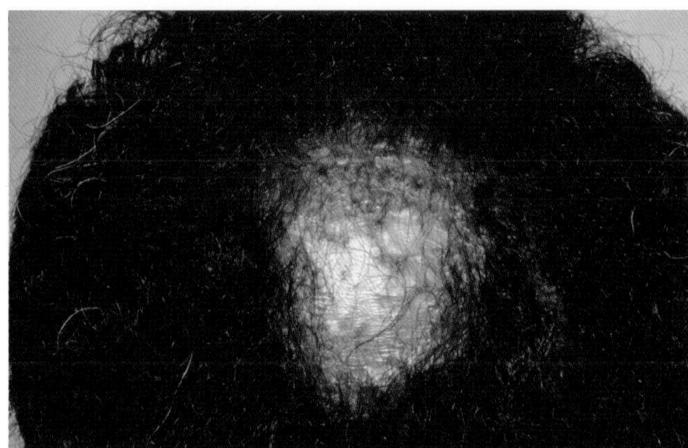

Figure 19.11 Folliculitis decalvans.

resulting in chronic tight pulling of the hair, for example, tight braiding, weaves or pony tails is causative.

Neutrophilic disorders

Dissecting folliculitis presents with multiple painless boggy nodules, typically on the vertex or occiput, which frequently discharge purulent exudate. Superficial pustules are often seen. This condition is mostly seen in young black males who may also suffer from acne and hidradenitis suppurativa. Treatment options include oral antibiotics (usually tetracyclines), oral corticosteroids, dapsone and isotretinoin.

Folliculitis decalvans is a rare form of recurrent folliculitis which leads to patches of scarring. Crusting and tufting of the hairs may be seen where multiple hairs emerge from a single follicle (Figure 19.11). Topical and oral antibiotics with antistaphylococcal activity are the mainstay of therapy, supporting the hypothesis that this condition is due to an abnormal host response to *S. aureus*. Rifampicin 300 mg twice daily and clindamycin 300 mg twice daily for 12 weeks is often effective.

Table 19.2 Causes of scarring alopecia.

Primary
Lichen planopilaris
Discoid lupus erythematosus
Pseudopelade of Brocq
Central centrifugal cicatricial alopecia and traction
Dissecting folliculitis
Folliculitis decalvans
Secondary
Post-traumatic
Burns
Radiotherapy
Neoplasia (e.g. squamous cell carcinoma, lymphoma and sarcoma)
Infection
Bacterial (e.g. folliculitis, acne keloidalis and syphillis)
Viral (e.g. herpes zoster)
Fungal (e.g. with kerion formation)

Secondary causes of scarring alopecia

Many well-recognised secondary causes of scarring alopecia exist (Table 19.2). Treatment is directed at the cause.

Excessive hair

Two patterns of hair overgrowth are recognised: hirsutism and hypertrichosis.

Hirsutism

This is defined as increased growth of the terminal hairs in androgen-sensitive areas such as the beard and moustache regions in females (Figure 19.12). The presence of terminal hair in a male distribution is not necessarily a sign of disease, and the determination of whether a patient has hirsutism must take into account the normal pattern of hair growth for the patient's racial origin. The patient's cultural and social background plays a major factor in determining how much facial and body hair is cosmetically acceptable. While hirsutism is most noticeable on the face, it may also affect other androgen-responsive areas such as the thighs, the back and the abdomen.

The assessment of the patient with hirsutism must include a general examination to identify an underlying endocrine abnormality, particularly if there is a relatively short history associated with amenorrhoea and signs of virilisation. Features suggestive of virilisation in addition to hirsutism include deepening of the voice, increased muscle bulk and cliteromegaly, an extremely sensitive sign. These features suggest a more sinister underlying cause. A list of the causes of hirsutism is given in Table 19.3.

Management

As a general rule, if the menstrual cycle is normal, so are the hormone levels. Over-investigation should be avoided once it is clear that there is no significant endocrine abnormality. Measurement of serum testosterone alone is sufficient for basic screening. Urgent referral to a specialist clinic is indicated if the concentration of serum testosterone is more than twice the upper limit of normal. More than 90% of premenopausal patients with hirsutism will have polycystic ovarian syndrome.

Treatments include suppression of androgens, peripheral androgen blockade and mechanical or cosmetic treatment. The use of eflornithine cream is a useful new adjuvant licensed for facial hirsutism that inhibits ornithine decarboxylase, an enzyme involved in controlling hair growth and proliferation. It is most effective when combined with local cosmetic or depilatory treatments, including laser hair removal.

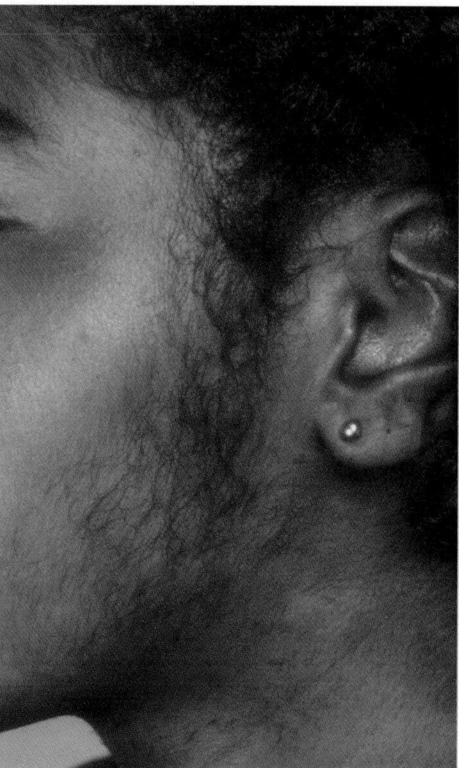

Figure 19.12 Hirsutism.

Table 19.3 Causes of hirsutism.

Ovarian
Polycystic ovarian syndrome
Ovarian tumours
Adrenal
Congenital adrenal hyperplasia
Cushing's disease
Prolactinoma
Gonadal dysgenesis
Androgen therapy
Idiopathic (racial and familial, with a wide spectrum of normal variation)

Hypertrichosis

This describes the excessive growth of hair in any part of the body and may be localised (e.g. Becker's naevus) or generalised

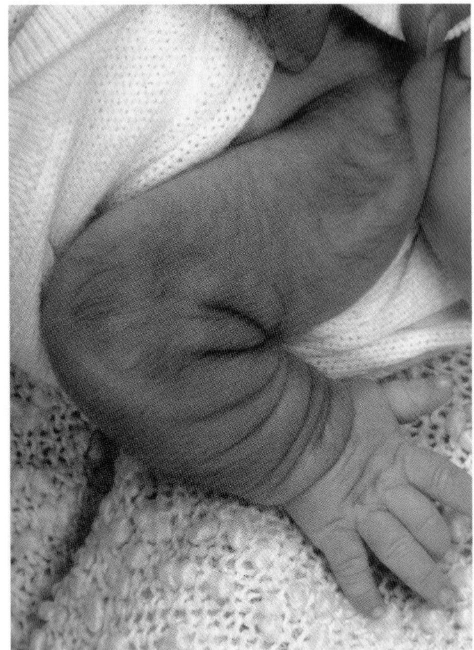

Figure 19.13 Hypertrichosis.

Table 19.4 Hypertrichosis due to drugs.

Streptomycin
Ciclosporin
Minoxidil
Diazoxide
Phenytoin
Penicillamine
Psoralens

(Figure 19.13). Causes may be congenital or acquired; important systemic diseases associated with hypertrichosis include hyperthyroidism, porphyria and anorexia nervosa. Drugs which commonly cause hypertrichosis are listed in Table 19.4.

Treatment is directed at the underlying cause and stopping any implicated drug, where possible. Symptomatic approaches include depilation using creams, shaving and waxing.

Skin disease involving the scalp

Scalp involvement is a prominent feature of numerous skin conditions. The most common inflammatory dermatoses which manifest in this way are psoriasis and seborrhoeic dermatitis (Figure 19.14). Reassuringly, these conditions are rarely associated with permanent hair loss. Thick adherent scales develop in pityriasis amiantacea and may represent the first manifestation of psoriasis (Figure 19.15), usually seen in children. Patients with scalp psoriasis benefit from combination treatments including coal tar, topical steroids (+/− vitamin D analogues) and keratolytics such as salicylic acid.

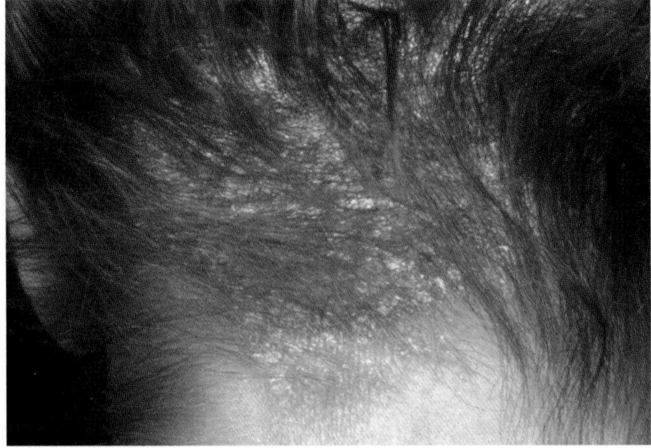

Figure 19.14 Seborrhoeic dermatitis.

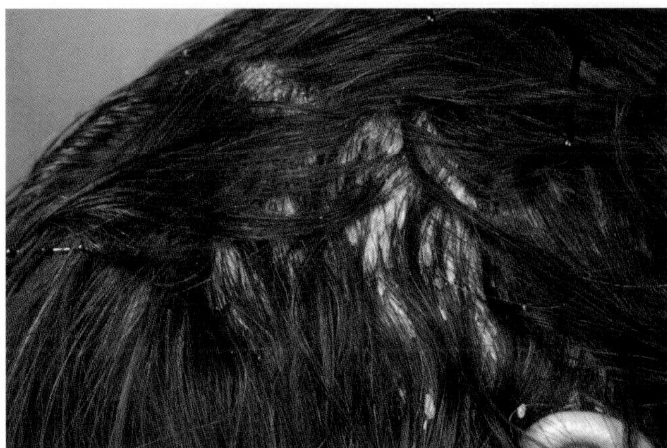

Figure 19.15 Pityriasis amiantacea.

Seborrhoeic dermatitis is probably due to an altered host immune response to *Malassezia furfur* yeast, which lives in hair follicles. This causes erythema and scaling of the scalp. Removing the yeast with antifungal agents such as topical ketoconazole shampoo and treating inflammation with topical steroids provides benefit.

Atopic eczema, allergic contact dermatitis commonly to paraphenylenediamine (PPD) found in black hair-dye and immunobullous disorders such as pemphigus vulgaris may also involve the scalp.

Further Reading

Dawber RPR and Van Neste D. *Hair and Scalp Disorders: Common Presenting Signs, Differential Diagnosis and Treatment*, 2nd Edition, Taylor and Francis, London, 2004.

McMichael AJ and Hordinsky MK. *Hair and Scalp Diseases: Medical, Surgical and Cosmetic Treatments (Basic and Clinical Dermatology)*, Informa Healthcare, New York, 2008.

CHAPTER 20

Diseases of the Nails

David de Berker

Dermatology Department, United Bristol Healthcare Trust, UK

> **OVERVIEW**
> - Nails are ectodermal derivatives composed of keratin which grow forward from a fold of epidermis over the nail bed. Finger nails grow at approximately 1 mm per week and toe nails 1 mm per month.
> - The attachment of the nail plate to the underlying nail bed can be affected by excess keratin, inflammatory changes or infection, which causes the nail plate to lift: onycholysis.
> - Thickening of the nail plate may occur as a result of inflammatory, traumatic and infective conditions.
> - Transverse ridges are seen in psoriasis and eczema. Beau's line is a transverse depression affecting most of the nails due to a severe illness or physiological stress.
> - Changes in the shape of the nail include clubbing, which is due to swelling and increased vascularity of the tissues surrounding the nail. Koilonychia is a 'spoon-shaped' deformity of the nail that may be associated with iron deficiency.
> - Infection and inflammation adjacent to the nail results in paronychia that may be acute or chronic.
> - Colour changes in the nail can arise through alteration of the nail bed or the nail plate and sometimes both. These include leukonychia (whitening of the nails) and black discolouration from subungual bleeding.
> - Longitudinal brown streaks often occur in those with racially pigmented skin. In Caucasians, isolated brown streaks in the nail may be due to a dysplastic naevus, and involvement of the nail fold suggests a subungual melanoma.

Introduction

In humans, the main function of the nails is to protect the distal soft tissues of the fingers and toes from the physical trauma of everyday life.

The nail is derived from the ectoderm and is composed of keratin (Figure 20.1). The nail plate grows forward from a fold of epidermis over the nail bed, which is continuous with the matrix proximally. Nail keratin is derived mainly from the matrix with contributions from the dorsal surface of the nail fold and the nail bed.

ABC of Dermatology, Sixth Edition. Edited by Rachael Morris-Jones.

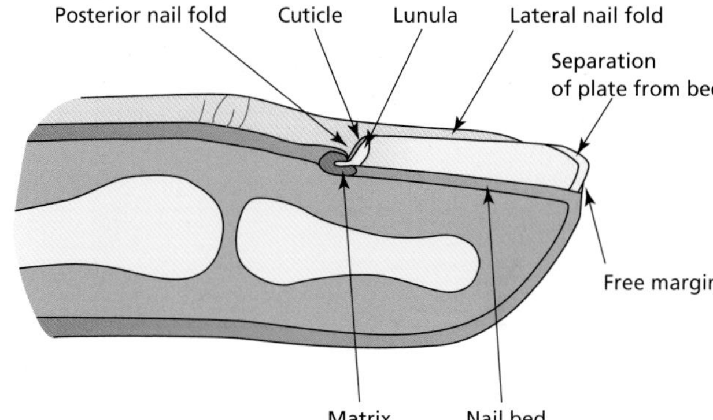

Figure 20.1 Section through finger.

The nail grows slowly for the first day after birth and then more rapidly until it slows in old age. The rate of nail growth is greater in the fingers than the toes, particularly on the dominant hand. It is slower in women but increases during pregnancy. Finger nails grow at approximately 0.8 mm per week and toe nails 0.25 mm per week.

Changes of shape and attachment

Pitting

This is seen clinically as small surface depressions of the nail plate that result from a loss of the parakeratotic scale such as occurs in psoriasis (Figure 20.2a and b showing nail pitting and appearances with a dermatoscope). The scale develops through inflammatory diseases affecting the proximal nail matrix including psoriasis, eczema, lichen planus and alopecia areata.

Subungual hyperkeratosis

Where scaling occurs beneath the nail in the distal nail bed, the compacted scales build up to produce dense subungual hyperkeratosis. This is most commonly seen in psoriasis, eczema and fungal nail disease. In the toes, it may be part of a reaction to trauma or generalised hyperkeratosis.

Oily spot

This sign is specific to psoriasis and reflects the presence of a patch of psoriasis in the nail bed with no connection to the free edge. There is discolouration of the nail, giving an oily appearance.

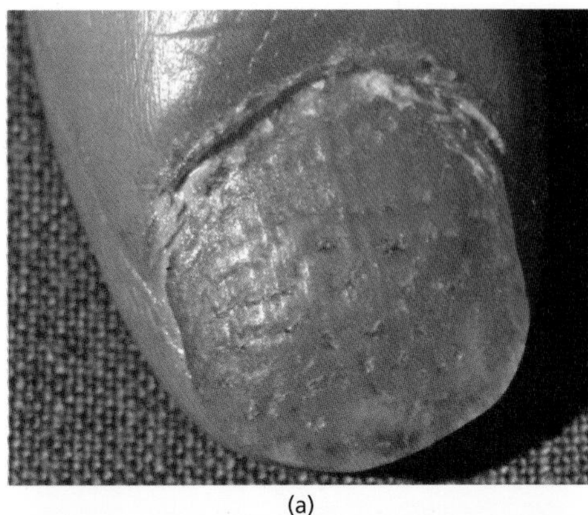
(a)

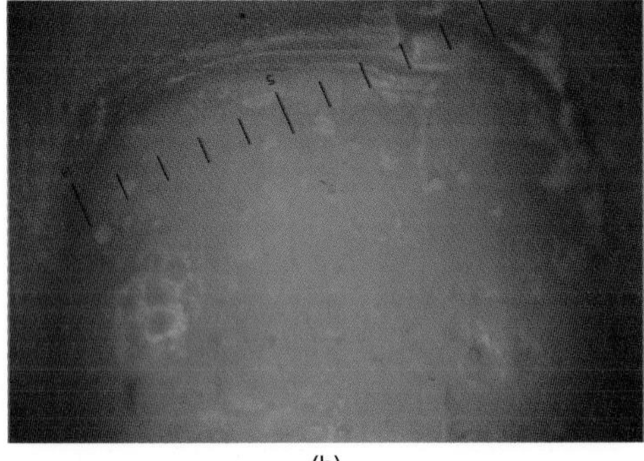
(b)

Figure 20.2 (a) Pitting of nail and (b) pitting of nail appearance with dermatoscope.

Onycholysis

Nail plate attachment to the nail bed may be lost by various degrees. This can be due to an inflammatory, traumatic or infective process affecting the distal nail bed, altering its biological function allowing nail plate attachment. Acute trauma usually settles with re-adherence. Forms of chronic trauma include manicure where the person uses a sharp instrument to remove subungual debris from beneath the nail (Figure 20.3). This form of trauma may be a sole cause of onycholysis, or may be a factor in association with a skin disease, such as psoriasis. Systemic causes of onycholysis include thyrotoxicosis.

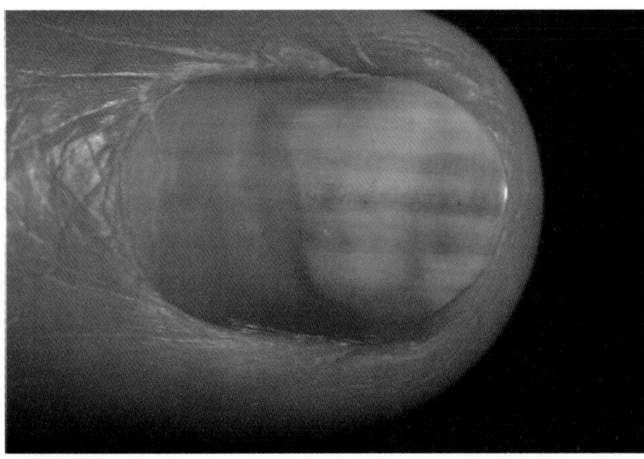

Figure 20.3 Onycholysis due to manicure beneath the nail.

Chronic onycholysis becomes vulnerable to secondary infection with microbes that thrive in warm damp spaces. These are mainly *Candida* spp. and *Pseudomonas pyocyanae*. Such microbes may contribute to the persistence of the split from the nail bed and will increase discomfort and malodour.

Nail plate thickening

The nail plate thickens and becomes yellow in a wide range of diseases and also as part of normal ageing on the toes. Eczema, psoriasis, lichen planus and yellow nail syndrome are the main inflammatory diseases with this effect. Fungal infection can result in the same problem, although as in all the inflammatory diseases it may be possible to make a distinction between thickening due to increase of subungual keratin and thickening due to change in the nail plate (Figure 20.4). Chronic trauma can cause thickening, where the response of the nail is analogous to that of the skin in general. This is seen in hammer toe, where the free edge of the toe is directed downwards to act like a piano string hammer at each step. This force transmits back to the nail matrix and results in thickening of the nail.

Transverse ridges

These are most commonly seen in psoriasis and eczema where there is inflammation of the proximal nail fold and secondary change of nail matrix function. Isolated digital trauma may cause a similar, but solitary, transverse ridge.

Irritant dermatitis (eczema)

This is a significant cause of chronic paronychia. Common factors are a low threshold for an irritant reaction, such as background atopy or skin problems elsewhere, in combination with an occupational irritation of the skin at the base or sides of the nail. This resulting inflammation spreads to involve the nail matrix. When further combined with damp or wet work (which is a common form of irritant) there is a disposition to secondary infection with *Candida* spp.

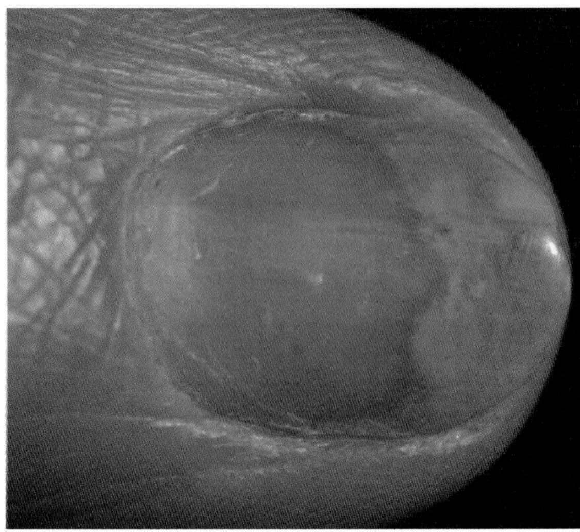

Figure 20.4 Onycholysis and hyperkeratosis of nail plate in psoriasis.

Beau's line

A substantial general physiological disturbance can result in a solitary episode of reduced nail matrix function. If this reduction falls short of complete matrix shut down, then there is a partial thickness transverse break in the nail plate. This will normally affect many nails at once, with subsequent nail growth marking out the time of recent disturbance such as a date in a calendar record of the preceding months. This was originally identified by Joseph Beau, a Parisian cardiologist who termed it *retrospective semeiology*, from the Greek, meaning to study signs and symbols. While it is most commonly thought to be an indicator of past physiological changes, it is also seen in people who have a severe deterioration in their eczema or psoriasis as well as less common diseases, such as bullous pemphigoid.

Nail loss (onychomadesis)

Where the nail matrix inflammation is global and severe, it may be sufficient to precipitate nail shedding and interruption of nail matrix nail plate production entirely. This can be a result of severe inflammatory skin disease or an episode of trauma. The latter is particularly the case when there is substantial bleeding beneath the nail, which separates the nail from the nail bed.

Longitudinal splits

A single split on one nail with no other nail or skin disease is most likely to represent an area of focal matrix damage (Figure 20.5). This can be due to acute trauma with scarring, chronic trauma from underlying or overlying mass or a dysplastic process destroying a small area of nail matrix such that it does not produce nail. Such presentations need close examination and imaging and may require surgical exploration and sampling. Where longitudinal splits are multiple, they are usually a result of a generalised inflammatory or degenerative process. The most typical of these are lichen planus and ageing, respectively. Ageing is a non-specific process, where there is a loss of nail substance and increased fragility, giving rise to splits. These are usually only manifested in the distal few millimetres of nail. A hybrid between inflammation and degeneration is seen in the genodermatosis Darier's disease where distal nicks in the nail may extend proximally to be markedly destructive (Figure 20.6). This is usually seen in combination with other signs specific to this disease.

Transverse (lamellar) splits

This is seen in childhood mainly in the big toes and where there is thumb sucking. It can also be seen in middle age and beyond, probably as part of a degenerative process. It represents a loss of adherence between the lamellae of the nail plate, which is made up of a tier of over 100 cells in the vertical axis. As the nail reaches the free edge, it is vulnerable to the action of solvents penetrating the free edge and promoting loss of cohesion between the lamellae.

Pustules in the periungual skin

This is more strictly a periungual sign, but with significance to the nail. Pustules can be sterile or reflect infection. In the acute presentation, it is always wise to assume infection until proven otherwise. Infective causes are typically through minor trauma and pyogenic bacteria such as *Staphylococcus aureus* where the red and swollen digit will also have one or more pustules. This is an acute paronychia.

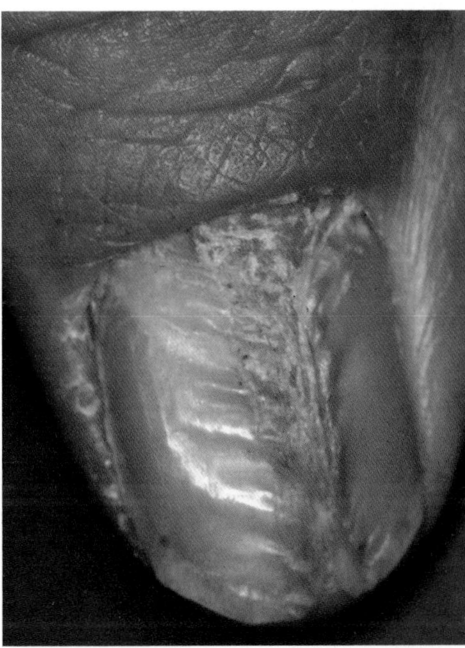

Figure 20.5 Longitudinal ridge and partial split termed canaliform dystrophy of Heller. Matrix inflammation with nail fold trauma can play a part.

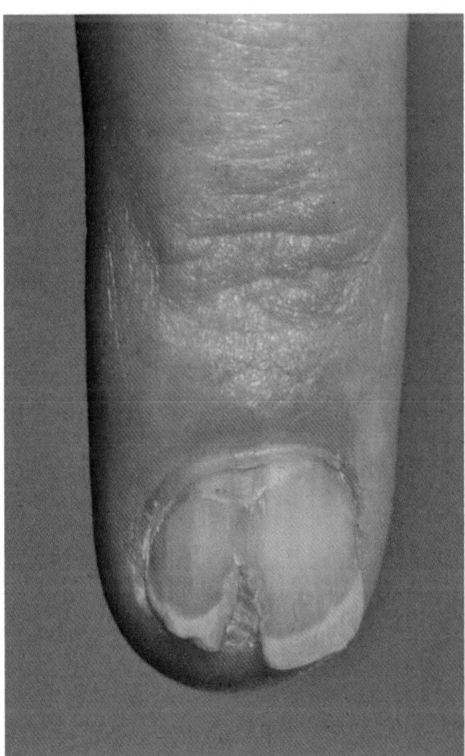

Figure 20.6 Darier's disease.

Herpes simplex can produce a similar appearance although the pustules are smaller, more numerous and clustered and have a vesicular character. *Candida* can also result in pus, but usually with a more indolent course. Sterile pustules are usually due to psoriasis. There may be less pain and associated inflammation than with the acute infective disease and multiple digits might be involved as well as other body sites. The pustules gradually resolve, leaving a brown residue. In some instances, sterile psoriatic pustules can affect the nail unit either as part of more generalised pustular psoriasis or as variants of palmoplantar pustulosis or acrodermatitis or Hallopeau.

Koilonychia

This term refers to a 'spoon-shaped' deformity of the nail. This is seen in normal infants, mainly of their toe nails. In older people, it may be a manifestation of iron-deficiency anaemia. It is also a non-specific feature of diseases where there is atrophy of the nail unit. Where the nail plate is thin, it can dip centrally, which is seen in variants of lichen planus.

Clubbing

Clubbing is a change in the shape of the nail secondary to chronic swelling of periungual tissues with increased vasculature. There is an increase in the transverse and longitudinal curvature (Figure 20.7). At the base of the nail, where it meets the proximal nail fold, the angle with the nail fold is lost because of the swelling and the consistency is 'boggy'. It is a change due to systemic or inherited factors, which means that it affects all nails, although the changes in the toes are less obvious than in the digits of the hands. Where cyanotic heart disease or fibrotic or cavitating pulmonary disease is the underlying cause, the nail bed may be cyanosed. Idiopathic variants, or where inflammatory bowel and liver disease are causal, can be a normal pink colour.

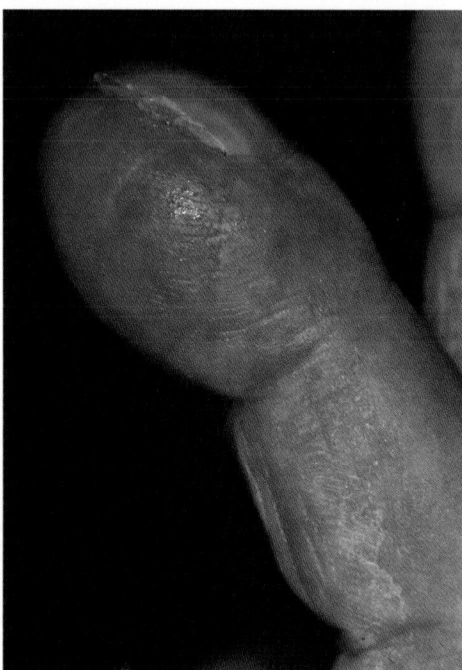

Figure 20.7 Clubbing with loss of the angle between the proximal nail fold and the base of the nail.

Changes of colour

Colour changes in the nail can arise through alteration of the nail bed or the nail plate and sometimes both. Dermoscopy is a useful tool for evaluating pigment of the nail unit.

Nail bed changes

Leukonychia

Whitening of the nail is classified according to the origin of the colour change. Apparent leukonychia (Figure 20.8) reflects changes in the vascular state of the nail bed. Most commonly, this is oedema or loss of normal vascular pigment, as seen in hypoalbuminaemia with cirrhosis of the liver. True leuconychia is where the substance of the nail plate is altered so that it appears white whether it is *in situ* or avulsed. Biologically, this comes about for two reasons.

Firstly, there may be alteration of the nail after it has been formed and the most common cause of this is fungal infection. Secondly, abnormal nail plate production may result in white nail. This occurs most commonly in a punctuate or transverse linear pattern, and has little significance. It does not represent lack of calcium. There is also a familial variant where the entire nail may be white.

Apparent leukonychia occurs in hypoalbuminaemia and old age.

Red lunula is seen in inflammatory joint disease, cardiac failure, blue cyanotic heart or respiratory diseases.

Grey colour can be caused by mepacrine.

Purple/black discolouration results from subungual bleeding.

Nail plate changes

Patchy brown discolouration is seen in the 'yellow nail syndrome', fungal infection and psoriasis. Drugs may cause more uniform changes in colour; for example, tetracycline may produce yellow nails, antimalarials a blue discolouration and chlorpromazine a brown colour.

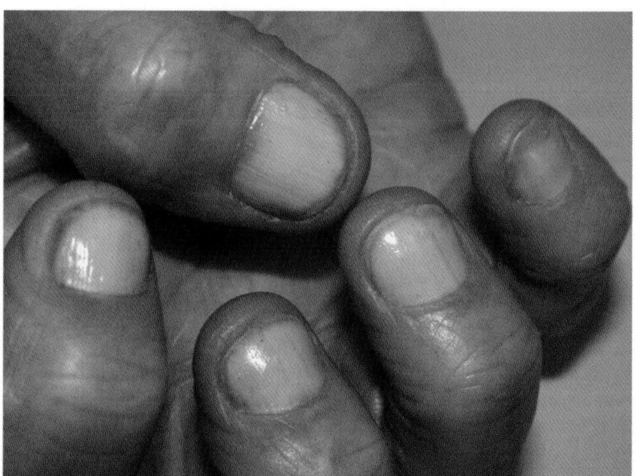

Figure 20.8 Apparent leuconychia.

True leukonychia is seen with fungal infection (superficial white onychomycosis), trauma and autoimmune nail disease. Mees lines are a form of true leukonychia seen as white transverse band on the nail. They arise when poisons such as chemotherapy are administered on an intermittent basis. The rhythm and approximate timing of doses of chemotherapy can be determined by the position of the white transverse line.

Yellow nail syndrome is associated with respiratory and sinus disease. Prolonged repeated use of nail varnish causes alteration of nail keratin, termed *granulation*. This gives a yellow appearance (Figure 20.9).

Thickened nail occurs from trauma or fungal infection.

Brown colour or melanonychia refers to a brown streak in the nail due to pigment production in the nail matrix (Figure 20.10). The melanin source may be benign or malignant. Dark-skinned races have prominent benign multiple brown streaks. Pale-skinned people have a higher chance of a melanonychia, representing a malignant process (melanoma). Slight discolouration of the nails may be seen in Addison's disease caused by adrenal insufficiency.

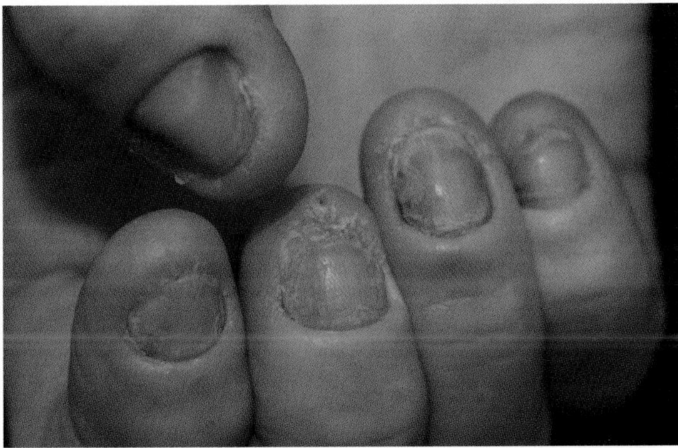

Figure 20.9 Yellow nail syndrome.

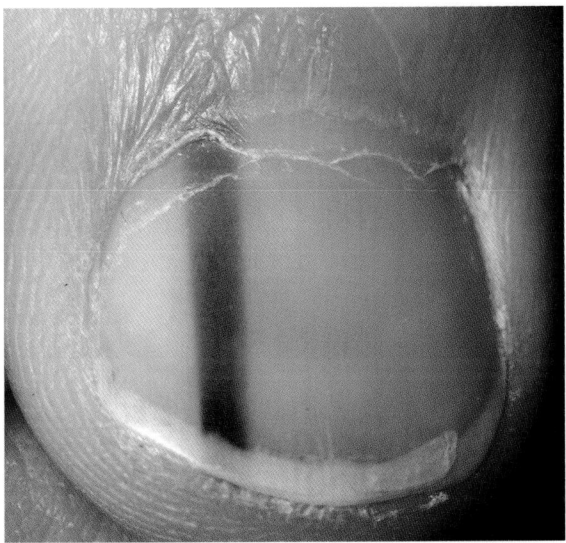

Figure 20.10 Linear melanonychia.

Minocycline and zidovudine can result in melanonychia.

Longitudinal pigmented streaks result from increased melanin deposition in the nail plate (Box 20.1).

Box 20.1 **Pigmented streaks in nails**

Single

Melanocytic naevi or lentigo
Subungual melanoma
Trauma

Multiple

Racial
Drugs
Addison's

Longitudinal brown streaks are frequently seen in individuals with racially pigmented skin. This is rare in Caucasians and while it may still represent a benign process it is important that isolated brown streaks in the nail of pale-skinned people are seen by a specialist for an expert diagnosis to exclude the possibility of subungual melanoma. This is associated with Hutchinson's sign in which pigmentation extends into the surrounding tissues, particularly the cuticle. Adrenal disease may rarely be associated with longitudinal streaks.

Common dermatoses and the nail unit

Psoriasis is one of the most common dermatoses with nail involvement. About 80% of people with psoriasis will have some nail features at some point in the course of their disease. The features include pitting, transverse ridges, onycholysis, oily spots, subungual hyperkeratosis (Figure 20.11) and chronic paronychia. At times, disease may be sufficiently severe as to result in loss of function through pain and the inability to sustain pressure or undertake fine manipulation.

Eczema may be associated with brittle nails that tend to split. Thickening and deformity of the nail occurs in eczema or contact

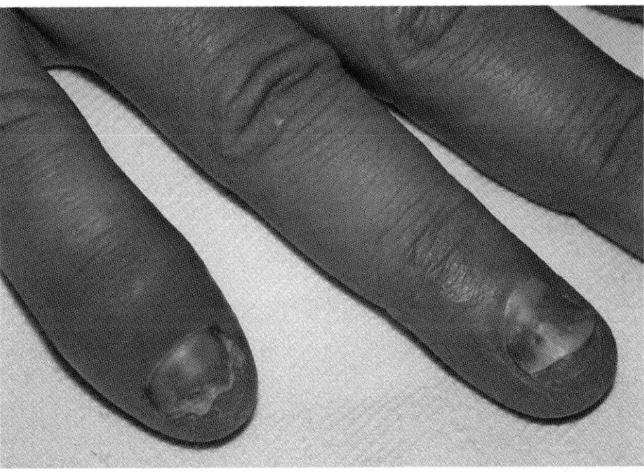

Figure 20.11 Nail psoriasis with onycholysis, pitting and arthritis of the distal interphalangeal joint of the little finger.

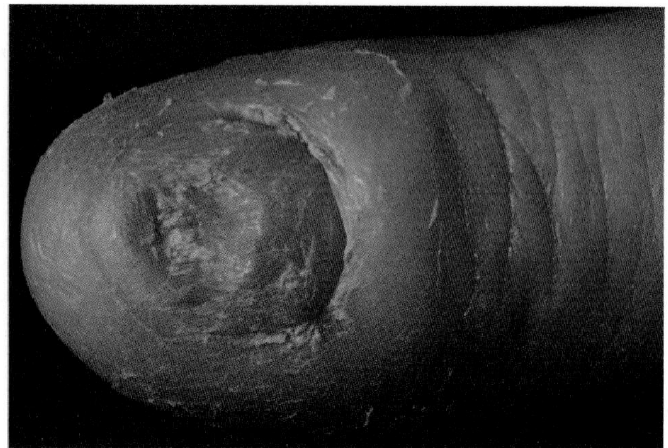

Figure 20.12 Eczema causing inflammatory matrix changes and compounded by picking with surrounding eczema and loss of intact nail.

dermatitis, sometimes with transverse ridging. Pitting can also be seen. Nail bed changes are less common than in psoriasis, although allergic contact sensitivity where allergen is sequestered beneath the nail can produce dramatic acute and chronic nail bed disease (Figure 20.12).

Lichen planus can result in many features mimicking psoriasis, but in its most characteristic form produces atrophy of the nail plate which may completely disappear. The cuticle may be thickened and grow over the nail plate, known as *pterygium formation* (Figure 20.13).

Alopecia areata is associated with changes in the nails in about 30% of cases. Features include ridging, pitting, leuconychia and friable nails. Where the nails are friable, it is referred to as *trachyonychia* and may involve any or all of the nails – known as *20-nail dystrophy* (Figure 20.14).

Darier's disease is associated with dystrophy of the nail and longitudinal streaks which end in triangular-shaped nicks at the free edge (see Figure 20.6). On the skin, there may be the characteristic brownish scaling papules on the central part of the back, chest and neck. These are made worse by sun exposure.

Autoimmune conditions such as pemphigus and pemphigoid may be associated with a variety of changes including ridging, splitting of the nail plate and atrophy and shedding in some or all of the nails.

Discolouration of the nail and friability are associated with *lupus erythematosus* (Figures 20.15 and 20.16).

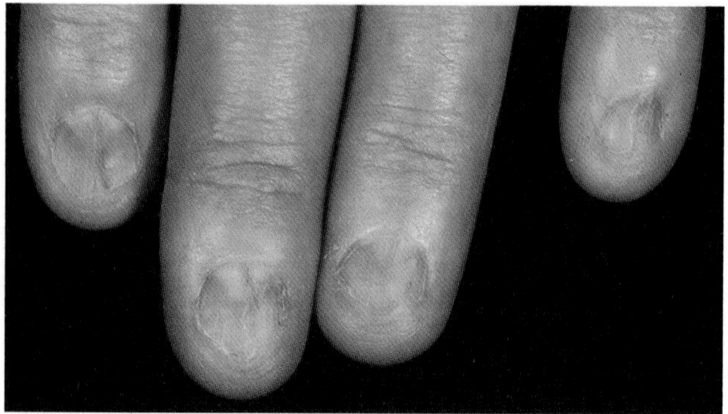

Figure 20.13 Lichen planus.

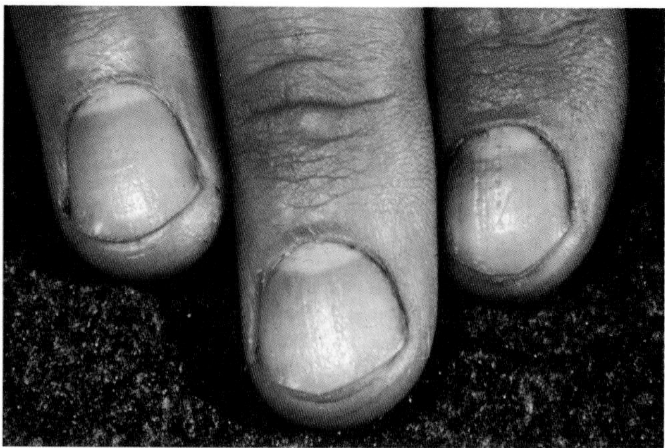

Figure 20.14 Nail dystrophy with alopecia areata comprising multiple small, regular, pits.

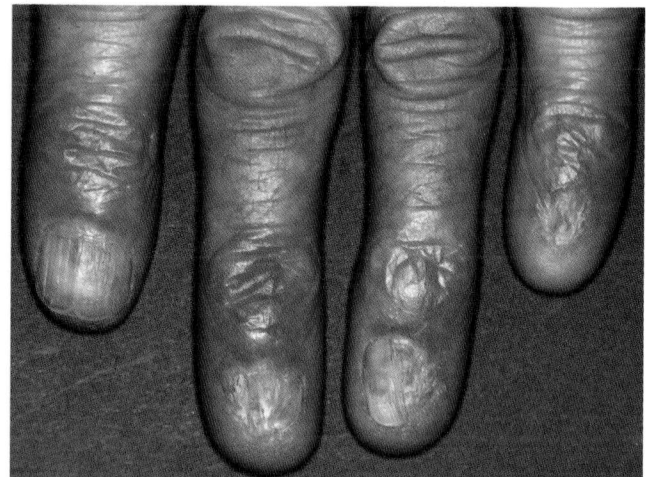

Figure 20.15 Dystrophy due to lupus.

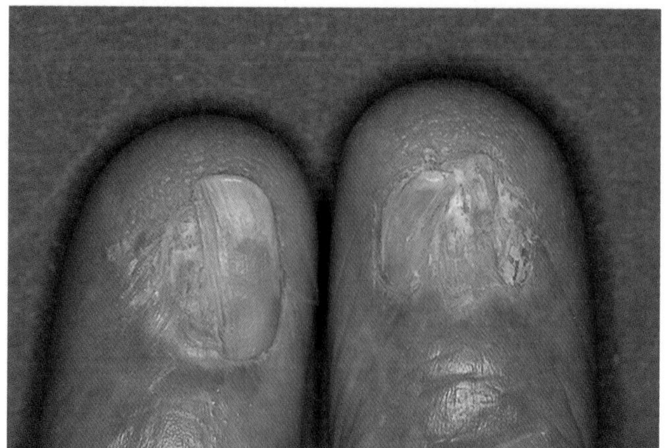

Figure 20.16 Pterygium formation with lupus.

Infection

Bacterial infection of periungual tissues

Infection of the nail unit may affect the soft tissues or the nail plate. The proximal and lateral nail folds are typically affected by *S. aureus* or less commonly *Streptococcus* or gram-negative organisms. Treatment is with drainage of any pus collection and systemic antibiotics, modified after initiation depending on culture results.

The nail bed may become infected as a result of onycholysis (Figure 20.17). *Candida* and *Pseudomonas* are the most common agents, where their growth is promoted by the damp warm character of the onycholytic space. Treatment may entail clipping back the nail to expose the nail bed, avoidance of wet work, drying beneath the nail with a hair dryer daily and the use of antimicrobials. Topical antimicrobial treatment can be the use of gentamicin eye drops beneath the nail, or as part of a long-term regimen to prevent relapse, undertaking daily 5-min soaks with vinegar or sodium hypochlorite solution. Ultimately, cure relies on management of the onycholysis.

Fungal nail infection

Nail plate infection with dermatophyte fungi is mainly associated with nail bed involvement and typically occurs in a previously traumatised nail. Dermatophyte nail fungal infection is usually of the toe nails rather than the finger nails and involvement of nearby skin should be sought and treated, especially between the fourth and fifth toes. It is important to confirm the presence of fungus before considering treatment as nail psoriasis, eczema and trauma can all look similar. The diagnosis is confirmed by taking generous clippings of the nail plate and subungual debris for microscopy and culture (Figure 20.18). Positive culture is a prerequisite for systemic treatment. In some settings, polymerase chain reaction is used to identify the fungus, although it will not determine whether the fungus is alive and hence viable.

Culture will determine if the fungus is a dermatophyte such as *Trichophyton rubrum*, or a non-dermatophyte. The latter are

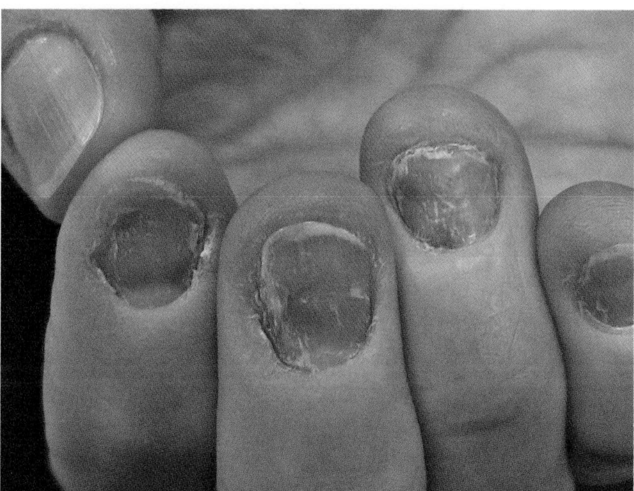

Figure 20.17 Chronic paronychia with alteration of nail plate shape and discolouration secondary to nail fold inflammation and microbial colonisation.

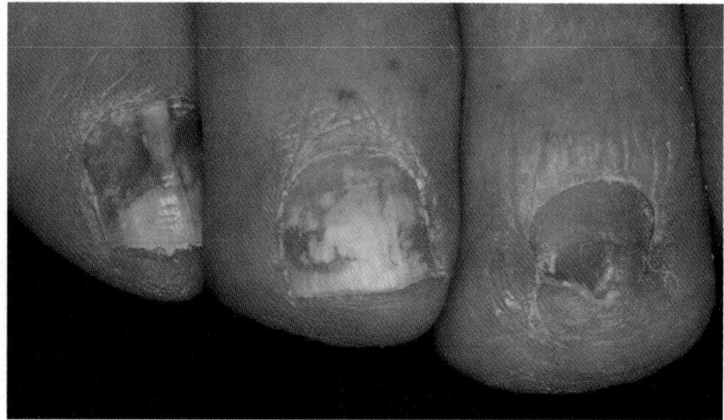

Figure 20.18 Fungal infection with superficial pattern (fourth toe) and distal and subungual pattern on the little toe.

more difficult to treat effectively and therapy should be guided by a dermatologist or someone with specialist knowledge of onychomycosis.

Treatment of dermatophyte onychomycosis is optional based on patient preference and clinical factors. Systemic treatment with terbinafine is likely to ultimately achieve a normal nail in about 50% of patients. This figure will be slightly increased by concomitant use of topical amorolfine lacquer weekly.

Trauma

Acute trauma is usually either a crush or leverage injury. Crush injury is typically associated with subungual bleeding. Where this involves more than 50% of the nail area, drainage is indicated to relieve pain and reduce the risk of compression. An opened red hot paper clip or a nail drill, usually available in emergency departments, can be used. Leverage injuries lead to complete or partial lifting of the nail plate, with nail avulsion in the latter instance. It is best to clean the nail and return it *in situ* to act as a dressing to the wounded nail bed. It will need to be held in place by a dressing or cyanoacrylate glue. It will eventually drop off when the new nail generates beneath.

Chronic trauma of the toe nails is typically due to poorly fitting footwear, where the free edge of the nail is brought into repeated contact with the shoe. This is most marked when the footwear is pointed or there is a high heel, creating a force on the foot downwards into the toe of the shoe. Trauma between toes and footwear can also arise with well-fitting shoes in activities such as step aerobics, hill walking (downwards), skiing and long-distance running. The initial effect of chronic trauma is asymptomatic bleeding. Later, there is thickening and yellow discolouration of the nail. Over many years, the shape of the nail matrix is altered and the nail may grow upwards and lose nail bed attachment. With marathon running, it is not uncommon for people to shed nails after the event.

Chronic trauma of the fingernails arises through 'habit tic' picking (Figure 20.19), manicure or occupational repetitive trauma, such as cardboard box assembly.

In all instances of chronic trauma, management relies on identification of the cause and its avoidance. For some patterns of self-inflicted trauma, it is not easy to persuade the patient of their role in the process. Physical protection of the nail and nail fold with

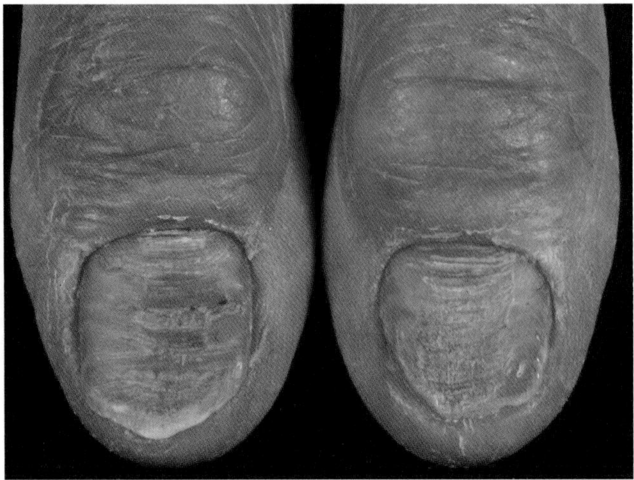

Figure 20.19 Chronic rubbing trauma to the proximal nail fold leads to a 'habit-tic' pattern of longitudinal dystrophy.

occlusive dressing, sometimes supplemented with steroid ointment, can be helpful in instances of fingernail problems.

General diseases affecting the nails

Nail changes in systemic illness

Acute illness

Acute illness results in a transverse line of atrophy known as a *Beau's line*. Shedding of the nail, onychomedesis, may occur in severe illness.

Chronic illness

Clubbing affects the soft tissues of the terminal phalanx with swelling and an increase in the angle between the nail plate and the nail fold. There is chronic swelling of periungual tissues with increased vasculature associated with an increase in the transverse and longitudinal curvature of the nail (see Figure 20.7). At the base of the nail, the angle with the nail fold is lost due to the swelling, and the nail fold has a 'boggy' consistency. It is due to systemic or inherited factors, which means that it affects all nails, although the changes in the toes are less obvious than in the digits of the hands. It is associated with chronic fibrotic, infective or malignant respiratory disease, cyanotic heart disease and occasionally inflammatory bowel disease. It can be hereditary and may be unilateral in association with vascular abnormalities.

Cyanosis – Where cyanotic heart disease or fibrotic or cavitating pulmonary disease is the underlying cause, the nail bed may be cyanosed. In idiopathic variants, or where there is underlying inflammatory bowel and liver disease, it can be a normal pink colour.

Splinter haemorrhages occur beneath the nail and are usually the result of minor trauma. They are also associated with a wide range of general medical conditions including subacute bacterial endocarditis and severe rheumatoid arthritis.

Lesions adjacent to the nail

Viral warts are the most common tumour arising in the nail folds (see Chapter 14) and nail bed with secondary effects on the nail plate. In childhood, these usually resolve without treatment. In adults, resolution is less predictable. Topical, surgical, laser and chemotherapeutic options are available but all have a significant failures rate with possible complications of pain, infection and scarring in the more aggressive treatments.

Myxoid pseudocysts arise through damage to the synovial capsule, which allows escape of synovial fluid in the subcutaneous tissue. This is usually secondary to osteoarthritis although it can be caused by specific trauma. The fluid collects on the dorsal aspect of the digit, beneath the proximal nail fold but above the matrix, or beneath the matrix. Where the location impinges on the nail matrix, nail plate growth will be altered to reflect the pattern of pressure (Figure 20.20). Careful ligature of the defect in the synovial capsule can be curative, but has a relatively high failure rate in the toes.

Naevi may occur adjacent to the nail and a benign melanocytic naevus can produce a pigmented streak.

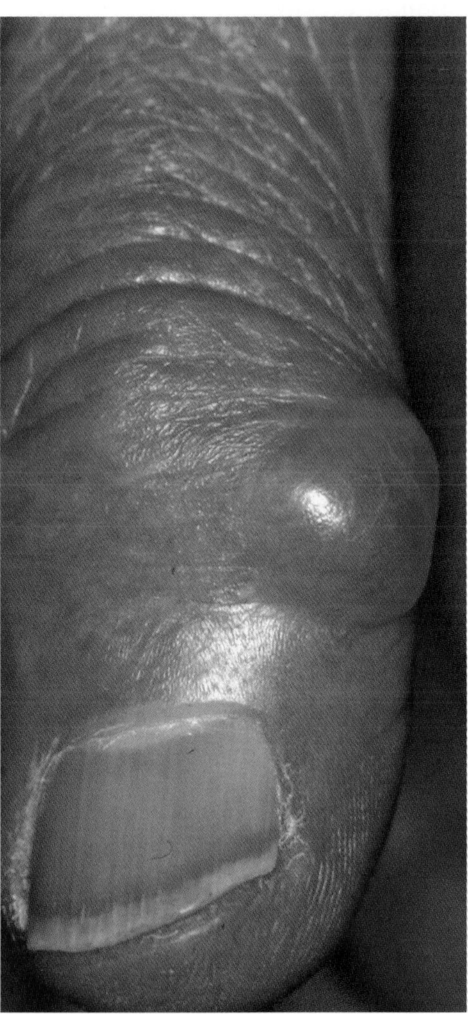

Figure 20.20 Mucoid cyst, also called *myxoid pseudocyst*.

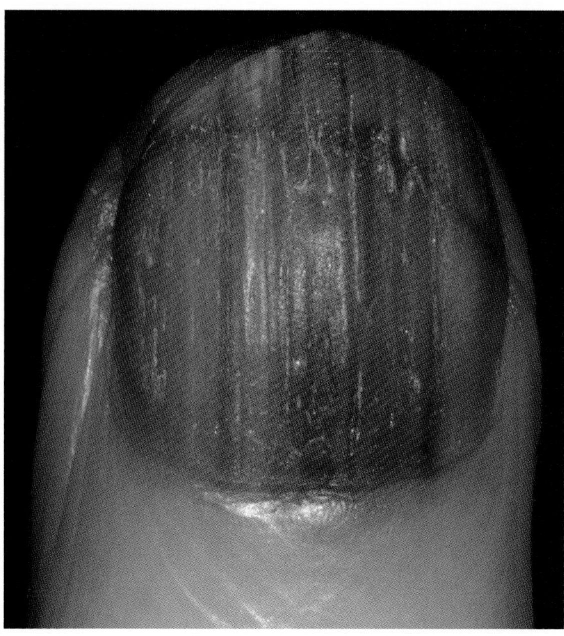

Figure 20.21 *In situ* melanoma with progressive pigmentation of nail plate.

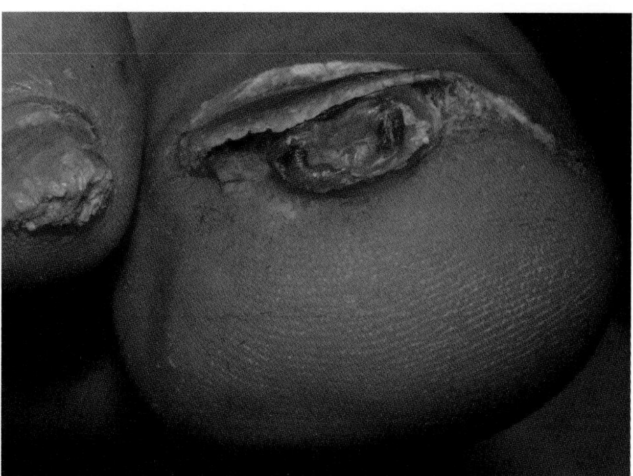

Figure 20.22 Subungual exostosis of the big toe.

Melanoma (Figure 20.21) typically arises from a pigmented lesion located in the nail matrix, which contributes pigment to the nail plate and consequently creates a dark longitudinal streak in the nail. It can be difficult to distinguish from a benign naevus in the early stages. As it progresses, it often causes pigmentation of the cuticle, Hutchinson's sign. Further evolution is associated with destruction of the nail plate such that it causes nail splits or loss. Sometimes, subungual melanoma is amelanotic so that there are no pigmentary changes, and any rapidly growing soft tumour should raise suspicions of this condition. There are some similarities with pyogenic granuloma, which means all pyogenic granulomas should be histologically confirmed as such. Melanoma of the nail unit is usually detected later than melanoma at other sites such that it is thicker and hence more advanced. This lends it a worse prognosis.

Subungual exostosis can cause a painful lesion under the nail (Figure 20.22). It is confirmed by X-ray examination. Lateral and plane views are needed to ensure that a subtle bony protuberance is not missed. A large part of the pathology is the cartilaginous cap which is radiolucent.

Glomus tumours arise as dermal tumours beneath the nail. They are characterised by pain which is worse in the cold and at night. Pain can be diminished by elevating the limb. When the tumour is in the nail bed there may be minimal or no clinical changes. When it is located beneath the matrix, pressure upon the matrix will alter matrix function. This causes a red streak in the nail, which ultimately may wear through the nail and produce a split. Treatment is by surgical excision.

Periungual fibrokeratomas appear as firm fibrous lumps that may be spherical or elongated. Nail growth is altered by pressure on the nail matrix. They are associated with tuberous sclerosis but this is unlikely with single lesions in an adult. However, a full examination and family history should be carried out to ensure that the diagnosis has not been missed. Patients presenting with multiple tumours are more likely to have tuberous sclerosis. Surgery can be effective in fibromas causing functional impairment or pain.

Treatment of nail conditions

Inflammatory and infective nail conditions often occur when there has been inadequate hand or foot care. The principles of care of the nails are as follows.

- Keep nails short. Do not cut toe nails too short for fear of precipitating in-growing nail.
- Dry hands and feet carefully after washing, especially between digits and under rings.
- Wear gloves when undertaking wet work, gardening or work entailing contact with solvents or abrasive materials.
- Ensure well-fitting footwear with a high 'box' (the space at the end to accommodate the toes).
- Use emollients to prevent drying of the skin and treat tinea pedis early with topical antifungal creams.

Tumours require surgical management, which is best provided by a dermatological surgeon or a plastic or orthopaedic surgeon with expertise in hand or foot surgery.

Severe systemic inflammatory diseases can be associated with nail changes that may be severe enough to affect function and quality of life. In these instances, systemic therapies such as ciclosporin, methotrexate, retinoids, prednisolone or biologics may be warranted. The nature of nail growth suggests that benefit of therapy may not be seen for 2–3 months, but once the inflammatory disease is suppressed it is possible to discontinue therapy and await further improvement. Systemic therapy may be given as pulses which make it possible to reduce the risk of side effects and to maximise cost benefit.

Nail Cosmetics

Nail cosmetics can provide a useful means of concealing aspects of nail disease not responding to treatment. Pitting can be hidden by coloured nail lacquer or filled with acrylic gel. Lacquer will also conceal onycholysis. However, once the nail plate starts to have structural changes such as splits or reduction in nail bed attachment, any form of artificial nail is at risk of causing additional problems. The most common is exacerbation of onycholysis as the adherent artificial nail acts as a lever that pulls the residual nail further from the nail bed. Other problems include subungual infection due to the crevices created with the imperfect adherence of the artificial nail. Removal of the artificial nail can also result in further disintegration of the diseased nail plate.

Further Reading

Baran R, de Berker DAR, Holzberg M and Thomas L, eds. *Baran and Dawber's Diseases of the Nails and Their Management*, 4th Edition, Wiley-Blackwell, Oxford, 2012.

de Berker DA, Baran R and Dawber RP. *Handbook of Diseases of the Nails and their Management*, Blackwell Scientific Publications, Oxford, 1995.

CHAPTER 21

Benign Skin Tumours

Rachael Morris-Jones

Dermatology Department, Kings College Hospital, London, UK

> **OVERVIEW**
>
> - Skin cells can proliferate in a benign controlled manner, known as *hyperplasia*, or as an uncontrolled, dysplastic growth to produce cancer.
> - Benign skin lesions are common and generally have a well-defined appearance. Any sudden increase in size, irregularity or bleeding may suggest malignant change.
> - Benign skin lesions are usually asymptomatic but may bleed persistently (pyogenic granuloma) or cause pain (poroma). Some benign tumours are disfiguring and cause psychological problems.
> - Benign pigmented tumours include seborrhoeic keratoses, which are well defined with a warty rough dull surface, freckles (lentigines) and skin tags.
> - Pigmented naevi may be congenital or acquired. The vast majority remain benign. However, change in colour, texture, size or new satellite lesions developing may indicate malignant change.
> - Benign vascular lesions include port wine stain, cavernous haemangioma and naevus flammeus neonatorum.
> - The most common acquired vascular lesions are spider naevi, Campbell de Morgan spots (cherry haemangiomas) and pyogenic granulomas.

Introduction

Any cell within the skin can proliferate to form a benign lump or skin tumour. In general, a proliferation of cells can lead to hyperplasia (benign overgrowth) or dysplasia (malignancy/cancer). This chapter considers benign lesions, which by definition are harmless, but may cause symptoms such as pain, itching and bleeding or may be a cosmetic nuisance. Many benign skin lesions are pigmented, which can lead to a high level of anxiety for patients and occasionally medical staff as they may be confused with melanoma.

Pattern recognition plays a valuable role in the correct diagnosis of benign skin lesions. The clinical features of any lesion can be a useful guide to distinguishing the benign from the malignant. However, if there is uncertainty as to the nature of any skin lesion after clinical examination then a diagnostic biopsy for histology is essential. The old adage 'if in doubt cut it out' may be appropriate if there is diagnostic uncertainty and skin experts are not available locally to see the patient.

Benign cutaneous lesions are almost universally present on the skin of adults and are therefore so common that most are ignored and are never brought to medical attention. Nonetheless, the sudden appearance of new lesions, symptoms such as itching, pain or bleeding or the unsightly nature of lesions may bring them to the attention of the affected individual and thus the local practitioner. Reassurance is usually all that is needed. However, in some instances benign skin lesions need removal, for example, if they bleed persistently (pyogenic granulomas), they repeatedly catch on clothing (protuberant benign moles) or they cause pain (poroma on the foot). Some individuals are deeply affected by the cosmetic appearance of their benign skin lesions and these may therefore need removal on psychological grounds.

From a medical practitioner's point of view, we need to decide whether a lesion can be safely left or should be treated. This chapter concentrates on the correlation between clinical and pathological features of common benign tumours which should ease their diagnosis (Table 21.1). Chapter 22 examines premalignant and malignant skin tumours.

Table 21.1 Differential diagnosis of common benign skin tumours.

Clinical features	Differential diagnoses
Pigmented	Seborrhoeic keratoses, dermatosis papulosa nigra, freckles (lentigines), solar lentigo, melanocytic naevus, blue naevus, Mongolian blue spot, dermatofibroma, apocrine hidrocystomas
Vascular	Naevus flammeus, strawberry naevus, port-wine stain, spider naevi, Campbell de Morgan spots, pyogenic granuloma
Papules	Skin tags (fibroepithelial polyps), milia, sebaceous gland hyperplasia, dermatosis papulosa nigra, syringomas, trichoepitheliomas, apocrine hidrocystomas
Nodules	Dermatofibroma, lipoma, angiolipoma, epidermoid cyst, pilar cyst, pilomatrixoma, poroma, intradermal naevus, apocrine hidrocystomas
Plaques	Naevus sebaceus, epidermal naevus, inflammatory linear verrucous epidermal naevus (ILVEN), seborrhoeic keratoses

ABC of Dermatology, Sixth Edition. Edited by Rachael Morris-Jones.

Pigmented benign tumours

Seborrhoeic keratoses

Seborrhoeic keratoses are increasingly common with increasing age. Lesions are most frequently seen on the trunk, face and neck in sizes varying from 0.5 to 3.0 cm in diameter. Seborrhoeic keratoses may be barely palpable, protuberant or pedunculated. They always have a warty dull surface. Colours are highly variable from pale tan through to dark brown (Figure 21.1). When deeply pigmented, inflamed or growing they can appear to have some malignant characteristics which may cause anxiety. Seborrhoeic keratoses, however, have some characteristic features which include

- well-defined edge (Figure 21.2)
- warty, papillary surface, often with keratin plugs
- raised above surrounding skin to give a 'stuck on' appearance.

Dermatosis papulosa nigra (DPN)

These lesions are usually multiple small pigmented papules seen on the face of adults with black skin (Figure 21.3). Dermatosis papulosa nigra (DPN) is very common with up to one-third of individuals with skin type VI affected. Frequently, there is a strong familial tendency towards the condition. Typically the lesions occur on the cheeks, forehead, neck and chest. Histologically they resemble seborrhoeic keratoses; however, some experts think they arise from a developmental defect in the follicular unit. No treatment is needed, but if patients find the lesions cosmetically unacceptable then light electrodesiccation and gentle curettage can effectively remove lesions. New ones will inevitably form, however (see Chapter 23).

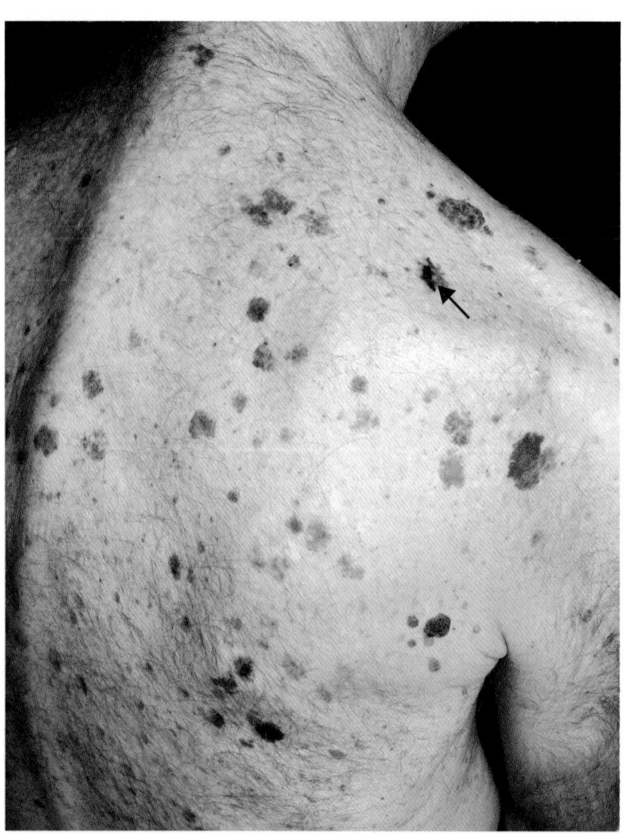

Figure 21.1 Seborrhoeic keratoses on the trunk, there is a melanoma on the right upper shoulder (shown by the arrow).

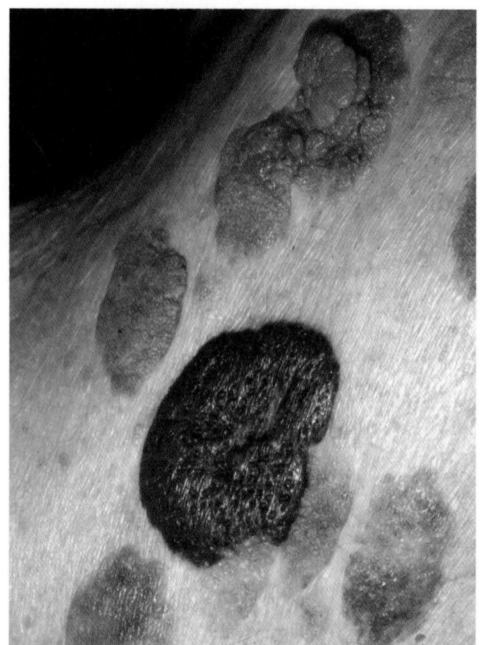

Figure 21.2 Seborrhoeic keratoses.

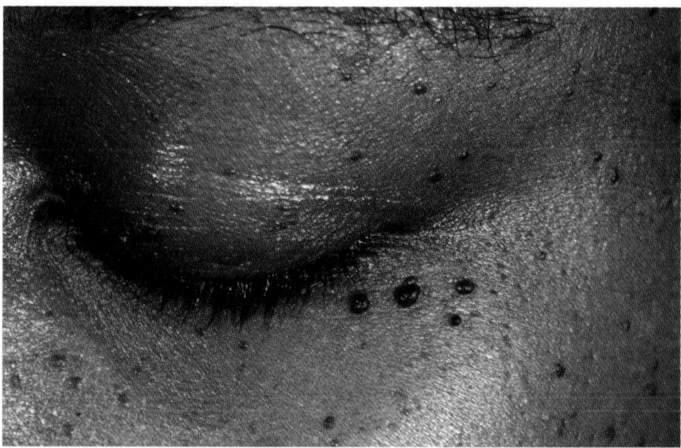

Figure 21.3 Dermatosis papulosa nigra.

Skin tags

Skin tags may be pigmented but are usually straightforward to diagnose. They are frequently multiple and more commonly occur at sites of occlusion where the skin may be rubbed by skin or clothing/jewellery in the axillae, neck, groin and under the breasts (Figure 21.4). If they are catching on clothing and so on, they can be removed by 'snip/shave' under local anaesthetic.

Lentigines (freckles)

Patients often refer to solar-induced freckles as 'sun spots' or 'liver spots'. Lentigines are small macular well-demarcated pigmented lesions that usually occur on sun-exposed skin (Figure 21.5). They

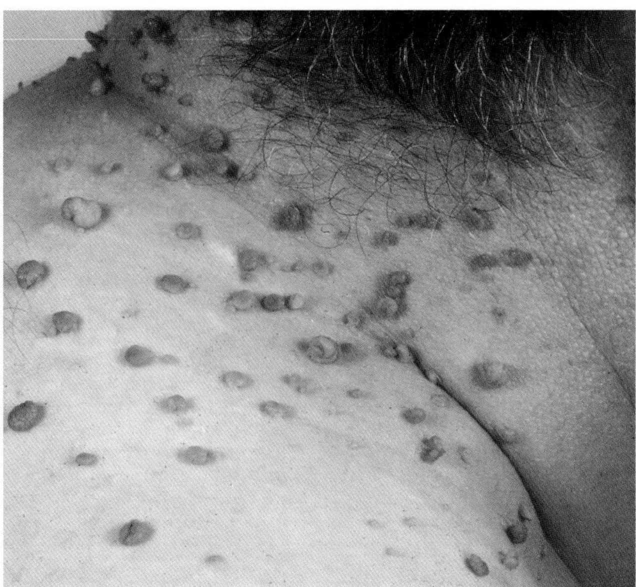

Figure 21.4 Skin tags.

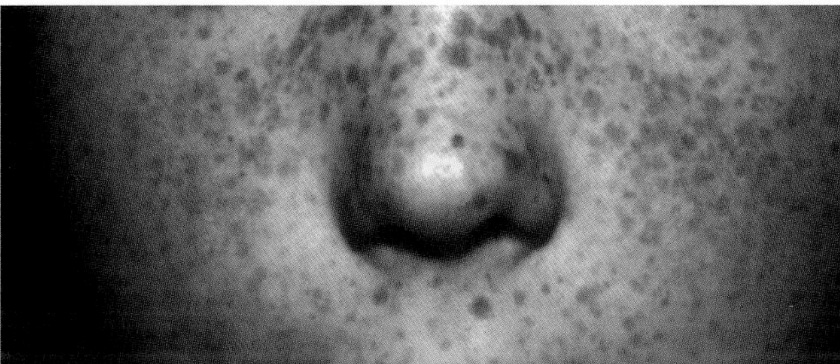

Figure 21.5 Lentigines.

first appear in childhood and generally increase in number with increasing age. Lentigines are more common in individuals with fair rather than dark skin types. The colour of the lentigines varies from pale tan to almost black, which usually corresponds to the amount of melanin pigment produced by the increased number of melanocytes. In contrast to moles where the melanocytes form nests (naevi), the melanocytes in lentigines line up along the basement membrane.

Benign lentigines may also occur on the lip and genital mucosa. Labial lentigines may be associated with Peutz–Jeghers syndrome (an inherited condition with gastrointestinal polyps), Laugier–Hunziker syndrome (which has associated nail pigmentation) and LAMB (lentigines, atrial myxoma, mucocutaneous myxomas and blue naevi). In LEOPARD syndrome (lentigines, electrocardioconduction defects, ocular hypertelorism, pulmonary stenosis, abnormal genitalia, retardation of growth and deafness) lentigines are characteristically seen on the neck and trunk. No treatment is usually required for lentigines; however, treatment with liquid nitrogen may help them fade.

Melanocytic naevi

The majority of moles are benign and can be safely ignored. However, knowing which are potentially harmful or malignant can be difficult for inexperienced practitioners. Clinical features of benign moles will be considered in this chapter to aid their diagnosis. Malignant moles are considered in Chapter 22.

The term *naevi* is derived from the Greek word meaning 'nest'. A proliferation of melanocytes forms these nests at different levels in the skin resulting in moles. If the nests of melanocytes are confined to the dermoepidermal junction, then the mole is referred to as *junctional naevus*, if they are in the dermis only, 'intradermal naevus' and if present in the epidermis and dermis, 'compound naevus'. Naevi may be congenital ('birth mark') or acquired, usually in early childhood. The number of moles usually remains static in adulthood with a decline after the sixth decade.

Congenital melanocytic naevi

Between 1% and 2% of neonates have a congenital naevus present at birth. Similar lesions can appear during the first 2 years of life that look histologically identical to congenital moles. Melanocytes are derived from neural crest cells; during embryogenesis they migrate into the skin and the central nervous system. Congenital naevi are thought to result from an anomaly of melanocyte development or migration. Congenital naevi are classified according to their size: small are less than 1.5 cm, medium 1.5–19.9 cm and giant greater than 20 cm in diameter. Congenital naevi usually grow in proportion to the growth of the child, and their colour varies from pale brown to black. With increasing age congenital naevi often develop hair and become more protuberant (Figure 21.6).

Giant lesions can cover a considerable area of the trunk and buttocks, such as the bathing trunk naevi, and these are the most likely to undergo malignant change (~5%). The majority of congenital naevi are, however, benign. If malignancy is suspected due to a sudden change in size, colour, border and development of new satellite lesions, then surgical excision would be indicated. Surgical removal of very large lesions may be difficult, and tissue expanders, staged operations and skin grafting are often needed. Attempts at curettage or laser removal have both been advocated as alternatives to excision, but recurrence is more likely.

Mongolian blue spots are congenital skin lesions that result from collections of melanocytes deep in the skin, usually present on the back. The lesions are macular and large and may be multiple. The condition is most common in black and Asian skin (Figure 21.7).

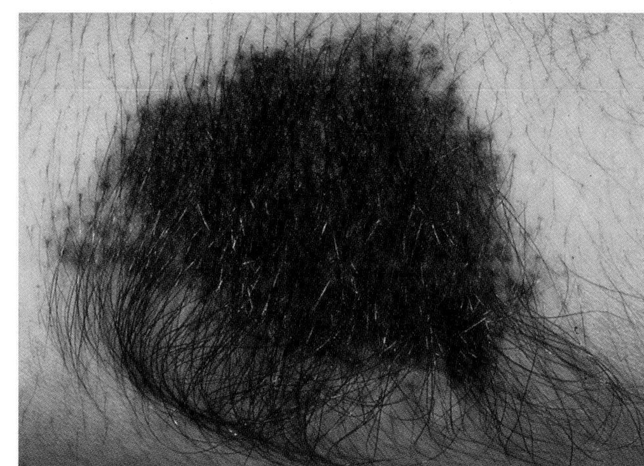

Figure 21.6 Congenital melanocytic naevus.

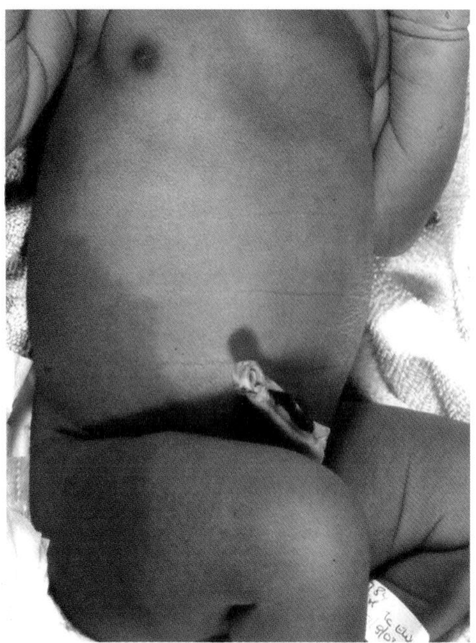

Figure 21.7 Mongolian blue spot.

Acquired melanocytic naevi

These are moles acquired during childhood. The main stimulus to their formation is thought to be solar radiation and a genetic susceptibility. These moles have a variable appearance determined by the depth of the melanocytes and the cellular type.

Junctional naevi are flat macules with melanocytes proliferating into nests that sit along the dermoepidermal junction (Figure 21.8).

Compound naevi have clusters of melanocytes at the dermoepidermal junction and within the dermis. These naevi are raised and pigmented (Figure 21.9). The surface of the naevus may be thrown into folds because of the melanocyte proliferations, giving a papillary appearance.

In a purely *intradermal naevus*, the junctional element is lost, and nests of melanocytes are found within the dermis alone. These naevi are frequently non-pigmented and most commonly occur on the face (Figure 21.10). These moles are raised from the skin surface and may catch on clothing or may cause a cosmetic problem – they may be treated by 'shave' of the top portion of the mole under local anaesthetic.

Blue naevus is a collection of deeply pigmented melanocytes situated deep in the dermis, which accounts for the deep slate-blue colour (Figure 21.11).

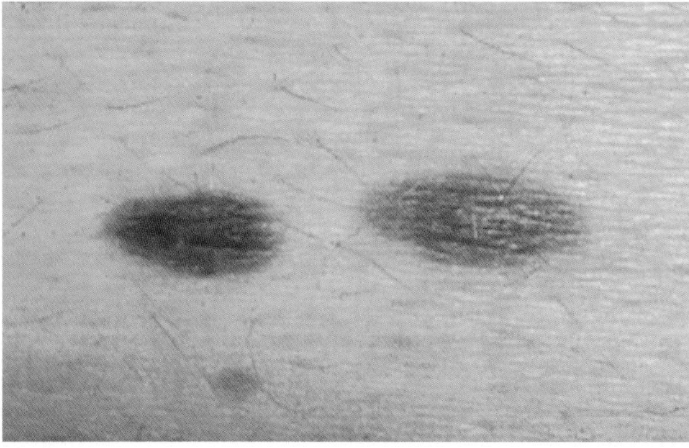

Figure 21.8 Junctional naevus.

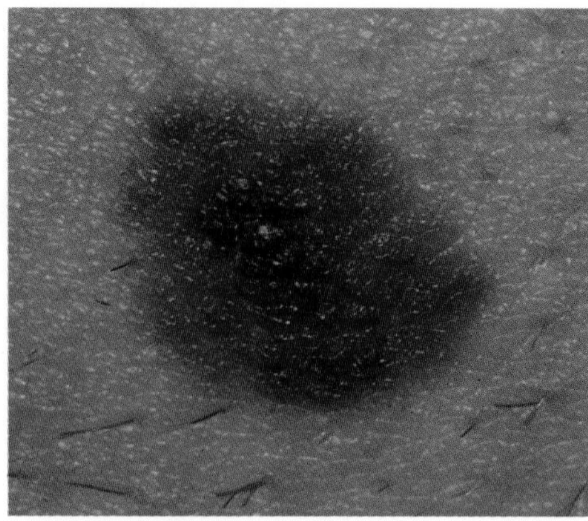

Figure 21.9 Compound naevus.

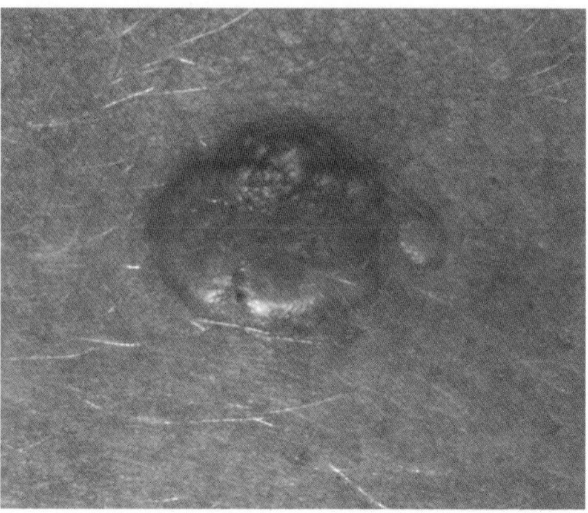

Figure 21.10 Intradermal naevus.

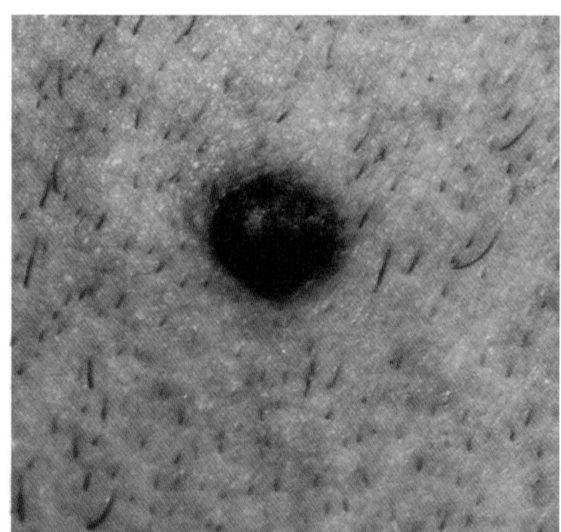

Figure 21.11 Blue naevus.

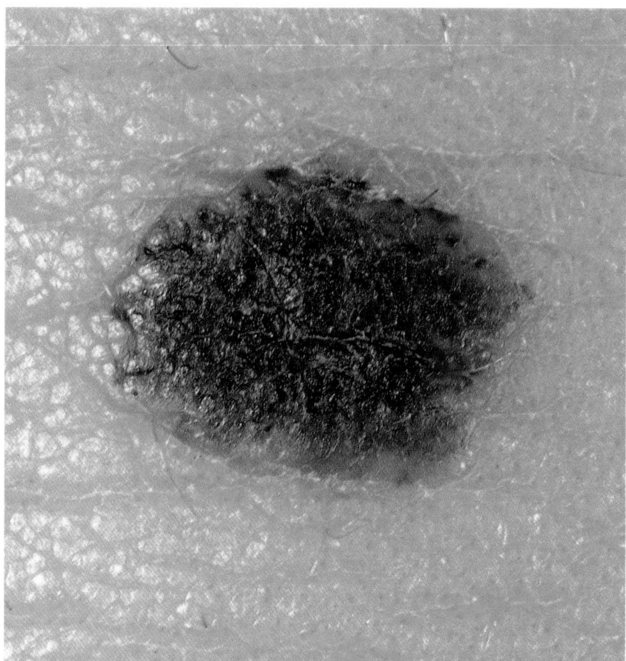

Figure 21.12 Spitz naevus.

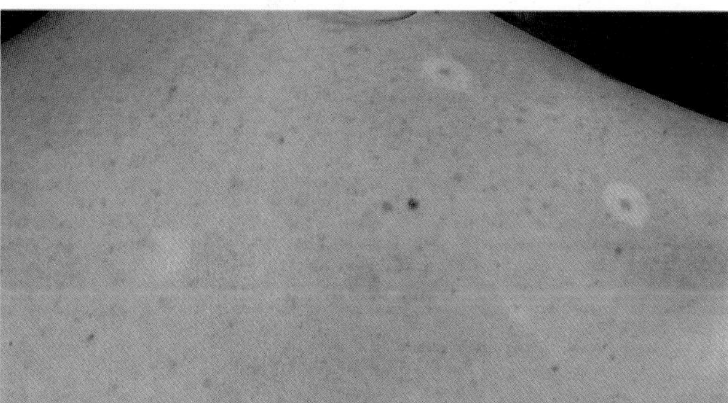

Figure 21.13 Halo naevus.

Spitz naevus presents as a fleshy pink or pigmented papule in children. It is composed of large spindle cells and epitheloid cells with occasional giant cells, arranged in nests (Figure 21.12).

Halo naevus consists of a melanocytic naevus with a surrounding halo of depigmentation (Figure 21.13). Patients may have several halo naevi simultaneously. They are thought to be associated with the presence of antibodies against melanocytes, which can cause the entire naevus to disappear eventually.

Becker's naevus is an area of increased pigmentation, often associated with increased hair growth, which is usually seen on the upper trunk or shoulders (Figure 21.14).

Dermatofibroma

These are firm discrete nodules arising in the dermis, usually on the legs of women. Initially lesions may appear red or light brown but usually mature into a firm brown papule with a ring of darker peripheral pigment (Figure 21.15). Lesions may be itchy or even painful. The underlying pathophysiology is poorly understood; some authors believe they arise at the site of insect bites or minor trauma while others believe them to be a true benign tumour of fibroblasts. They can be excised under local anaesthetic if they are problematic but a linear scar will result from surgery.

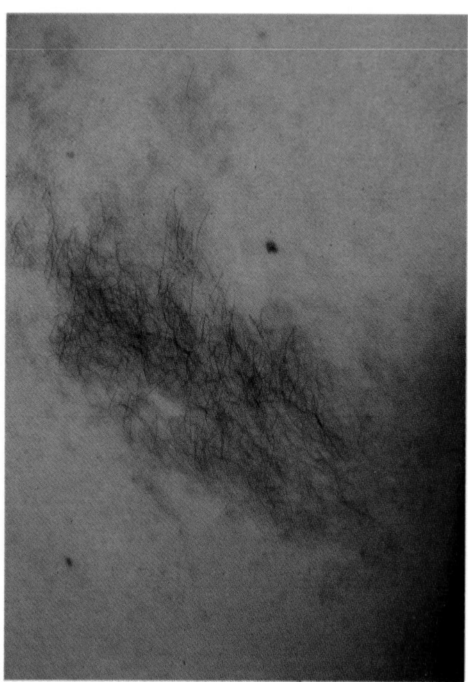

Figure 21.14 Becker's naevus.

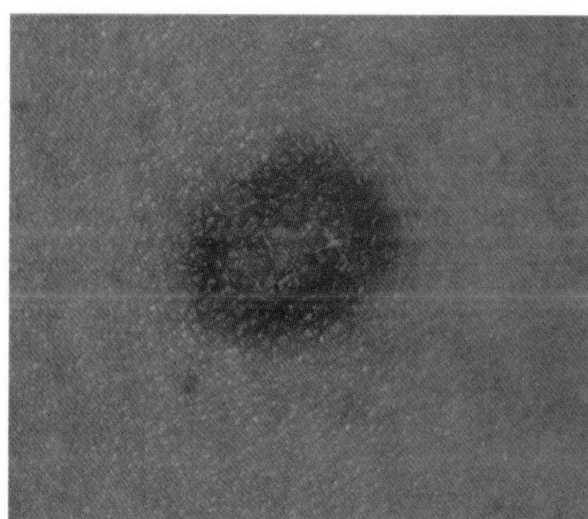

Figure 21.15 Dermatofibroma.

Benign vascular tumours

The most common benign vascular malformations and tumours are described and their management options discussed.

Naevus flammeus neonatorum refers to 'stork marks' or 'salmon patches' present at birth most commonly at the glabella, eyelids and nape of the neck (Figure 21.16). Up to one-third of neonates are affected. Lesions on the neck persist for life; however, facial lesions usually fade or completely disappear by the age of 2 years.

Port-wine stains are capillary malformations of the superficial dermal blood vessels that are present at birth. Therefore, they are not strictly neoplasms but are discussed here for convenience. They most commonly occur on the head and neck. Lesions may

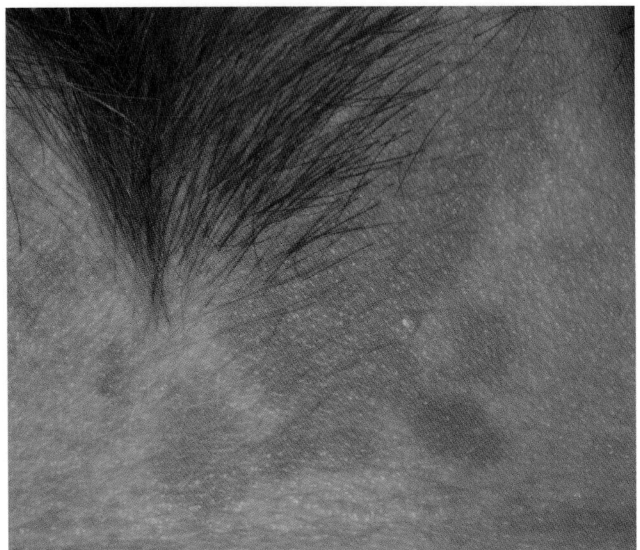

Figure 21.16 Naevus flammeus neonatorum.

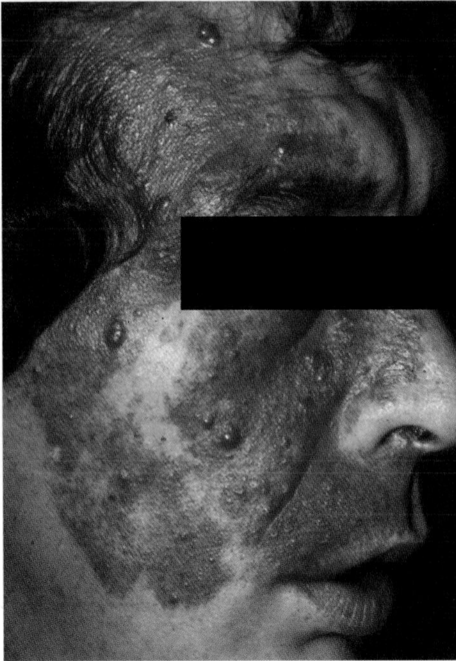

Figure 21.17 Sturge–Weber syndrome.

initially be of a pale pink colour but darken with increasing age through red to purple. Capillary malformations increase in size proportionally with the growth of the child and tend to persist. Port wine stains on the face are usually unilateral with a sharp midline border (Figure 21.17). In time, the affected area becomes raised and thickened due to a proliferation of vascular and connective tissue. If the area supplied by the ophthalmic or maxillary divisions of the trigeminal nerve is affected, there may be associated angiomas of the underlying meninges with epilepsy – Sturge–Weber syndrome. Patients should have an magnetic resonance imaging (MRI) scan with gadolinium enhancement to visualize neural involvement. Klippel–Trenaunay syndrome usually presents with a capillary malformation associated with limb overgrowth and varicosities. In addition, lesions of the limb may be associated with arteriovenous fistulae: the so-called Parkes–Weber syndrome.

Capillary malformations may be treated with a pulsed-dye laser which targets oxyhaemoglobin (see Chapter 24). The ideal age for treatment is difficult to determine. Some experts feel laser treatment should be undertaken before the first birthday, but a general anaesthetic may be necessary. The outcome of laser treatment depends on the size, location and depth of vessels in the skin, but most lesions require multiple treatments. Patients can be offered cosmetic camouflage.

Cavernous haemangiomas/strawberry naevi are true benign vascular neoplasms which grow out of proportion to the growing neonate. These lesions usually appear at birth or during the first few weeks of life and rapidly enlarge at around 6 months of age (Figure 21.18a). The exact cause is unknown; however, several theories exist including speculation that they may arise from endothelial cells breaking away from the placenta. Lesions may be single (80%) or multiple and are more common in infants whose mothers underwent chorionic villous sampling. Clinically, a soft vascular swelling is found, most commonly on the head and neck. The lesions resolve spontaneously in time and do not require intervention unless recurrently bleeding or interference with visual development occurs. Oral propranolol (1–3 mg/kg/day) or atenolol is the current treatment of choice to shrink down haemangiomas that are life threatening, affect function/development or are ulcerated and bleeding (Figure 21.18b). The first dose is usually given with cardiac monitoring. The site and size of the haemangioma will determine the length of the treatment course needed to shrink the lesion; however, up to age 12 months may be needed to prevent regrowth. Alternative interventions include laser treatment, prednisolone and sclerotherapy (see Chapter 24).

Spider naevi consist of a central vascular papule with fine lines radiating from it (Figure 21.19). They are more common in children and women. Large numbers may raise the possibility of liver disease or an underlying connective tissue disorder such as systemic sclerosis. They may be treated with a pulsed dye laser or hyfrecation.

Campbell de Morgan spots (cherry haemangiomas) are discrete red papules 1–5 mm in diameter. They occur in up to 50% of adults, are usually multiple and occur most frequently on the trunk (Figure 21.20).

Pyogenic granuloma is poorly named as it is not infectious but a lobular capillary haemangioma. The usually single vascular lesion grows rapidly and easily bleeds with minor trauma (Figure 21.21). The bleeding can be profuse and recurrent. Lesions may arise at the site of trauma, often on the digits. Distinction from amelanotic melanoma is important. Although benign, pyogenic granulomas need to be removed surgically by curettage and cautery (under

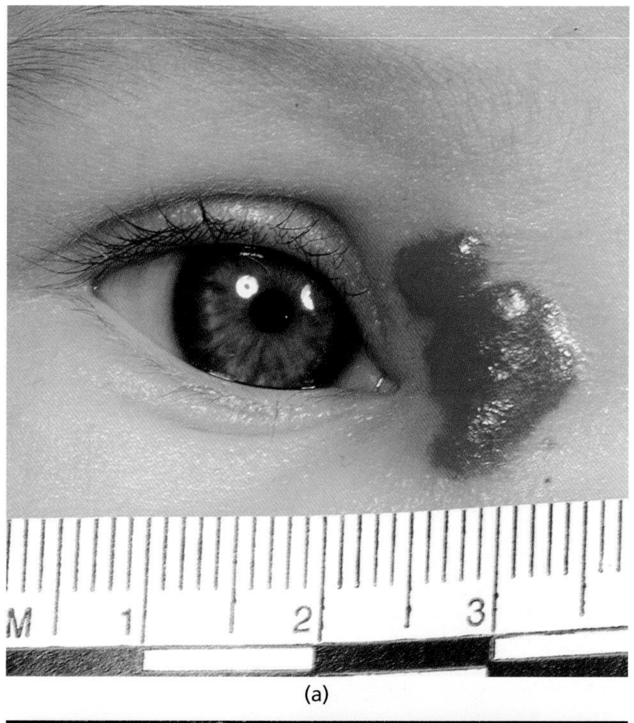

(a)

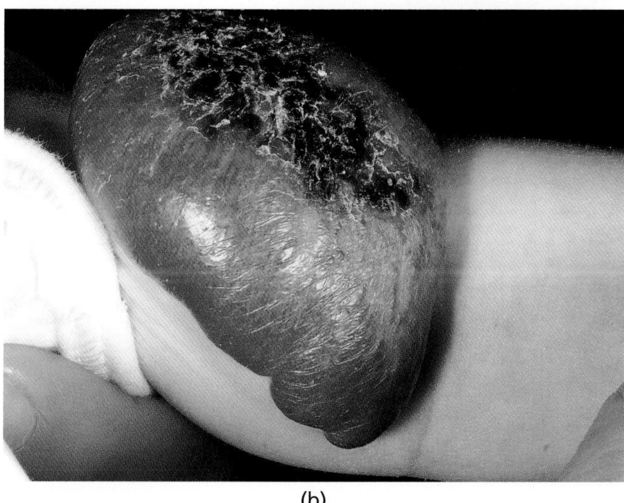

(b)

Figure 21.18 (a) Cavernous (strawberry) haemangioma and (b) ulcerating and bleeding cavernous haemangioma suitable for treatment with systemic β blockers.

plain lignocaine local anaesthetic at digital sites) as they rarely resolve spontaneously (see Chapter 23).

Benign tumour papules

These commonly include skin tags (fibroepithelial polyps – see above), DPN (see above), syringomas, trichoepitheliomas, apocrine hidrocystomas, milia and sebaceous gland hyperplasia.

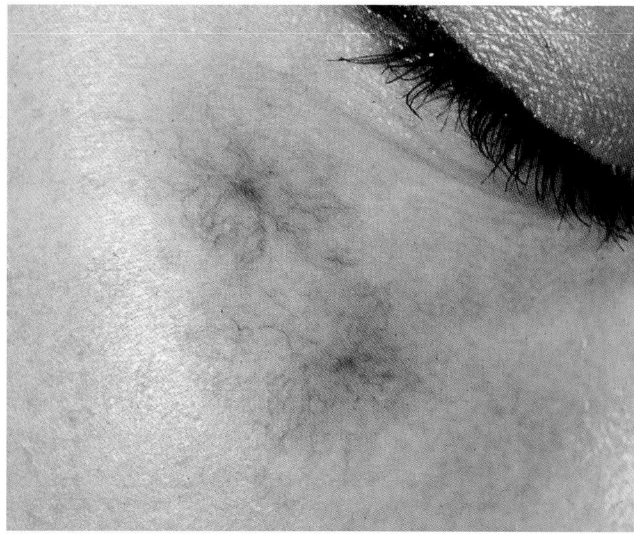

Figure 21.19 Spider naevi.

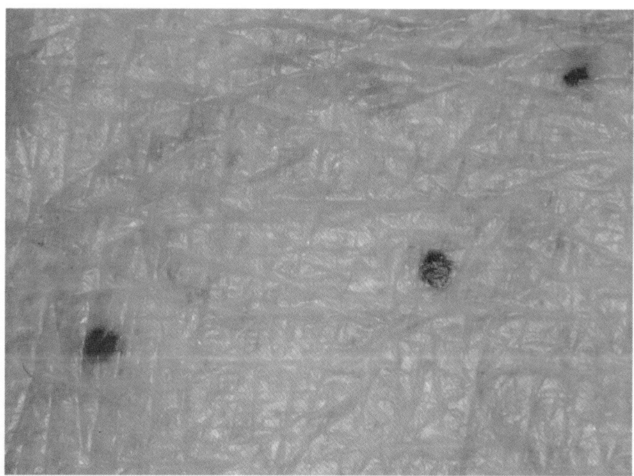

Figure 21.20 Campbell de Morgan spots.

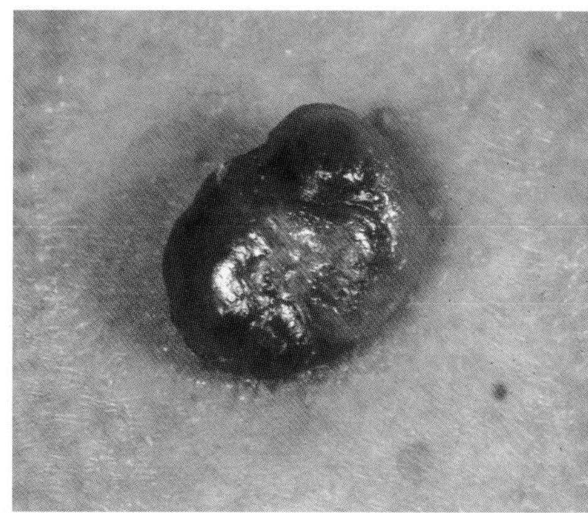

Figure 21.21 Pyogenic granuloma.

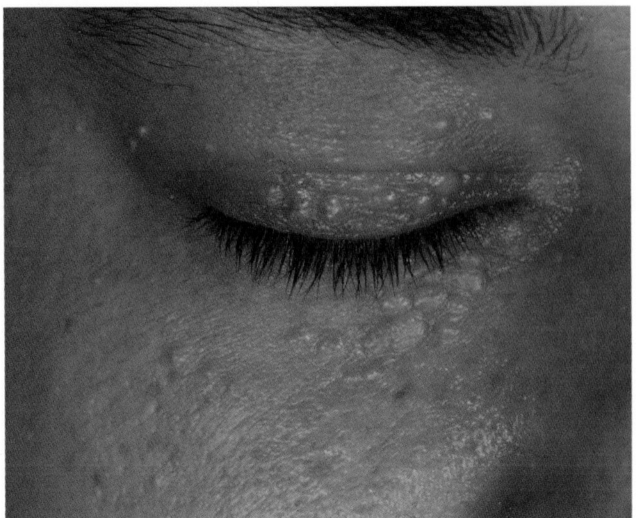

Figure 21.22 Syringomas.

Syringomas are benign adnexal tumours of the eccrine glands. Lesions are usually multiple, slow-growing, small and flesh coloured and usually appear on the face around puberty (Figure 21.22). The trunk and groin areas may also be affected. Treatment on cosmetic grounds is surgical with shave removal or cautery of the lesions.

Trichoepitheliomas are benign adnexal tumours of hair follicle origin. These may resemble syringomas as they are also small, often multiple and occur on the face and scalp (Figure 21.23). Surgical removal or laser treatment can help to alleviate the cosmetic appearance but lesions tend to be multiple and may recur.

Apocrine hidrocystoma are benign adnexal tumours of apocrine glands that form papules or nodules around the eyes. Lesions are solitary or multiple and may be translucent (Figure 21.24) or pale through to black (lipofuscin pigment).

Milia are small keratin cysts consisting of small white papules found on the cheek and eyelids. Milia are common on the cheeks of newborns, and secondary milia may occur following skin trauma or inflammation (Figure 21.25). These minute cysts are harmless and require no treatment. They can be removed under topical anaesthetic with a sterile needle.

Sebaceous gland hyperplasia is a benign hamartomatous enlargement of the sebaceous glands and therefore not a tumour. However, these small papules are not infrequently confused with benign skin tumours and basal cell carcinomas, and therefore are discussed here (Figure 21.26). Turnover of sebocyte cells within the glands decreases with increasing age, leading to hyperplasia. This is particularly prominent in patients who are immunosuppressed with ciclosporin. There is an increased frequency of sebaceous gland hyperplasia reported with Muir–Torré syndrome. Patients develop sebaceous adenomas/carcinomas in association with systemic malignancies.

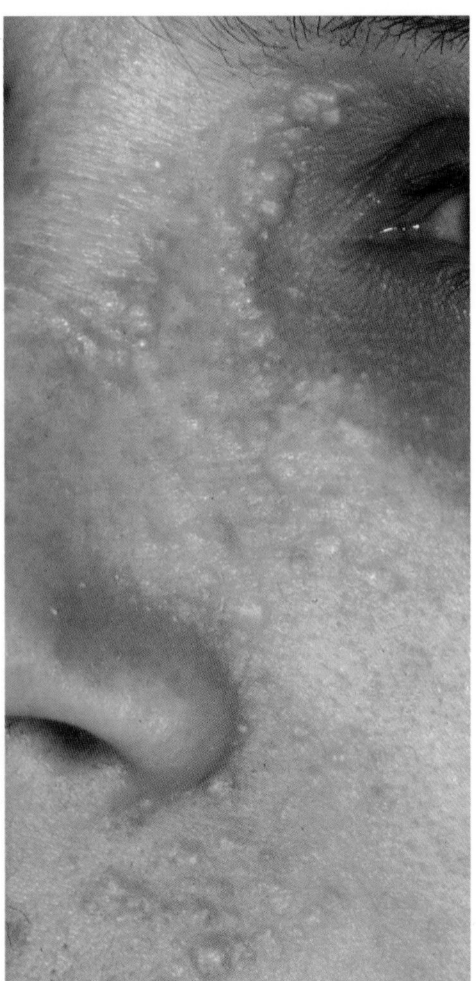

Figure 21.23 Trichoepitheliomas.

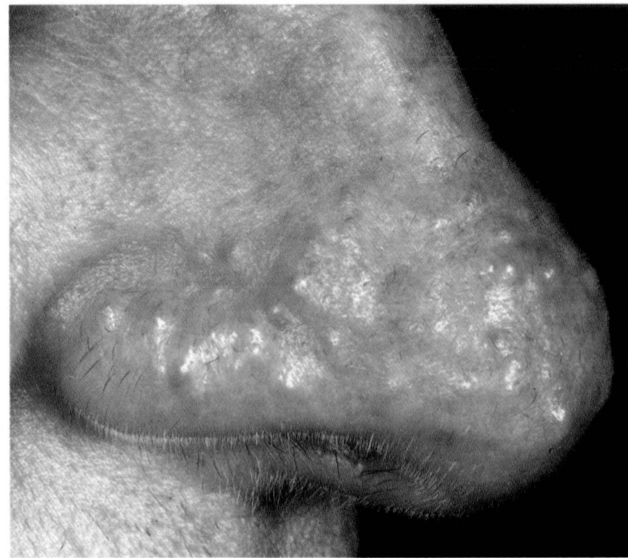

Figure 21.24 Apocrine hidrocystomas.

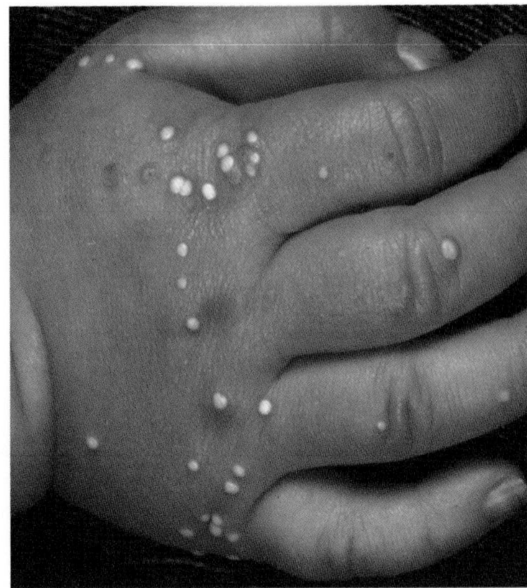

Figure 21.25 Milia.

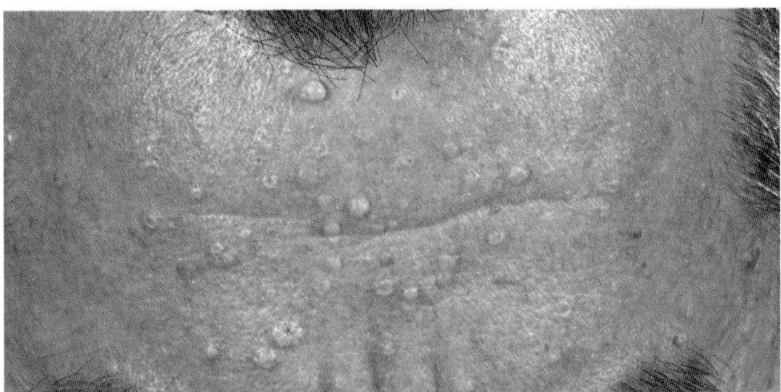

Figure 21.26 Sebaceous gland hyperplasia.

Benign tumour nodules

Lipomas are common slow-growing benign subcutaneous tumours of fat. They may be congenital or acquired, single or multiple (Figure 21.27). Lipomas are usually asymptomatic but they may classically cause pain when they are associated with Dercum's disease (postmenopausal women who may be obese, depressed or alcoholic with multiple painful lipomas on the lower legs). *Angiolipomas* may also be painful.

Benign painful tumours in the skin: 'BENGAL'

- *B*lue rubber bleb naevus
- *E*ccrine spiradenoma
- *N*eurilemmoma/neuroma
- *G*lomus tumour
- *A*ngiolipoma
- *L*eiomyoma (Figure 21.28).

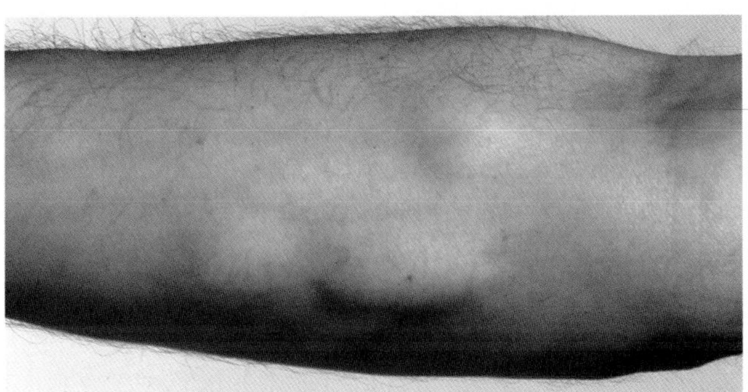

Figure 21.27 Lipoma.

Epidermoid cysts (previously called *sebaceous cyst*) are common. They are soft, well-defined, mobile swellings usually on the face, neck, shoulders or chest. There may be an obvious central punctum (Figure 21.29). Epidermoid cysts arise due to a proliferation of epidermal cells in the dermis derived from the hair follicle. They may become inflamed or infected causing discomfort and discharge (thick yellow material that has a bad odour) but are generally

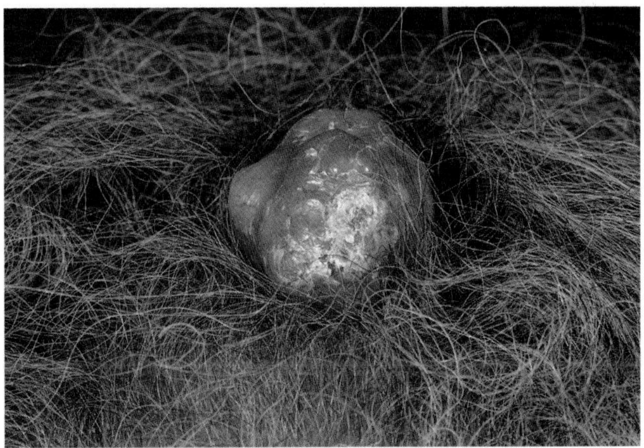

Figure 21.28 Leiomyoma on scalp vertex.

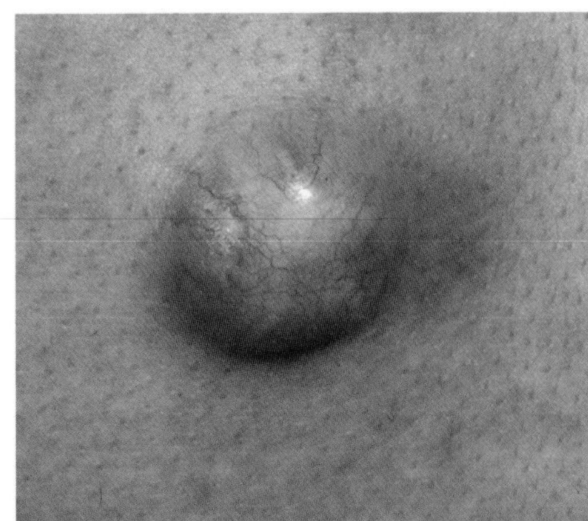

Figure 21.29 Epidermoid cyst.

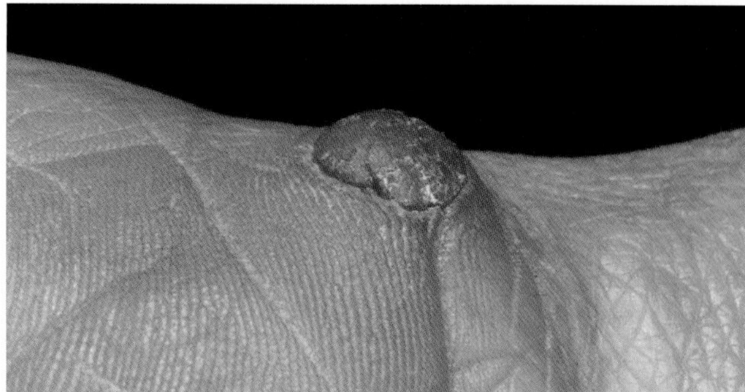

Figure 21.30 Eccrine poroma.

asymptomatic. If cysts are troublesome they can be completely excised or removed by punch extrusion (see Chapter 23).

Pilar cysts on the scalp are very common and frequently multiple. Clinically, they can resemble epidermoid cysts but they do not have a punctum. They are derived from hair follicles. Surgical removal may be necessary in some cases, when the tumour usually 'shells out' very easily.

Pilomatrixoma is a benign tumour of the hair matrix. A very hard slow-growing lump usually presents on the head/neck of a child. Lesions may be a few centimetres in diameter. Spontaneous regression is not usually observed, and although they are benign most tumours are excised for histology.

Poromas may be apocrine- or eccrine-derived benign tumours of the skin. These nodular lesions are slow growing but may be painful (Figure 21.30). Rarely lesions may undergo malignant transformation. Surgical excision of poromas is the treatment of choice.

Keloid scars is a benign tumour of dermal fibroblasts that form at the sites of skin trauma – which may be minor such as a graze/burn, or secondary to inflammatory conditions such as chicken pox/acne or may result from deliberate skin piercing (Figure 21.31) or indeed any kind of surgery. Keloid scars proliferate beyond the site of the injury and they do not regress, unlike hypertrophic scars.

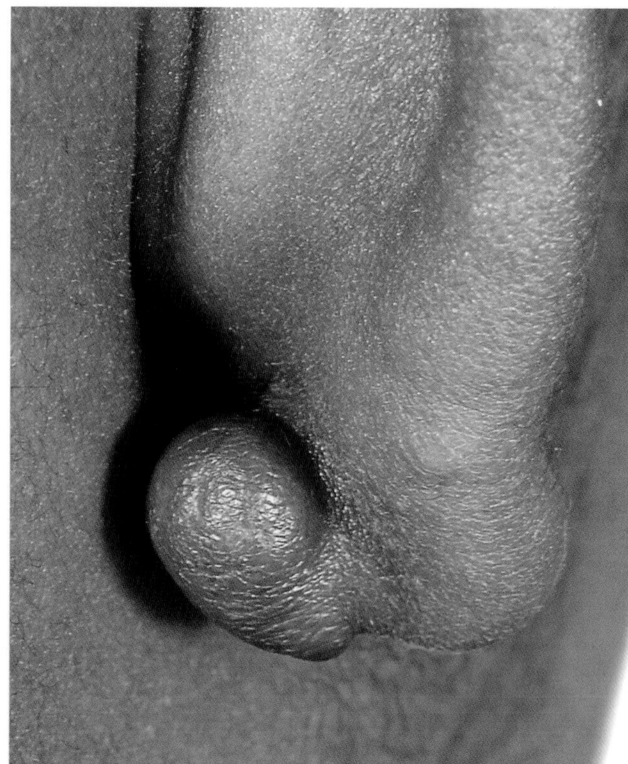

Figure 21.31 Keloid scar secondary to ear piercing.

Benign tumour plaques

Naevus sebaceous is a warty, well-defined plaque of 0.5–2 cm in diameter that mainly occurs on the scalp. Lesions may be present at birth or appear during childhood and slowly increase in size. In neonates, a hairless yellow plaque may be seen on the scalp (Figure 21.32). As the lesion matures, it may become verrucous and occasionally a trichoblastoma may develop within it. This is

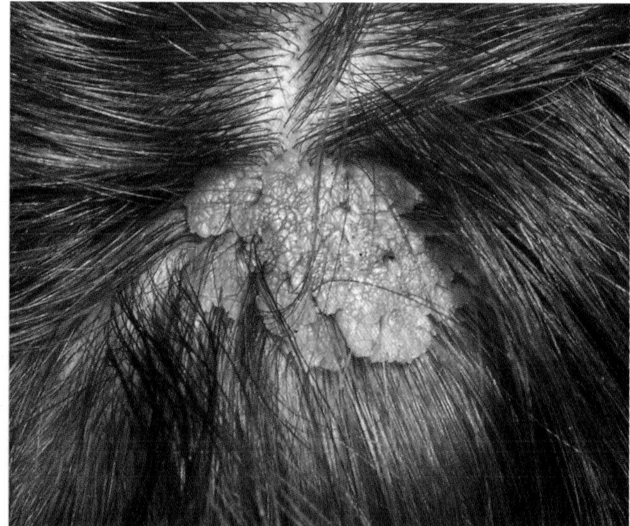

Figure 21.32 Naevus sebaceous.

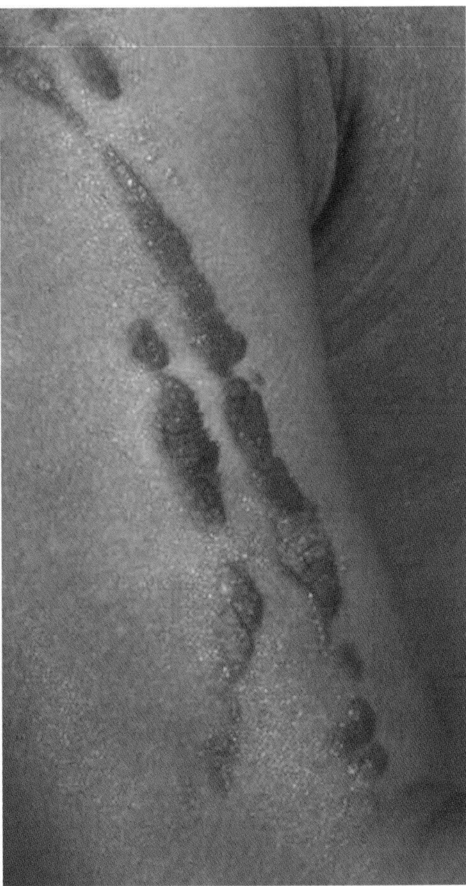

Figure 21.33 Epidermal naevus.

a benign tumour that may be misdiagnosed histologically as a basal cell carcinoma. Very large lesions may be associated with internal disorders.

Epidermal naevi are congenital lesions that may be linear or clustered and appear as warty brown papular lesions on the skin (Figure 21.33).

Inflammatory linear verrucous epidermal naevus (ILVEN) may be present at birth or appear during the first 5 years of life, most commonly on the lower limb or trunk. Lesions are warty and brown and are usually linear or clustered. Lesions may become red and inflamed and may be mistaken for eczema (Figure 21.34). Topical steroids and emollients may help to relieve itching and dryness.

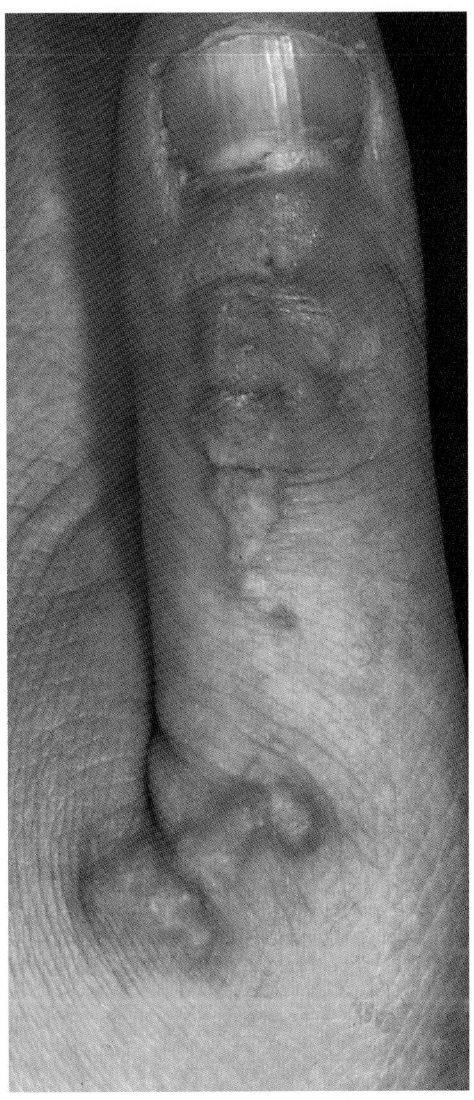

Figure 21.34 Inflammatory linear verrucous epidermal naevus (ILVEN).

Further Reading

Leboit PE, Burg G, Weedon D and Sarasin A. *Pathology and Genetics of Tumours of the Skin* (IARC WHO Classification of Tumours), WHO, Lyon, 2005.

Mackie RM. *Skin Cancer: An Illustrated Guide to the Etiology, Clinical Features, Pathology and Management of Benign and Malignant Cutaneous Tumours*, 2nd Edition, Martin Dunitz, London, 1996.

CHAPTER 22

Premalignant and Malignant

Rachael Morris-Jones

Dermatology Department, Kings College Hospital, London, UK

Skin tumours

OVERVIEW

- Skin cancers are among the most common malignancies and arise when there is an uncontrolled proliferation of undifferentiated dysplastic cells.
- In premalignant lesions, there is abnormal growth of cells but not complete dysplastic change. This occurs in actinic keratoses and Bowen's disease.
- Squamous cell carcinoma (SCC) develops in previously normal skin or pre-existing lesions such as actinic keratoses or Bowen's disease.
- Basal cell carcinoma (BCC) is the most common cancer in humans. Clumps of dysplastic basal cells form nodules that expand and break down to form an ulcer with a rolled edge.
- The carcinogenic effect of the sun is an important cause of skin cancer and is a major factor in the high incidence of melanoma.
- Pigmented naevi or moles are usually benign but the signs of malignant change must be recognised.
- Melanoma is a malignant tumour of melanocytes. A major risk factor is high intensity UV exposure, particularly in childhood.
- Melanoma occurs in various forms; superficial spreading melanoma is the most common. Other types include lentigo maligna melanoma, nodular melanoma, acral melanoma and amelanotic melanoma.
- The prognosis of melanoma depends on the depth of invasion.

Introduction

Malignancies of the skin are among the most common cancers known to man. In benign tumours, there is a proliferation of well-differentiated cells with limited growth, whereas in a malignant tumour, the dysplastic cells are undifferentiated and expand in an uncontrolled manner. The carcinogenic effect of the sun is thought to play an important role in many types of skin cancer. One hundred years ago, a tanned skin indicated outdoor work. Nowadays, many individuals deliberately seek the sun for the purposes of tanning. Longer holidays, cheap flights and a fashion to be tanned may all have contributed to the doubling of melanoma incidence over the past decade.

ABC of Dermatology, Sixth Edition. Edited by Rachael Morris-Jones.

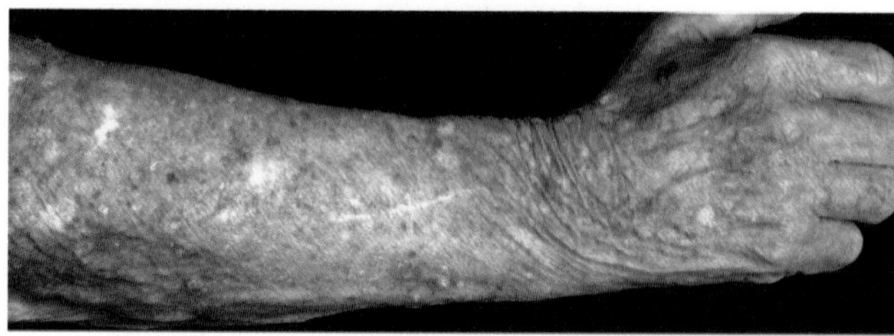

Figure 22.1 Sun-damaged skin with multiple actinic keratoses.

However, recently there has been an increasing global awareness concerning the dangers of strong sunlight. Public health campaigns such as 'slip slop slap' ('*slip* on a shirt, *slop* on sunscreen and *slap* on a hat') in Australia have been very successful at modifying people's behaviour in the sun. High-intensity ultraviolet (UV) light can lead to sun-burning episodes in fair-skinned individuals, and this is thought to be a risk factor for melanoma, the most serious form of skin cancer.

The visible nature of skin cancer means detection should be straightforward by the trained eye, although histological confirmation is essential. Early recognition of malignant skin tumours by medical practitioners is essential in order that patients suffer minimal morbidity and avoid skin-cancer-induced mortality.

Premalignant skin tumours

Actinic keratoses

Actinic keratoses (AKs) occur on exposed skin, particularly in those who have worked outdoors or have been exposed to short intervals of high-intensity UV. AKs occur on the face (including the lip), dorsal hands, distal limbs and bald scalp, particularly in those with fair/sun-damaged skin and increasing age (Figure 22.1). Clinically, their appearance varies from a rough area of skin to a raised keratotic lesion. The edge is irregular and they are usually less than 1 cm in diameter. Histologically, AKs have altered keratinisation, which may lead to dysplasia and eventually invasive squamous cell carcinoma (SCC). Malignant change may be suspected in an AK that suddenly grows rapidly, becomes painful or inflamed.

Management

Treatment with liquid nitrogen (cryotherapy) by a medical practitioner is usually effective for individual lesions with cure rates of around 70% (see Chapter 23). Various topical preparations that can be applied by patients themselves are currently available. 5-Fluorouracil (5-FU) 5% cream (Efudix®) and 0.5% solution (Actikerall) are useful in treating large areas of sun-damage with multiple AKs, and is applied once daily for 4–6 weeks. The 5-FU kills any dysplastic keratinocytes and therefore produces brisk inflammation at the application site. Patients may therefore need to stop using the cream for a few days during the treatment course if discomfort is severe. Currently, 5-FU appears to be the most cost-effective treatment for AKs.

Imiquimod 5% (Aldara®) is an immunomodulatory preparation that recruits immune cells to the area of skin where it is applied, which then attack the dysplastic cells. Imiquimod is applied three times a week for 4 months. 3.75% imiquimod (Zyclara) has recently been launched and should be used daily for 2 weeks, 1 week off and then treatment repeated for a further 2 weeks. There is some evidence that memory T-cells are induced by this therapy, resulting subsequently in lower numbers of clinical AKs.

Topical non-steroidal anti-inflammatory diclofenac (Solaraze®) has been shown to be effective against small AKs if it is used regularly twice daily for 3 months. This treatment seems to produce less skin irritation than 5-FU or imiquimod.

Ingenol mebutate gel (Picato®) is a recent addition to the treatment choice for actinic keratosis. It is a cytotoxic agent derived from Milk Weed plants that is formulated in two concentrations 0.015% (for the face once daily for 3 consecutive days) and 0.05% (for the trunk and limbs once daily for 2 consecutive days). Its effects are mediated by a brisk inflammatory reaction at the site, and the rates of clearance are reported between 34% and 42%. At 1 year follow-up, relapse rates are reported to be around 50%.

Photodynamic therapy (PDT) (see Chapter 24) has been shown to be as effective as 5-FU in the treatment of AKs. PDT is carried out by a medical practitioner rather than the patients themselves and can treat large areas of skin. The main limitation of PDT is usually the patient's ability to tolerate the burning pain felt in the skin during delivery of the treatment.

Any lesions not responding to the above measures should be biopsied to check for invasive malignancy.

Bowen's disease

Bowen's disease is SCC *in situ*; SCC occurs in the epidermis with no evidence of dermal invasion. Bowen's disease is more common in the elderly and is seen most frequently on the trunk and limbs. Risk factors for Bowen's disease include solar radiation, human papillomavirus warts (HPV 16), radiotherapy, ingestion of arsenic in 'tonics' and exposure to chemicals. Clinically, Bowen's disease is characterised by well-defined, erythematous patches with slight crusting (Figure 22.2). Lesions enlarge slowly and may reach up to 3 cm in diameter. After many years, invasive carcinoma may develop. Bowen's disease may be confused with a patch of eczema or superficial basal cell carcinoma (BCC). Erythroplasia of Queyrat is a similar process occurring on the glans penis or prepuce.

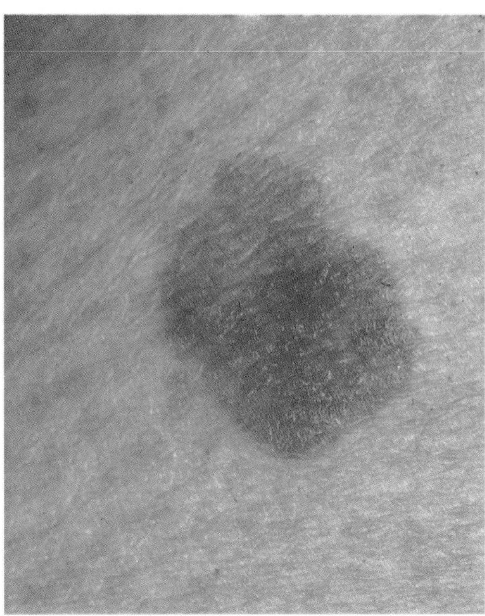

Figure 22.2 Bowen's disease

Skin biopsy can confirm the diagnosis histologically. Management includes excision, curettage and cautery, cryotherapy, 5-FU, imiquimod 5% and PDT (see Chapters 23 and 24).

Malignant skin tumours

Basal cell carcinoma (BCC)

This is the most common cancer in humans with a lifetime risk of around 30%. Known risk factors for BCC include increasing age, fair skin, high-intensity UV exposure, radiation, immunosuppression, previous history of BCCs and congenital disorders such as Gorlin's syndrome. Sun-exposed skin in the 'mask area' of the face is most frequently affected. Typically, lesions start as small papules that slowly grow. Lesions often have a 'pearly' shiny translucent quality. Colour varies from clear to deeply pigmented. The tumour is composed of masses of dividing basal cells that have lost the capacity to differentiate any further. As a result, no epidermis is formed over the tumour and the surface breaks down to form an ulcer, the residual edges of the nodule forming the characteristic 'rolled edge'. Once the basal cells have invaded the deeper tissues the rolled edge disappears.

BCC types

Nodular lesions appear as small papules or nodules with a rolled edge (Figure 22.3) and frequently a central depression that may become ulcerated. The nodules are pearly and may have dilated telangiectatic vessels on their surface. The histological features of BCC show collections of basaloid tumour cells (Figure 22.4), the pattern of which determines the histological type (i.e. nodular, superficial, morphoeic, cystic, etc.). Determining the tumour type histologically prior to definitive treatment ensures that the most appropriate management plan can be devised for each patient. If the initial tumour is incompletely excised/inadequately treated then the BCC can recur (Figure 22.5). Many BCCs on the face

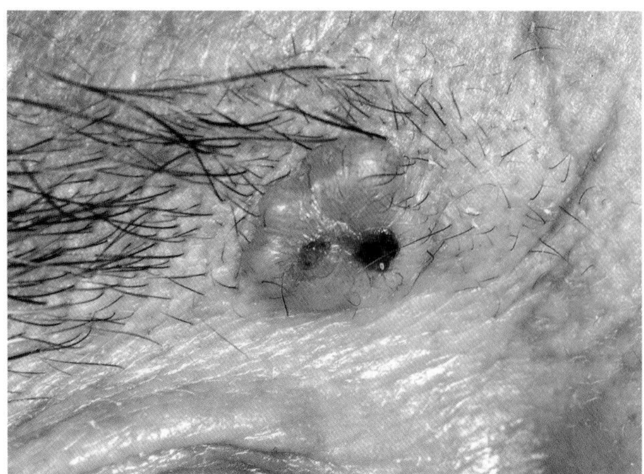

Figure 22.3 Nodular-type basal cell carcinoma above the eye.

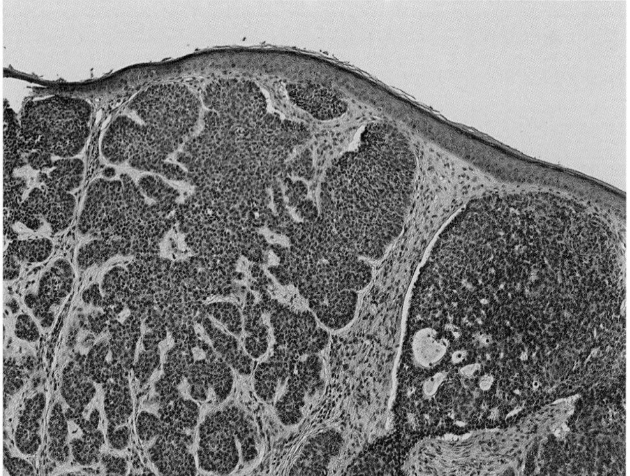

Figure 22.4 Nodular basal cell carcinoma histology.

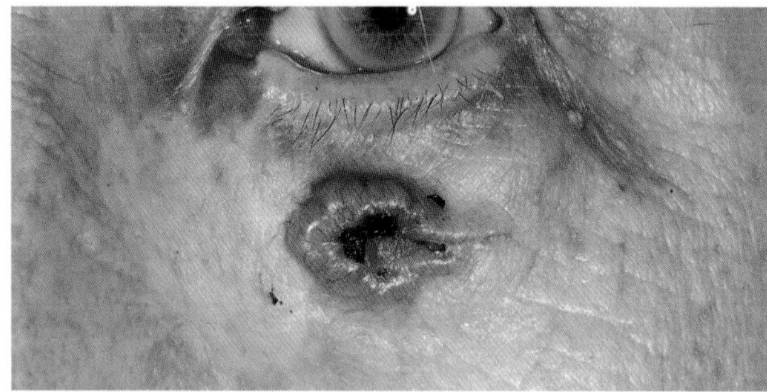

Figure 22.5 Recurrent nodular basal cell carcinoma.

are now treated routinely with Mohs' micrographic surgery to ensure that the tumour is fully resected (see Chapter 23) at the primary procedure.

Superficial lesions appear as an erythematous patch on the skin, often on the trunk. They may be mistaken for a patch of eczema or tinea, but are not usually pruritic and slowly enlarge (Figure 22.6). A firm 'whipcord' edge may be present.

Pigmented lesions can lead to confusion with naevi, seborrhoeic keratoses and melanoma (Figure 22.7).

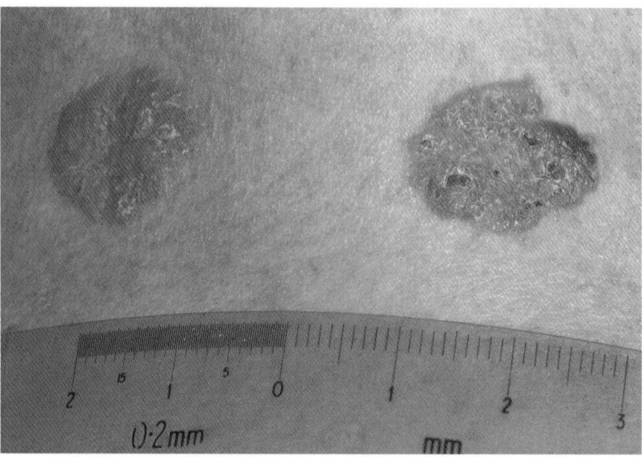

Figure 22.6 Superficial basal cell carcinoma.

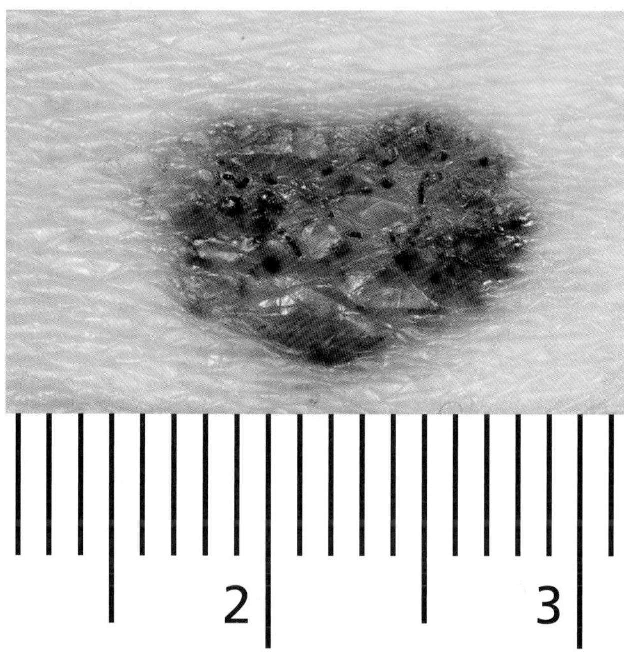

Figure 22.7 Pigmented basal cell carcinoma.

Morphoeic or sclerosing type appears as a superficial atrophic scar in the skin. There is loss of the normal skin markings and the edge is usually indistinct (Figure 22.8). This can lead to incomplete excision of these infiltrative BCCs and therefore Mohs' micrographic surgery may be indicated (see Chapter 23) to ensure surgical cure.

Management of BCC

The growth pattern determined histologically usually guides management, so most tumours are biopsied prior to definitive treatment. The site and the size of the BCC, co-morbidities and patient preference all guide what treatment option is most suitable. Treatment options include excision (including Mohs' micrographic surgery), excision and grafting, curettage and cautery, radiotherapy, cryotherapy, imiquimod 5% and PDT for large superficial BCCs (see Chapters 23 and 24). For advanced or metastatic BCCs

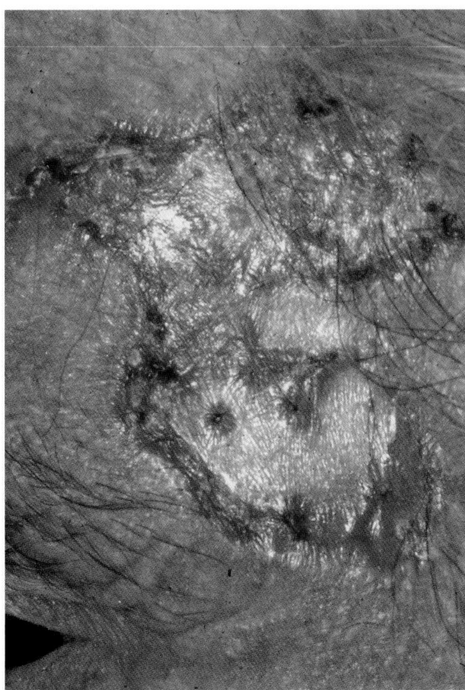

Figure 22.8 Morphoeic basal cell carcinoma.

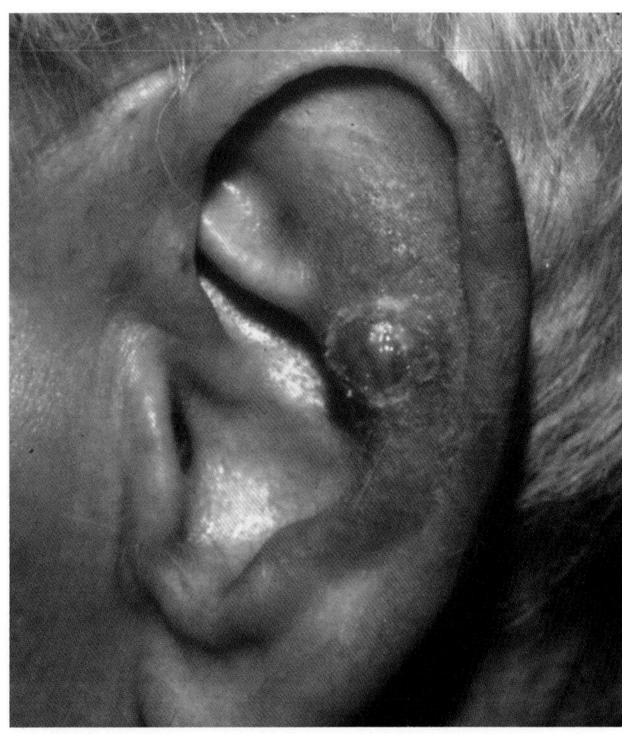

Figure 22.9 Squamous cell carcinoma: early stages on the pinna.

unsuitable for surgery/radiotherapy oral Vismodegib (Erivedge™) 150 mg daily can be taken. Erivedge has been shown to shrink 30–40% of tumours by blocking the abnormal signalling found in the Hedgehog pathway (present in 90% of BCCs).

Decisions as to the optimum therapy for each individual patient is complex and is therefore frequently discussed with the patient at a multidisciplinary skin cancer meeting including dermatologists, plastic surgeons, oculoplastic surgeons, oncologists and specialist cancer nurses.

As a general rule, surgical scars will improve with time compared to radiotherapy sites which tend to deteriorate cosmetically. Mohs' micrographic surgery is becoming the 'gold standard' for complete excision of BCCs on the face/scalp, particularly those near the eyes and other vital structures where identifying clear tumour margins is essential to preserve normal tissue and function. Large nasal tip lesions may be more optimally treated with radiotherapy as this can be a difficult site for grafting.

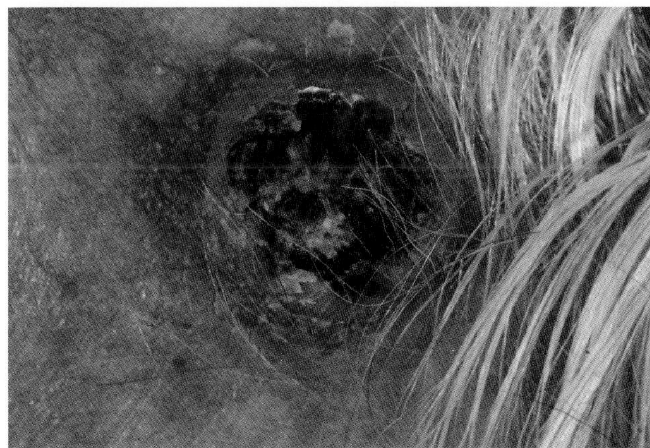

Figure 22.10 Hyperkeratotic rapidly enlarging squamous cell carcinoma.

Squamous cell carcinoma (SCC)

SCC is the second most common form of skin cancer after BCC. Risk factors for SCC are similar to those for BCCs but in addition SCC may develop in any chronic wound or scar (Marjolin's ulcer), and HPVs are thought to play a significant role in the pathogenesis. Transplant recipients who are medically immunosuppressed seem to be particularly susceptible to the development of SCCs which may be HPV mediated.

Dysplastic proliferations of abnormal keratinocytes may arise *de novo* or in pre-existing skin lesions such as AKs or Bowen's disease. By definition, SCCs have invasive tumour cells within the dermis. Seventy percent of lesions occur on the head and neck. Clinical suspicion of an SCC arises when lesions are rapidly growing, painful and markedly hyperkeratotic (Figures 22.9–22.11). SCCs are usually nodular with surface changes including crusting, ulceration or the formation of a cutaneous horn. Some lesions can be verrucous and therefore mistaken for viral warts, or indeed arise from a chronic viral wart.

Keratoacanthoma is thought to be a variant of SCC, and current thinking dictates these should be treated as if they are indeed SCCs. These lesions typically appear rapidly over a few weeks and have a characteristic central crater within the nodule (Figure 22.12). They may spontaneously regress, leaving a significant scar which has led to debate about their exact nature and how they should be managed. Histologically, they look malignant and most specialists feel comfortable treating them as for an SCC.

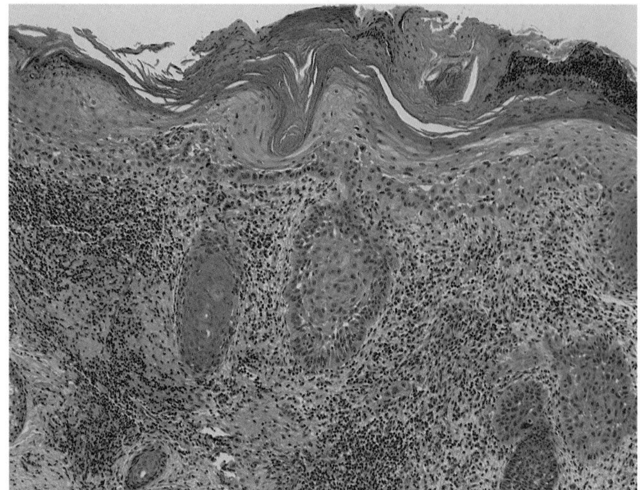

Figure 22.11 Squamous cell carcinoma histology.

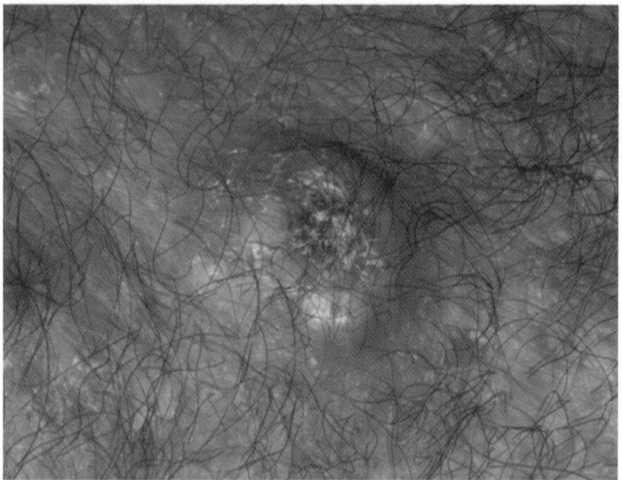

Figure 22.12 Keratoacanthoma.

Regional lymph nodes should be palpated to look for local metastases for any lesions suspicious of an SCC; in addition, involvement of other organs such as the liver, lung or brain may occur. A computed tomography (CT) scan may be indicated for very large or aggressive lesions before decisions concerning management.

Management of SCC

Management of these patients should ideally be discussed at a multidisciplinary team meeting with the patient (see section on management of BCC).

Surgical options. Ideally lesions should be excised with a 4–6 mm margin. Skin grafting may be required depending on the size of the lesion and the site. Tumour curettage and cautery (three passes over the affected area) can be highly successful in experienced hands.

Medical options. Radiotherapy can provide excellent results for tumours not amenable to surgery. Radiotherapy does, however, involve multiple trips to the hospital and symptoms of pain at the site during healing. In patients who develop multiple SCCs such as renal transplant patients, secondary prophylaxis with oral retinoids may be considered. These have been shown to reduce the number of new lesions appearing if taken indefinitely.

Moles/naevi: benign or malignant?

The term *naevus* (mole) is derived from the Greek word meaning 'nest', which is formed by a proliferation of melanocytes. Benign moles show little change and remain static for years. Any change may indicate that a mole is becoming more active or even transforming into a melanoma. Size, shape and colour are the main features, and it is change in these that is most important. The ABCDE acronym is a useful guide for assessing the malignant potential of a mole: *a*symmetry, *b*order (irregular), *c*olour (irregular), *d*iameter (>0.5 cm), *e*volving (Box 22.1). Any symptoms such as pain, crusting, ulceration or bleeding may also indicate malignant transformation. Patients can be educated about what changes to look for in their own moles so they can alert their local practitioner about any changes. Examine all of the patient's skin and look for any mole that 'stands out from the crowd'.

Box 22.1 **The ABCDE of malignant pigmented lesions**

- *Asymmetry* – if you draw an imaginary line through the centre of a mole in any axis and both halves match then the mole is symmetrical and likely to be benign.
- *Border* – benign moles usually have an even, regular outline. Any indentations such as scalloped edges may indicate malignant change, such that one part of the mole is growing.
- *Colour* – variation in colour may be a sign of dysplasia or malignant change in a mole. Melanomas may be intensely black and show variable colour within a single lesion from white to slate blue with all shades of black and brown. Amelanotic melanomas show little or no pigmentation.
- *Diameter* – apart from congenital naevi most benign moles are less than 1 cm in diameter. Any lesion growing to over 0.5 cm should be carefully checked. However some melanomas are small – 0.1–0.2 cm.
- *Evolving* – a mole changing over time.

Dysplastic naevi

- These are moles that look atypical ('funny-looking moles'). They are often deeply pigmented and have an irregular margin (Figure 22.13). Clinically and histologically, they have features of very early malignant change and therefore could progress to melanoma. Fifty percent of superficial spreading melanomas are thought to arise from pre-existing moles, many of which are atypical.

Some patients have multiple atypical moles and may have the so-called *dysplastic naevus syndrome.* Usually, there is a family history of dysplastic moles. During adolescence, these patients acquire multiple pigmented moles most frequently on the trunk. Compared to normal moles, these naevi are larger and their pigment more heterogeneous. These patients often need regular monitoring by a skin specialist.

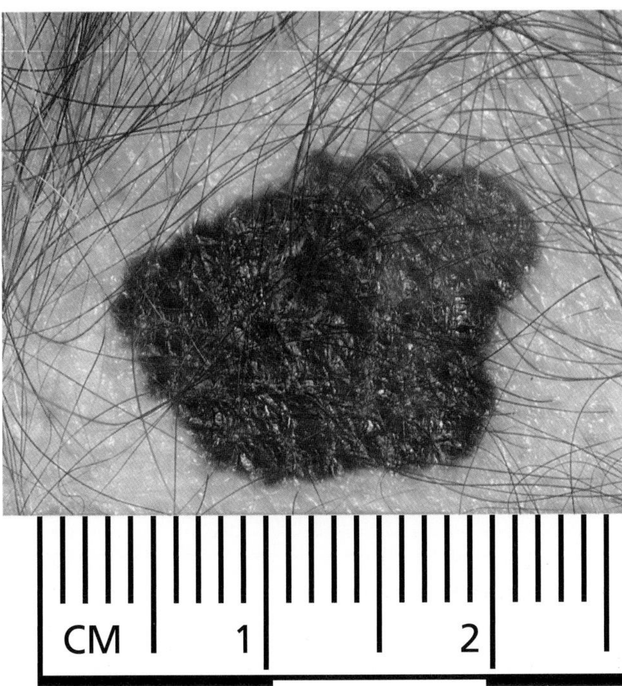

Figure 22.13 Dysplasic naevus.

Melanoma

Melanoma is an invasive malignant tumour of melanocytes. Melanoma accounts for 4% of skin tumours but is responsible for 75% of skin cancer deaths. Most cases occur in white adults over the age of 30. Females are more commonly affected than males in the USA but this trend is reversed in Australia. Solar radiation is a known carcinogen and is considered to be the main risk factor for melanoma, particularly intermittent unaccustomed and high-intensity UV exposure particularly in childhood. Other risk factors include light skin tones, poorly tanning skin, red or fair-coloured hair, light-coloured eyes, female sex, older age, a personal or family history of melanoma and congenital defect of DNA repair (xeroderma pigmentosum). The presence of giant congenital melanocytic naevi, one to four dysplastic naevi, multiple common moles, actinic lentigines and change in a mole are additional risk factors for melanoma.

Incidence

The incidence of melanoma has tripled over the past 20 years. In Australia, 1 in 35 women and 1 in 25 men will develop melanoma during their lifetime. In Europe, there are 63 000 new cases of melanoma diagnosed each year, accounting for 2% of all cases. In the USA, the lifetime risk of developing melanoma is estimated to be 1 in 60.

Sun exposure

The highest incidence of melanoma occurs in countries near the equator with high intensity UV throughout the year. However, skin type and the regularity of exposure to sun are also important. The incidence is higher in fair-skinned people who have concentrated high-intensity exposure on holiday than those with darker skin types who have regular exposure throughout the year. Sun-burning episodes are thought to be a risk factor for melanoma. The most frequent site of melanoma in women is the legs while in men it is the trunk. This is thought to be a direct consequence of behaviour in the sun, that is women expose their legs and men remove their shirts.

Pre-existing moles

It is rare for ordinary moles to become malignant but giant congenital naevi and multiple dysplastic naevi are more likely to develop into melanoma. Fifty percent of melanomas are thought to arise from pre-existing moles.

Types of melanoma

Clinically, there are five main types of melanoma.

Superficial spreading melanoma is the most common type. It is common on the back in men and on the legs in women. As the name implies the melanoma cells spread superficially in the epidermis, becoming invasive after months or years. The margin and the surface are irregular, with pigmentation varying from brown to black (Figure 22.14). There may be surrounding inflammation and signs of regression – pale areas within it. Nodules may appear within the tumour when it becomes invasive, which worsens the prognosis (Figure 22.15).

Lentigo maligna melanoma occurs characteristically on the face of elderly people. Initially, patients may have single or multiple solar lentigos which are benign and common but can look suspicious (Figure 22.15). However, over the years patients may develop a slowly growing, irregular and larger pigmented macule (lentigo maligna) (Figure 22.16a), which if very large can be treated with imiquimod over many months rather than extensive surgery (Figure 22.16b); however if a nodule/darker colour develops within the pigmented patch then suspect lentigo maligna melanoma (Figure 22.17).

Nodular melanoma presents as a dark nodule from the start without a preceding *in situ* epidermal phase (Figure 22.18). It is more

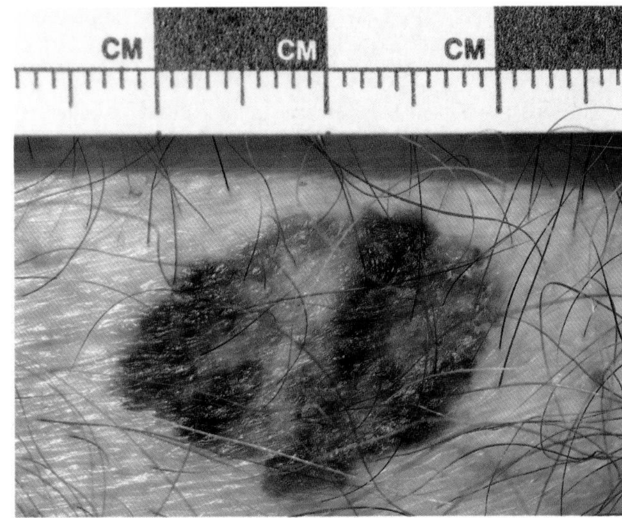

Figure 22.14 Superficial spreading malignant melanoma.

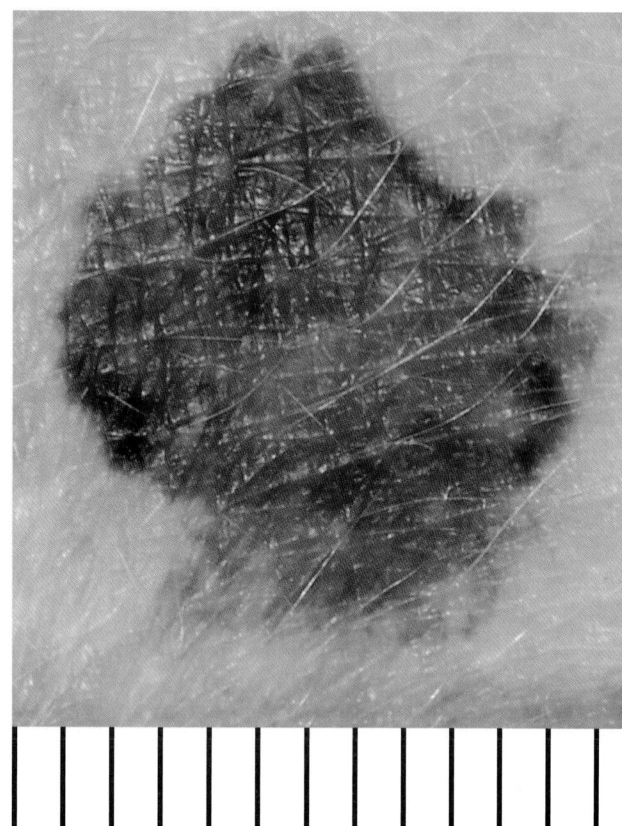

Figure 22.15 Benign solar lentigo.

common in men than in women and is usually seen in people in their fifties and sixties. This tumour is in a vertical growth phase from the start and therefore has a correspondingly poor prognosis.

Acral melanoma occurs on the palm and soles and near/under the nails. Benign pigmented naevi may also occur in these sites and it is important to recognise early dysplastic change (ABCDE – as above). A very important indication that discolouration of the nail is due to melanoma is 'Hutchinson's sign': pigmentation of the nail fold adjacent to the nail (Figure 22.19). It is important to distinguish talon noir, in which a black area appears on the sole or heel as a result of trauma – for example, sustained while playing squash – causing haemorrhage into the dermal papillae. Paring the skin gently with a scalpel will reveal distinct blood-filled papillae.

Amelanotic melanoma. As the melanoma cells become more dysplastic and less well differentiated they lose the capacity to produce melanin and form an amelanotic melanoma (Figure 22.20). Such non-pigmented nodules may be regarded as harmless but in fact are highly malignant. A rare form but also highly malignant is the dysplastic form of melanoma (Figure 22.21).

Prognosis

Prognosis depends on the depth to which the melanoma has penetrated below the base of the epidermis seen histologically: the so-called Breslow thickness of the lesion. This is measured

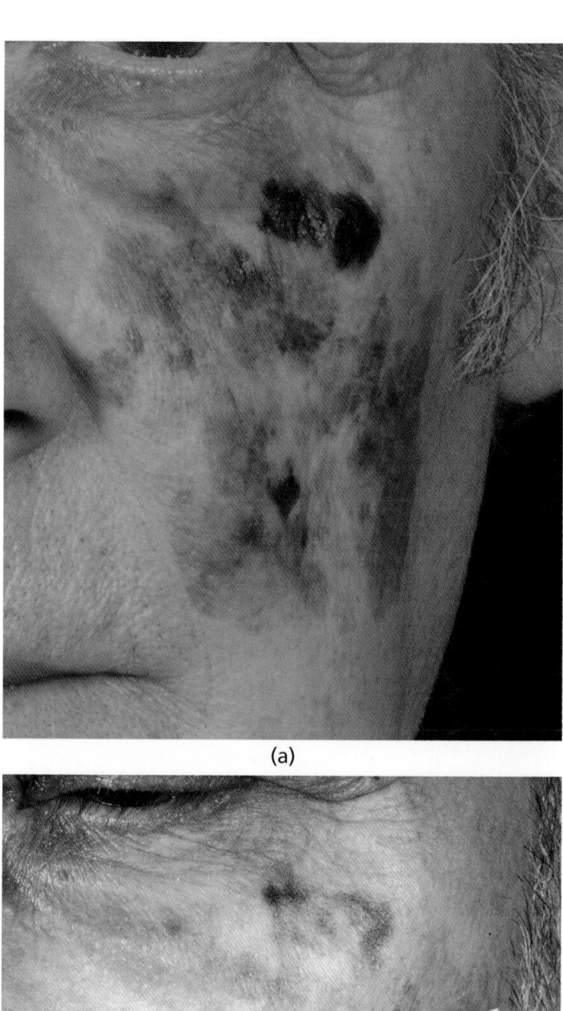

Figure 22.16 (a) Lentigo maligna pre-imiquimod treatment and (b) lentigo maligna midway through treatment with topical imiquimod.

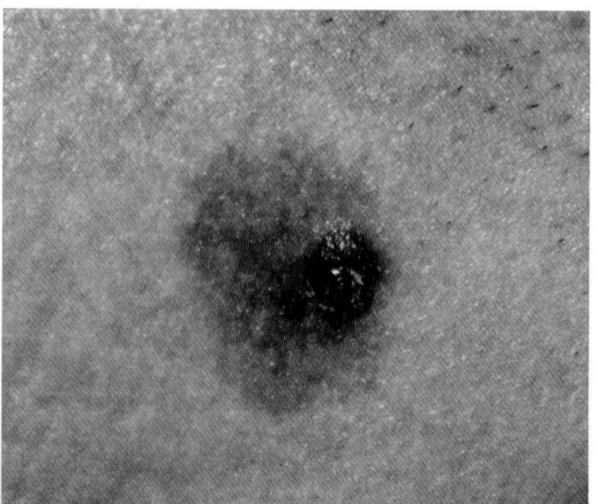

Figure 22.17 Lentigo maligna melanoma.

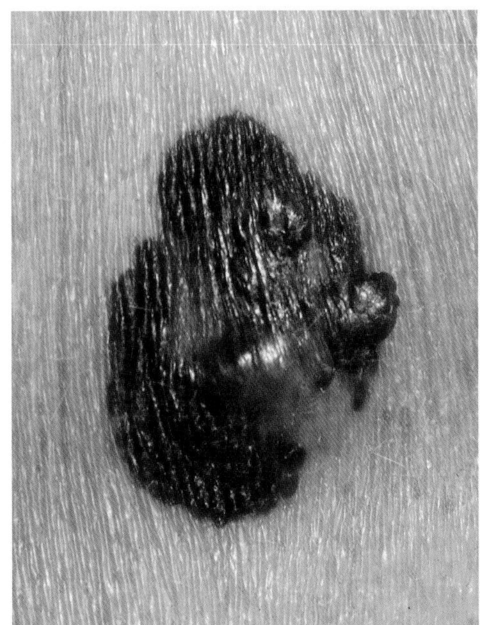

Figure 22.18 Nodular malignant melanoma.

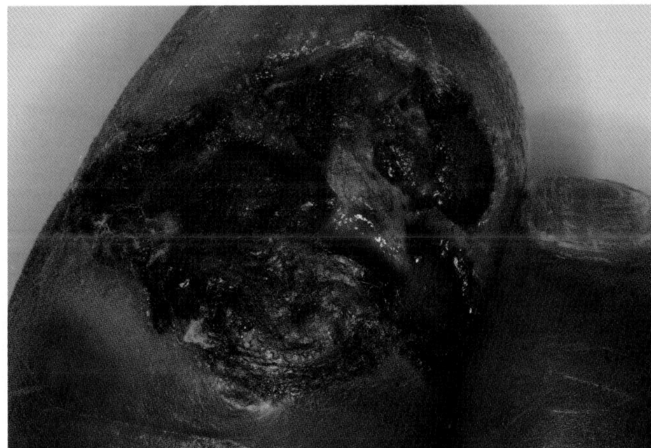

Figure 22.19 Acral malignant melanoma.

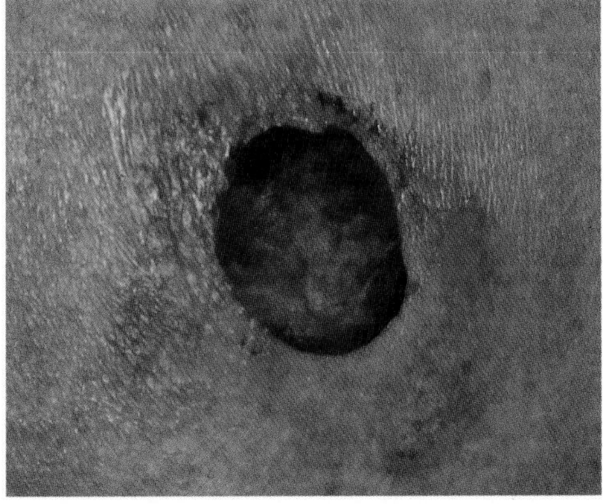

Figure 22.20 Amelanotic malignant melanoma.

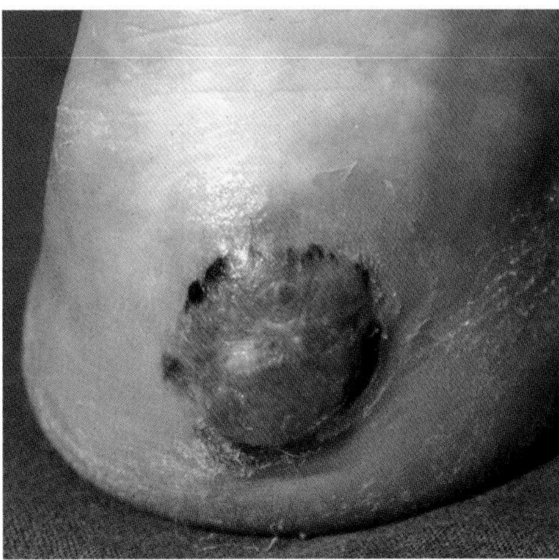

Figure 22.21 Dysplastic malignant melanoma.

histologically in millimetres from the granular layer to the deepest level of invasion. The depth alone can give an indication of prognosis: Breslow of less than 1.5 mm is associated with a 90% 5-year survival, 1.5–3.5 mm with a 75% 5-year survival and greater than 3.5 mm with only a 50% 5-year survival. These figures are based on patients in whom the original lesion had been completely excised. A recent study in Scotland has shown an overall 5-year survival of 71.6–77.6% for women and 58.7% for men. Ulceration, lymph node involvement and skin metastases are associated with a poorer prognosis and therefore accurate prognosis cannot be determined by Breslow thickness alone, Therefore, more accurate melanoma staging takes into account not only Breslow thickness but also ulceration, lymph node involvement and metastases to distant organs. If melanoma is not recognised and excised, then melanoma satellites (small islands of melanoma nearby) may develop (Figure 22.22a) and ultimately metastases in transit (local Figure 22.22b) and/or distant may spread haematogenously and via the lymphatics (Table 22.1).

Treatment of melanoma

If melanoma is suspected it should ideally be excised in its entirety with initially just a 2-mm margin for histological analysis. Definitive treatment including wide local excision margins will be guided by the Breslow thickness (determined histologically) as well as any potential risk for lymph node involvement. The higher the Breslow thickness the more likely that the draining lymph nodes may contain melanoma metastases. If a palpable lymph node is found on examination then a fine needle aspiration or lymph node removal for cytology/histology respectively should be undertaken. If no lymph nodes are palpable but the Breslow thickness is greater than 1 mm, then the patient may be offered sentinel lymph node biopsy (SLNB) (this is the first draining node from the melanoma skin site).

Sentinel lymph node biopsy (SLNB)

The presence or absence of nodal metastases is a significant prognostic indicator. SLNB is therefore currently offered in some centres to patients who have a melanoma of greater than 1 mm Breslow

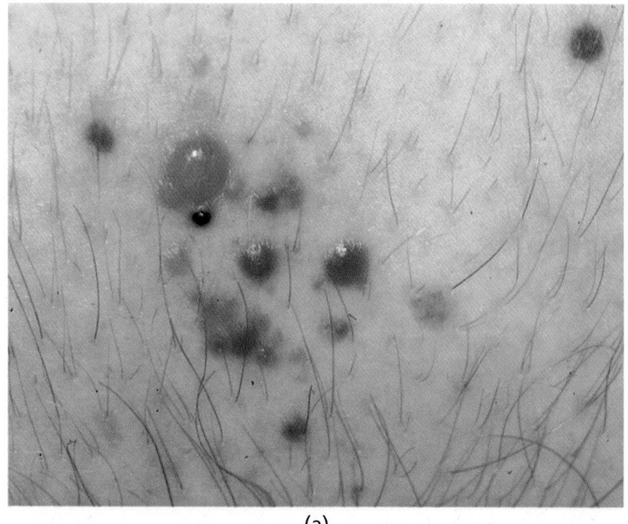
(a)

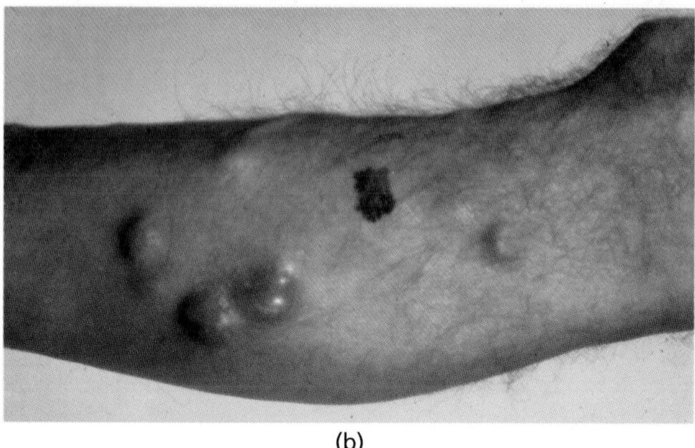
(b)

Figure 22.22 (a) Melanoma with surrounding satellites and (b) melanoma with local metastases in transit.

thickness. SLNB is usually undertaken simultaneously with the wide local excision. To detect the sentinel nodes lymphoscintigraphy (which maps the lymphatics using technetium-99m) is carried out, plus methylene blue dye is infiltrated around the excision scar and a gamma probe is used to identify positive nodes. All blue nodes and those with more than 10% radioactivity are identified as sentinel nodes. The sentinel lymph node/s are examined histologically for evidence of melanoma micrometastases. A false negative rate of between 4% and 12% is reported. If the sentinel lymph node is positive for melanoma then local lymph basin clearance and/or adjuvant therapy in a clinical trial is usually offered to the patient. Unfortunately, there is no evidence that undergoing SLNB and lymph basin clearance improves survival but it is the most accurate currently available staging method.

Adjuvant therapies for melanoma

Patients with stage 4 disease (i.e. where melanoma has spread from its original skin site as satellite lesions in the skin or distant metastases) may be suitable to have adjuvant non-surgical treatments. Currently, there are three main types: chemotherapy, targeted therapy and immunotherapy.

Table 22.1 Prognosis in melanoma.

Melanoma stage	5-year survival
Stage 1A melanoma with Breslow thickness ≤1 mm without ulceration/lymph node involvement	95%
Stage 1B melanoma with Breslow thickness ≤1 mm with ulceration/no lymph node involvement or 1.01–2 mm Breslow without ulceration/lymph node involvement	91%
Stage 2A melanoma with Breslow thickness >1 mm to <2.01 mm without ulceration/metastases or 2.01–4 mm without ulceration/lymph node involvement	77–79%
Stage 2B melanoma 2.01–4 mm Breslow with ulceration/no lymph nodes or >4 mm without ulceration/lymph nodes	63–67%
Stage 2C melanoma >4 mm Breslow with ulceration/no lymph nodes	45%
Stage 3A Any Breslow without ulceration/with 1–3 lymph node micrometastases	63–70%
Stage 3B Any Breslow with ulceration and 1–3 lymph node micrometastases or any Breslow without ulceration plus 1–3 lymph node macrometastases	46–59%
Stage 3C Any Breslow, without ulceration plus 1–3 macrometastases or ≥4 metastatic lymph nodes or melanoma satellites	24–29%
Stage 4 melanoma with metastases in the skin, subcutaneous tissue or lymph nodes at distant sites or metastases in visceral organs	7–19%

Chemotherapy with decarbazine or temozolomide kills rapidly dividing melanoma cells; however, side effects can be severe (hair loss, gastrointestinal (GI) upset, bone marrow suppression) and survival is only moderately enhanced.

Immunotherapy with interleukin 2 (IL-2) or ipilimumab enhances the patient's immune response to the melanoma resulting in tumour shrinkage or elimination. High dose IL-2 is given as an infusion three times a day for 5 days, twice per month. It has been reported in some cases to cure metastatic melanoma; however, adverse effects can be severe including hypotension, dysarrythmias and fever, which is often poorly tolerated by older patients. Ipilimumab is a humanised antibody that overcomes an immune suppressor protein produced by the melanoma. Cytotoxic T-lymphocyte-associated protein 4 (CTLA-4) produced by the melanoma mediates T-cell suppression, and it is this protein that ipilimumab blocks, leading to enhanced patient immune responses against the tumour. Ipilimumab is given IV (3 mg/kg) over 90 min once every 3 weeks for a total of four doses (total cost of four doses of 3 mg/kg for a 70 kg patient in the UK (2013) is £75 000). Side effects include colitis, hepatitis, rash and inflammation of endocrine glands (pituitary, adrenal and thyroid). Trials have shown that ipilimumab given at a dose of 3 mg/kg (four doses) to previously treated patients with melanoma overall survival was 18% at 4 years and for treatment-naïve patients who were given 10 mg/kg (four doses) overall survival was 37–49% at 4 years. Recent trials have reported the use of ipilimumab plus surgical resection of metastases leading to a 5-year survival rate of 50% (mean survival 60 months). Recent phase 1 studies have looked at giving patients combination therapies such as ipilimumab plus nivolumab (a PD1 blocking antibody), where overall they observed 40% tumour shrinkage and an estimated 1-year survival of 80%.

Targeted therapy currently involves detecting and targeting gene mutations within the patient's melanomas. 50% of melanomas have a single gene mutation in BRAF. BRAF is a human gene that makes a protein called B-Raf which is a cell growth signalling protein. Mutations in the BRAF gene therefore lead to switching on of tumour cell growth, and the melanoma becomes addicted to the actions of B-Raf, the so-called 'oncogene addiction'. These novel targeted therapies such as vemurafenib, dabrafenib and trametinib block the production of B-Raf protein resulting in tumour shrinkage prolonging survival by an additional 6 months. However, despite the continuation of therapy the melanomas eventually start to grow again by finding alternative pathways to stimulate tumour growth. Side effects of BRAF inhibitors include photosensitivity, joint pains/fatigue and an increase in non-melanoma skin cancers in about 30% of patients that usually require surgical excision.

Melanoma vaccines may provide hope for future patients with clinical trials currently underway in patients with stage 4 melanoma. Preliminary results show that by immunising patients with their own functionally mature dendritic cells that have been modified to produce interleukin-12p70 this switches on the production of cytotoxic T cells which are directed against gp100 tumour antigen. This vaccination process boosts the patient's ability to kill tumour cells in a very specific way. Further larger studies are needed to assess response rates and 5-year survival data.

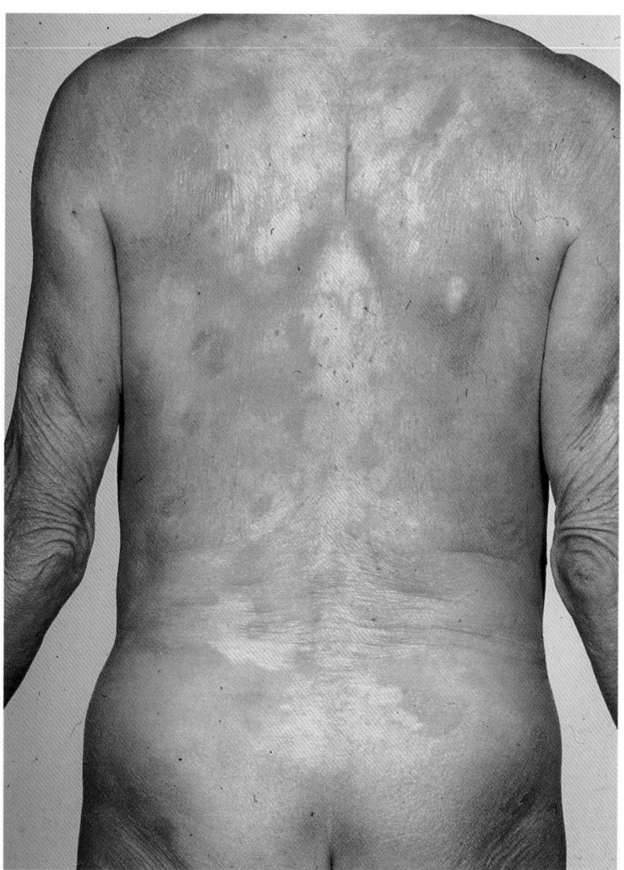

Figure 22.23 Mycosis fungoides.

Cutaneous lymphoma

Cutaneous lymphoma results from abnormal T or B lymphocytes invading the skin.

Cutaneous T-cell lymphomas (CTCLs) are a heterogeneous group of disorders that account for 80% of primary cutaneous lymphomas (B-cell types 20%). The most common form of CTCL is mycosis fungoides (MF), which is more common with increasing age, male sex and black skin. MF has a relatively good overall prognosis but some individuals may have more aggressive disease. Clinically, MF may initially resemble eczema, psoriasis or fungal infections. Patients have scaly erythematous patches and plaques on the skin, particularly on the trunk and buttock area (Figure 22.23). These may be itchy or asymptomatic. Lesions usually remain fixed and do not respond to mild topical steroids or antifungal creams. These lesions may remain stable for many years but eventually may transform to tumour stage disease when nodules may appear in longstanding plaques or arise *de novo*.

Five percent of MF patients develop a generalised exfoliative erythroderma with lymphadenopathy and atypical peripheral T cells (Sézary cells): the so-called Sézary syndrome. This can be considered to be a more aggressive form of MF. A clone of malignant T-cells can be demonstrated in the skin, lymph nodes and blood by T-cell gene rearrangement studies.

Management of early patch stage MF is usually with potent topical steroids, topical nitrogen mustard and phototherapy (PUVA). Plaque or tumour stage disease may be managed with localised radiotherapy. Results from multiagent chemotherapy regimens have been disappointing. Over the past decade, an oral synthetic rexinoid (a subclass of retinoid that activates retinoid X receptors) bexarotene has been used to treat more advanced CTCL with an overall response rate of 75%. Adverse effects may prohibit optimal dosing in some patients who may develop hypothyroidism, raised triglycerides, abnormal liver function tests, glucose abnormalities and neutropenia. Allogenic stem cell transplantation has been used in small numbers of patients with CTCL no longer responding to conventional therapies. High or conventional dose (non-myeloablative) chemotherapy with/without radiation therapy is given to patients prior to an infusion of donor stem cells. Small cases series report 75% of patients remaining disease free at 5 years; however, 25% of patients died from complications related to the stem cell transplant.

Primary cutaneous B-cell lymphomas (CBCLs) arise from a malignant transformation of B cells at different stages of their development leading to different types including follicular, marginal zone, diffuse large B-cell 'other' and diffuse large B-cell on the leg (the latter has a worse prognosis). Clinically, lesions present as firm indurated papules, nodules or plaques that may be erythematous, violaceous or brown (Figure 22.24).

Management of B cell lymphoma depends on the type but as a general rule low grade solitary lesions can be treated with surgical excision, localised radiotherapy, intralesional interferon alpha or intralesional rituximab. Multiple lesions can be treated

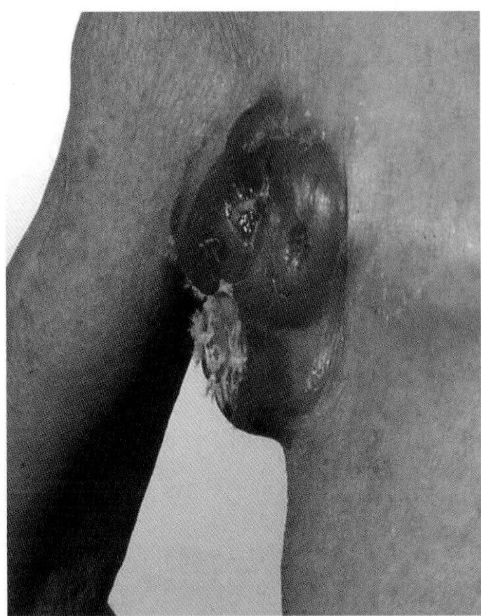

Figure 22.24 Primary cutaneous B-cell lymphoma.

with systemic rituximab. High grade poor prognosis CBCL may be managed with pegylated liposomal doxorubicin or CHOP chemotherapy (cyclophosphamide, hydroxydaunorubicin, oncovin (vincristine) and prednisolone).

Other cutaneous malignancies

Paget's disease of the nipple presents with unilateral non-specific erythematous changes on the areola/nipple spreading to the surrounding skin. The cause is an underlying adenocarcinoma of the ducts. It should be considered in any patient with eczematous changes in one breast that fail to respond to simple treatment (Figure 22.25). Extramammary Paget's can affect the axillae and groin.

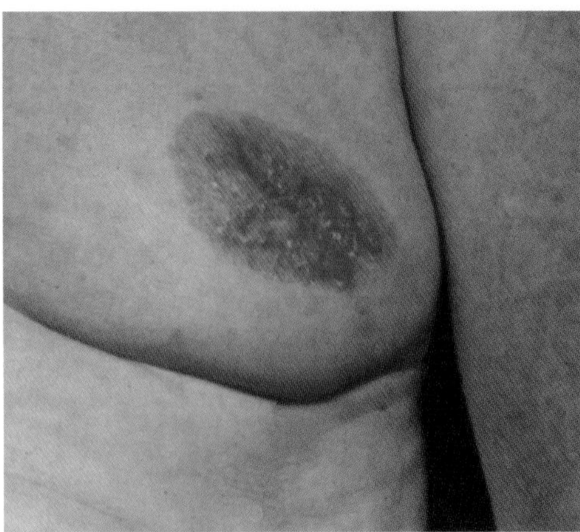

Figure 22.25 Paget's disease of the nipple.

Metastases from internal organs most commonly spread from cancers of the breast, lung, GI tract, renal tract, oral pharynx, larynx and melanoma (originating from the retina and leptomeninges). Early recognition of cutaneous metastases may allow accurate and rapid diagnosis of internal malignancy and expedite possible curative therapies.

Further Reading

Rajpar S and Marsden J. *ABC of Skin Cancer*, Wiley Blackwell, Oxford, 2008.

Rigel D et al. *Cancer of the Skin*, 2nd Edition, Sauders, 2011.

CHAPTER 23

Practical Procedures and Skin Surgery

Raj Mallipeddi

Cutaneous Laser and Surgery Unit, St. John's Institute of Dermatology, St. Thomas' Hospital, UK

OVERVIEW

- The object of physical treatments is to remove lesions and, if appropriate, to provide material for histological diagnosis.
- Destructive methods of treatment include cryotherapy, electrocautery and laser treatment. Curettage both destroys the lesion and provides fragmented material for histology.
- Cryotherapy involves the use of extreme cold to destroy the affected tissue. Solid carbon dioxide, nitrous oxide and ethyl chloride can all be used but liquid nitrogen is the most effective and commonly employed. It produces inflammation and may cause ulceration.
- Electrosurgery is the use of electric current to destroy tissue by heat in two forms: electrocautery using a heated element and electrodessication using a high frequency alternating current.
- Curettage is suitable for superficial lesions and is usually combined with electrocautery.
- Specimens for histology can be part of a lesion or the entire sample. Usually only part of the lesion is obtained by incisional, shave and punch biopsies, and therefore, the resulting specimens do not give information on the extent of the lesion as compared to full excisions.
- Surgical excisions require adequate training and knowledge of the management of skin lesions and correct surgical techniques to completely excise lesions while causing the least possible scarring.
- This chapter focuses on the more conventional procedures undertaken in general practice.

Cryotherapy

This involves the destruction of tissues by extreme cold (Box 23.1). The tissue is frozen to subzero temperatures, which is then followed by sloughing of dead tissue. Several mechanisms are involved including the osmotic effects of intracellular water leaving the cell and causing dehydration, intracellular ice formation disrupting the cell membrane and ischaemic damage due to freezing of vessels. Liquid nitrogen is most commonly employed, although various freezing agents are available such as solid carbon dioxide, nitrous oxide and a mixture of dimethyl ether and propane. Unless otherwise stated the rest of this section relates to liquid nitrogen cryotherapy.

Box 23.1 **Cryotherapy – practical points**

- Be confident of the diagnosis before treating any lesion with cryotherapy and if in doubt perform a biopsy or refer the patient to a specialist.
- Monitor the freeze time, spray in short bursts to maintain an ice-ball and stop when the desired freeze time is over.
- Warn patients about potential side effects including pain, redness, swelling and blistering.
- Children do not tolerate cryotherapy well; therefore consider alternative treatments.

The low temperature of liquid nitrogen (−196 °C), ease of storage and relative low cost make it an effective and convenient cryogen. However, its low temperature also results in rapid evaporation and therefore it should be stored carefully in an adequately ventilated area and preferably in a pressurised container.

Application technique

The liquid nitrogen is best applied as a spray using a canister (Figure 23.1).

An alternative method is to use a cotton bud that is immersed in liquid nitrogen and then applied to the lesion being treated, using moderate pressure until frozen. More than one application may be needed. A fresh cotton bud should be used for each patient to diminish the risk of transferring human papillomavirus. However, with this method there in an increase in temperature partly due to poor thermal capacity of the cotton and also warming when the cotton tip is transferred from the liquid nitrogen container to the patient's skin. The freeze time is important, and will vary according to the lesion being treated.

Freeze time is counted from the moment the entire lesion becomes frozen white rather than simply from when spraying begins. Once spraying is complete, the rate of thawing of the tissue is an important factor as more tissue destruction occurs with rapid freezing and slow thawing. The 'freeze–thaw' cycle may be repeated to increase the degree of damage and the additional

ABC of Dermatology, Sixth Edition. Edited by Rachael Morris-Jones.

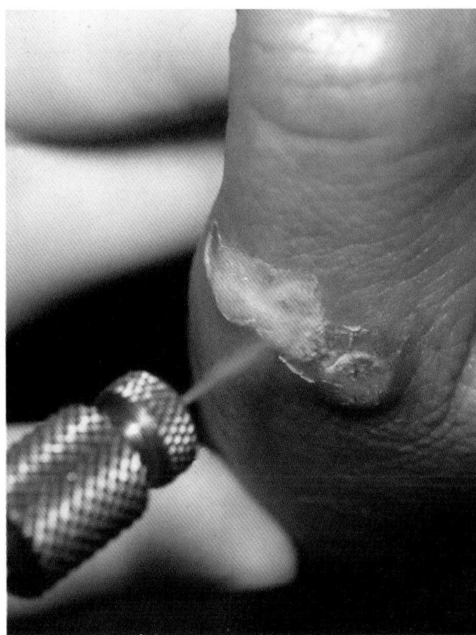

Figure 23.1 Cryotherapy.

freeze has a greater penetration due to improved cold conductivity of the previously frozen tissue. Freeze times and the number of freeze–thaw cycles depend on the type of lesion (i.e. whether benign or malignant) as well as the size and thickness.

Risks and precautions

- Patients should be warned about reactions which can occur within the first 48 h after treatment such as pain, redness, swelling and blistering, so that they are not unduly alarmed. A potent topical steroid cream applied over the affected area for a few days can be used to limit this.
- Ulceration may occur, particularly on the lower limb if there is poor perfusion.
- Although secondary bacterial infection is rare, increased pain, redness or swelling after 2–3 days may be indicative of this.
- Later risks include scarring and, particularly in darker skin types, hypopigmentation or hyperpigmentation. As might be expected, these are more of an issue with prolonged treatments.

Skin lesions suitable for freezing

Cryotherapy is usually initiated on the basis of a clinical diagnosis without prior histological confirmation, and therefore, the clinician must be confident of the diagnosis. If there is any diagnostic doubt, consider a biopsy first or alternative treatment modality where histology can also be obtained. The following lesions are frequently treated with cryotherapy.

Viral warts

A single freeze lasting 10–30 s per treatment, which includes a 1–2 mm margin of normal skin, is often sufficient, although a double freeze–thaw cycle may improve clearance, particularly for thicker warts. Usually several treatments at 2–3-week intervals are necessary and cryotherapy may be combined with topical therapies such as salicylic acid preparations for increased efficacy. Paring down the wart with a blade before cryotherapy can also be helpful.

Seborrhoeic keratoses

A single freeze of between 5 and 20 s including a 1- to 2-mm margin of normal skin should be effective for most lesions. A frozen lesion once thawed for a few seconds can also be curetted off. Larger, thicker lesions may require prolonged freezing or repeat freeze–thaw cycles, thereby increasing pain and inflammation. In these circumstances, it may be better to curette and gently cauterise the area.

Papillomas and skin tags

A single freeze of 5–10 s may be sufficient and it is helpful to stabilise the skin tag with metal forceps so that the liquid nitrogen is sprayed obliquely, avoiding non-lesional skin. An alternative method is to treat by compression with artery forceps dipped in liquid nitrogen.

Actinic keratosis

A single freeze of between 5 and 15 s including a 1- to 2-mm margin of normal skin is advised. When necessary, lifting away hard keratin to expose the underlying abnormal epithelium makes the freezing more effective. Rarely, a double freeze–thaw cycle may be needed but be aware that a lesion which does not respond to cryotherapy may be a squamous cell carcinoma.

Bowen's disease

This is an intraepidermal (*in situ*) form of squamous cell carcinoma, which can be effectively treated with a single freeze of up to 30 s including a 1- to 2-mm margin of normal skin. Again, a biopsy is necessary should there be any doubt about the diagnosis, and follow-up is essential to make sure the lesion has cleared and is not progressing.

Basal cell carcinoma

If cryotherapy is to be employed, it is best limited to the treatment of the superficial type of basal cell carcinoma (BCC), when lesions are primary (i.e. previously untreated), small (<1 cm in diameter) and well defined. The cure rate for other types of BCC is inferior with cryotherapy than with other forms of treatment such as excision. Two cycles of freezing lasting between 20 and 30 s, including a 3-mm rim of clinically normal skin, with a thaw time of 2 min is effective.

Electrosurgery

This term describes the use of electricity to cause thermal tissue destruction. There are two main forms of treatment: electrocautery and electrodessication.

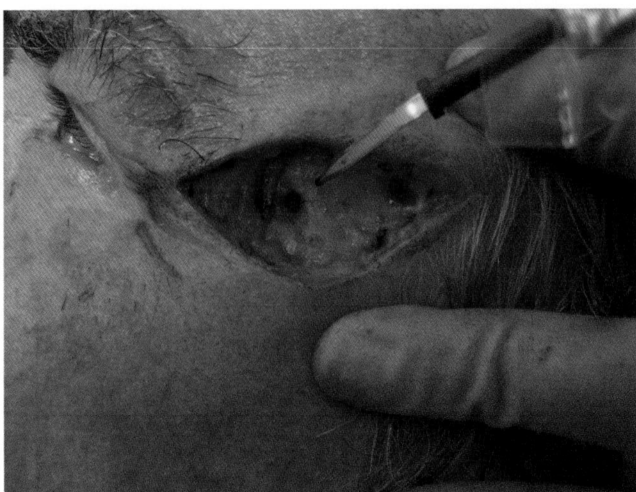

Figure 23.2 Electrodessication during surgery.

Electrocautery

Heat from an electrically heated element causes thermal damage by direct transfer of heat. Remember that in this situation, the treating element is hot.

Electrodessication (diathermy or hyfrecation)

High frequency alternating current energy is converted to heat because of tissue resistance. The treatment electrode is cold as heat generation occurs within the tissue. Electrode contact with skin causes superficial tissue dehydration. A variation of electrodessication is electrofulguration in which the electrode is held 1–2 mm from the skin surface to cause superficial epidermal carbonisation. Furthermore, depending on the voltage of current used and electromagnetic waveform, the degree of tissue cutting (electrosection) and coagulation (electrocoagulation) can be modified. If only one treatment electrode is present, then alternating current variably enters and exits the tissue, with electrons being randomly dissipated into the environment, and this is known as a *monopolar* procedure. However, if there is also a second indifferent electrode that completes an electrical circuit, the procedure is termed *bipolar*. With alternating current, the treatment electrodes are not truly positive or negative poles, and the terms *mono-* and *biterminal* are more accurate.

In routine dermatology, electrocautery or electrodessication can be used as the sole treatment for vascular lesions such as spider naevi and telangiectasia, although a vascular laser may produce better results with a lower risk of scarring. However, it is more commonly used for haemostasis during skin surgery (Figure 23.2) or in combination with curettage (see below).

Curettage

This is a simple method of removing superficial lesions, particularly in areas with thick underlying dermis such as the trunk and extremities (Box 23.2). A metal spoon or ring with a sharp edge is used to scrape away the lesion (Figure 23.3). The advantage over cryotherapy is that a sample can be sent for histology although completeness of removal cannot be accurately assessed. Curettage is combined with electrodessication or electrocautery to treat benign lesions such as seborrhoeic keratoses and xanthelasma as well as dysplastic lesions (actinic keratoses and Bowen's disease) and BCC. For curettage to work well, the lesion ideally should be softer than the surrounding unaffected skin.

Box 23.2 **Curettage – practical points**

- Use a curette which is of appropriate size for the lesion.
- Stretch the skin with the non-dominant hand and keep firm control of the curette to avoid unintended scraping of normal skin.
- Send the sample for histology but clearly state on the request that it is a curetted specimen.
- Consider shaving off the specimen first to provide a solid sample for diagnosis before commencing curettage and electrocautery. Pathologists prefer this to curetted fragments.

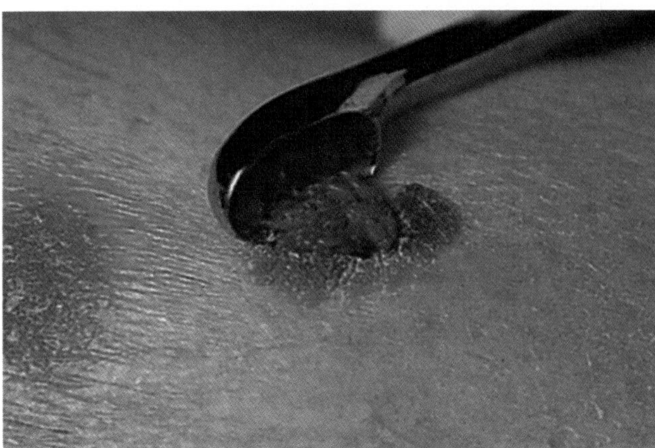

Figure 23.3 Spoon curettage.

Lesions suitable for curetting include

- seborrhoeic keratoses
- solitary viral warts
- actinic keratoses and Bowen's disease
- cutaneous horns
- small BCCs.

Technique

The area under and around the lesion is injected with a local anaesthetic. Next, using the thumb and index finger of the non-dominant hand ensure that the skin around the lesion is taut, so that there is a firm base on which to curette. Curette off the lesion and then cauterise the base to achieve haemostasis as well as to destroy any remaining tumour. Avoid curetting normal skin. For BCCs, the process is repeated so that a total of two or three cycles of curettage and electrocautery/electrodessication is performed.

Risks and precautions

- Patients should be warned that the wound may take 3–4 weeks to heal and that although the resultant scar will hopefully be a flat, white patch, it could ultimately become indented (atrophic) or even be pink and raised (hypertrophic), especially with more aggressive treatment causing a deep wound.
- Ulceration may occur, particularly on the lower limb if there is poor perfusion.
- The types of BCCs best treated with this method are primary, nodular, small (<1 cm diameter), well defined and in non-high risk or cosmetically sensitive sites. Sites generally to be avoided include the area around the eyes, nose, lips, chin, ears and hair-bearing scalp.
- If curettage results in exposure of subcutaneous fat then the procedure should be abandoned and the area excised down to fat and usually sutured. This is because firstly it is not possible to distinguish accurately between soft tumour and fat, and secondly the outcome will be suboptimal in terms of wound healing and scarring, once the fat layer has been breached.

Diagnostic biopsies

Although in many circumstances a diagnosis can be confidently made on clinical examination alone, often it is important to secure a diagnosis with the aid of histopathology. For example, a melanocytic naevus may be proved on histology to be completely benign or, by complete contrast, a malignant melanoma. There are different methods of performing a diagnostic biopsy, each with its own advantages and disadvantages. The area to be biopsied must be adequately infiltrated with local anaesthesia before commencing the procedure.

Shave biopsy

This is appropriate for sampling or removing lesions which are limited to the epidermis and papillary dermis including seborrhoeic keratoses, nodular BCCs and naevi. The skin is held taut and the lesion is gently sliced with either a scalpel blade or double-edged razor blade held horizontal to the skin surface. The angle of the blade controls the depth but the aim should be to reach the mid-dermis. Haemostasis can be achieved with electrosurgery or aluminium chloride but firm pressure may suffice. One advantage of this technique is that sutures are unnecessary. However, this technique is not recommended for any suspicious naevus, which should be excised entirely.

Punch biopsy

The biopsy tool comes in sizes varying from 2 to 8 mm (Figure 23.4) and consists of a small cylinder with a cutting rim which is used to penetrate the epidermis by rotation between the operator's finger and thumb. The skin is held taut at 90° to the orientation of the relaxed skin tension lines ('wrinkle lines') so that an oval defect results, which is easier to close (Figures 23.5–23.9). The resulting plug of skin is lifted out with forceps and cut off as deeply as possible. Pressure and/or electrosurgery is required for haemostasis. The advantage over a shave biopsy is that the specimen obtained is of full thickness containing epidermis, dermis and fat, but the area sampled is smaller. The punch biopsy tool can also be used to make holes over cysts and lipomas through which the contents can be extruded. Usually the defect left by the punch is

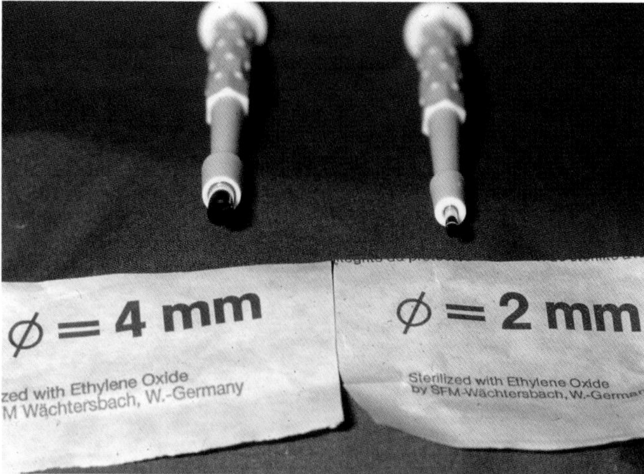

Figure 23.4 Punch biopsy tools.

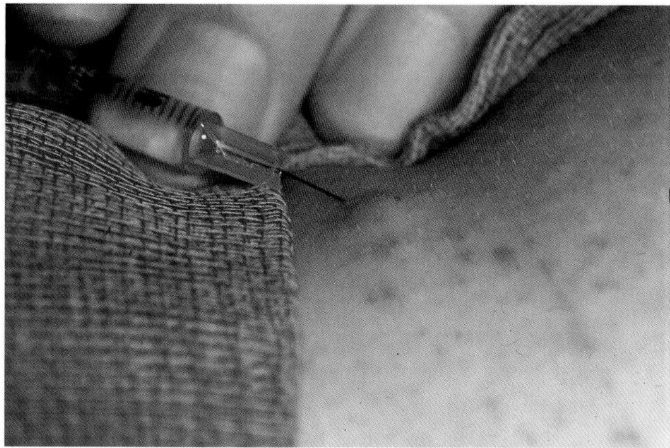

Figure 23.5 Punch biopsy: injecting local anaesthetic.

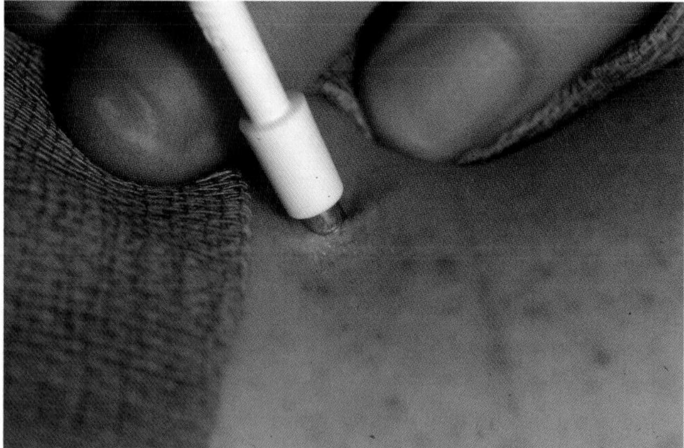

Figure 23.6 Punch biopsy: tool insertion.

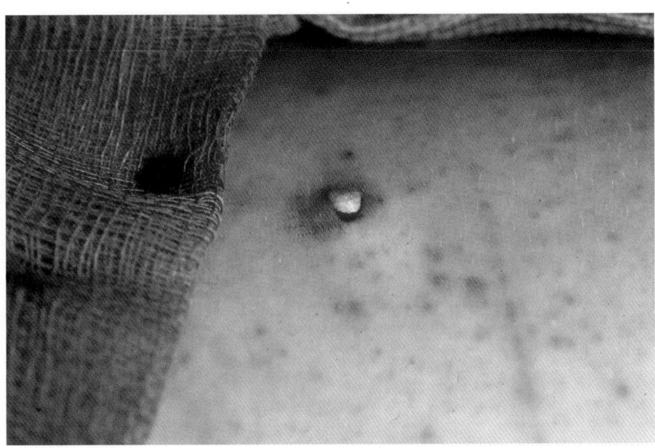

Figure 23.7 Punch biopsy: plug of skin.

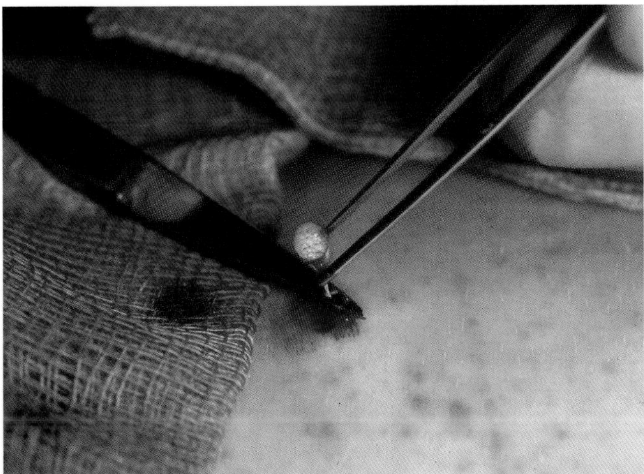

Figure 23.8 Punch biopsy: raising a plug of skin.

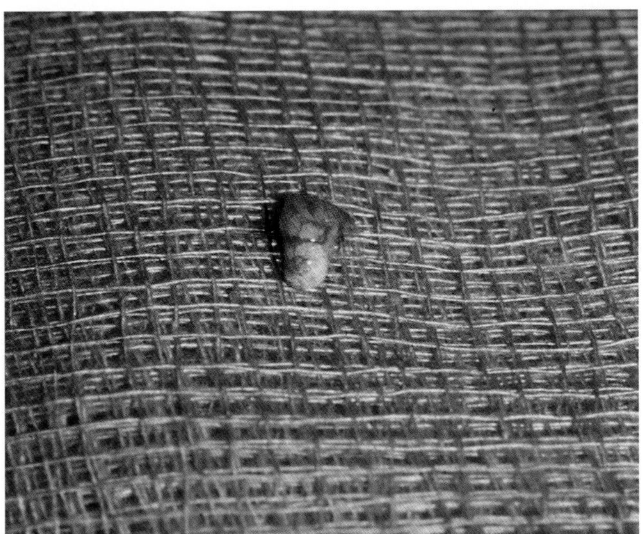

Figure 23.9 Punch biopsy: specimen taken.

sutured, although for smaller sizes (2 or 3 mm) secondary intention healing might be considered depending on the site.

Incisional biopsy

This is suitable for larger lesions and is taken across the margin of the lesion in the form of an ellipse. It is essential to include deeper dermis in certain conditions; for example, granuloma or lymphoid infiltrate may not be near the surface. An adequate amount of normal tissue should be included, so that this can be compared with the pathological area and this also means there is enough normal skin to suture the incision together (Figure 23.10).

Surgical excision

Excision of skin lesions is both curative and diagnostic. It may be the best way of making a diagnosis if there are multiple small papules or vesicles, one of which can be excised intact. Incisions should follow tension or wrinkle lines (Figures 23.11–23.13).

In the case of malignant lesions, it is particularly important that the whole lesion is adequately excised. The pathologist can report on the adequacy of excision, but this is hard to assess in lesions such

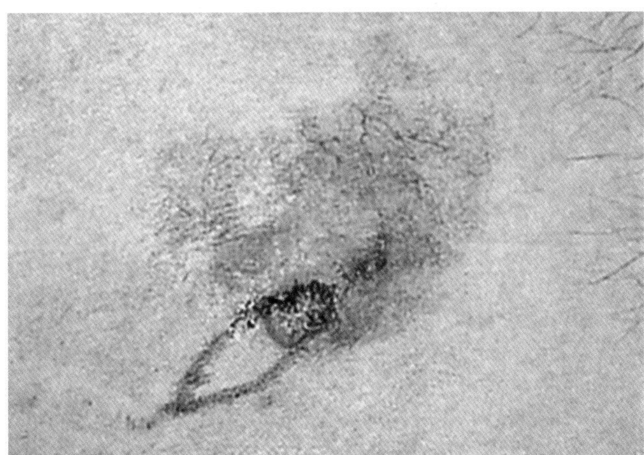

Figure 23.10 Incisional biopsy: marked area for sampling.

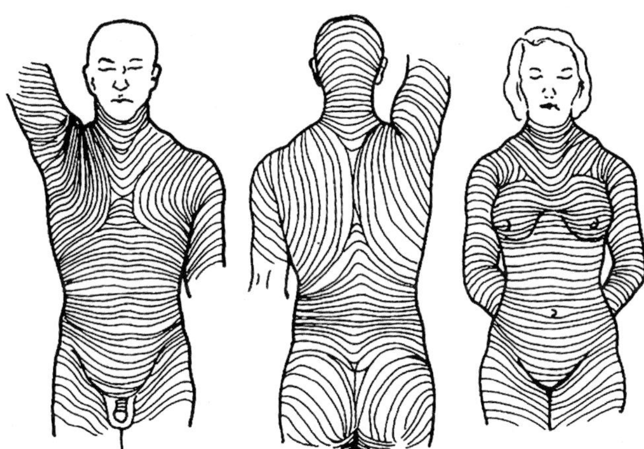

Figure 23.11 Surgical excision: 'skin wrinkle lines' of the trunk.

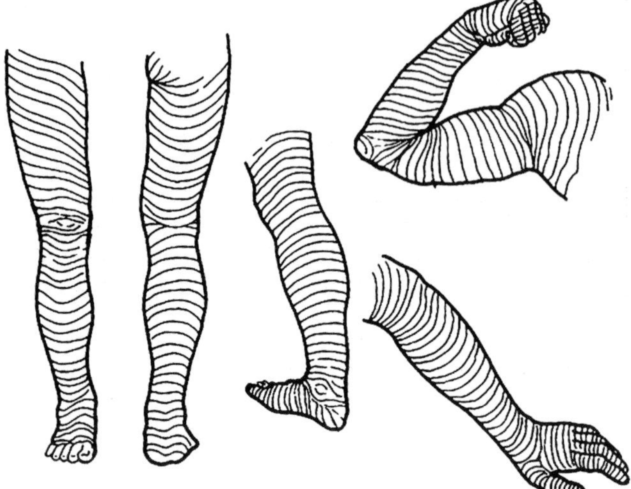

Figure 23.12 Surgical excision: 'skin wrinkle lines' of the limbs.

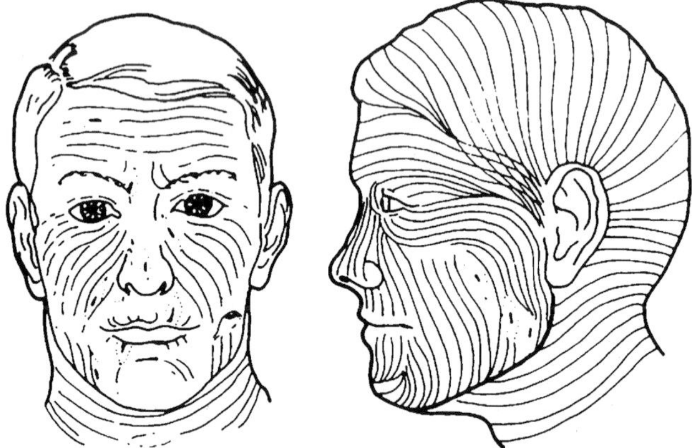

Figure 23.13 Surgical excision: 'skin wrinkle lines' of the face.

as multifocal BCC where there are scattered collections of cells. If there is likely to be any doubt about the excision being complete, it is helpful to attach a suture to one end of the excised specimen so that the pathologist can describe which border, if any, extends over the excision margin.

Technique

The basic technique consists of making an elliptical incision (Figures 23.14–23.16) with the length three times the width and the angles at the poles about 30° to minimise the formation of standing cones of tissue also known as *dog ears*. The long axis of the excision should be parallel to the 'wrinkle lines' of the skin or to the Langer lines. Although on most parts of the body these correspond closely, they are not exactly the same, as Langer lines correspond to the alignment of collagen fibres within the dermis. Scars parallel to these tend to heal better and be less obvious. Lesions excised on the sternal area, upper chest and shoulders are more likely to result in keloid scar formation and may be best referred to a dermatological or plastic surgeon.

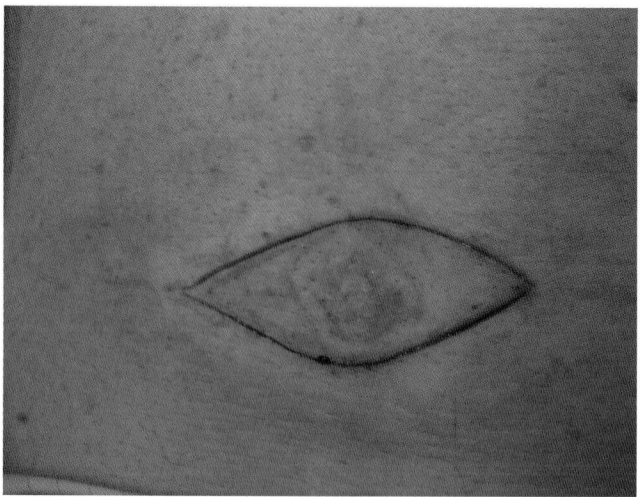

Figure 23.14 Surgical excision of BCC from lower back. Ellipse design including a 4-mm margin.

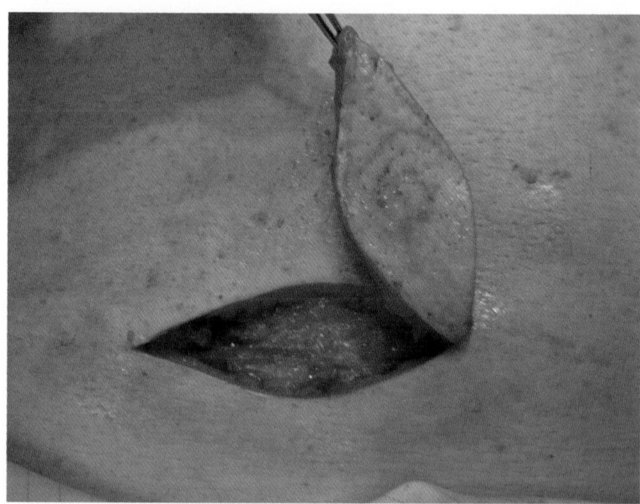

Figure 23.15 Surgical excision of BCC: removal of specimen illustrating the defect.

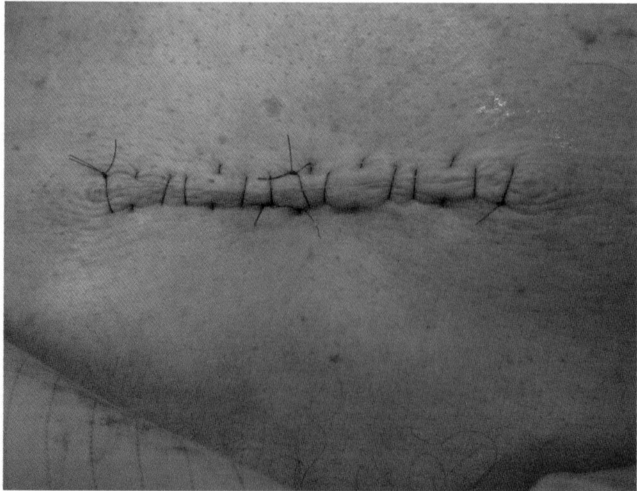

Figure 23.16 Surgical excision of BCC: after suturing, showing wound eversion.

Box 23.3 **Surgical excision**

- After initially inserting the needle, withdraw the plunger of the syringe to check that the needle has not entered the blood vessels. Raising a small 'bleb' of local anaesthetic ahead of the needle point helps to prevent this.
- It is important to learn appropriate suturing techniques for different sites of the body and size of lesion.
- Warn the patient about the resultant scar and be careful to avoid deformities such as displacement of the eyelid (ectropion).
- Always send an excised lesion for histology as a significant number of lesions considered likely to be benign clinically actually turn out to be malignant on histology.

Local anaesthetic is injected subcutaneously but close to the skin. The incision should be vertical rather than wedge shaped. Before suturing (Box 23.4) of the wound, undermining is often required to reduce wound tension. This involves dissection of the skin subdermally (blunt and/or sharp), although the depth will depend on the body site.

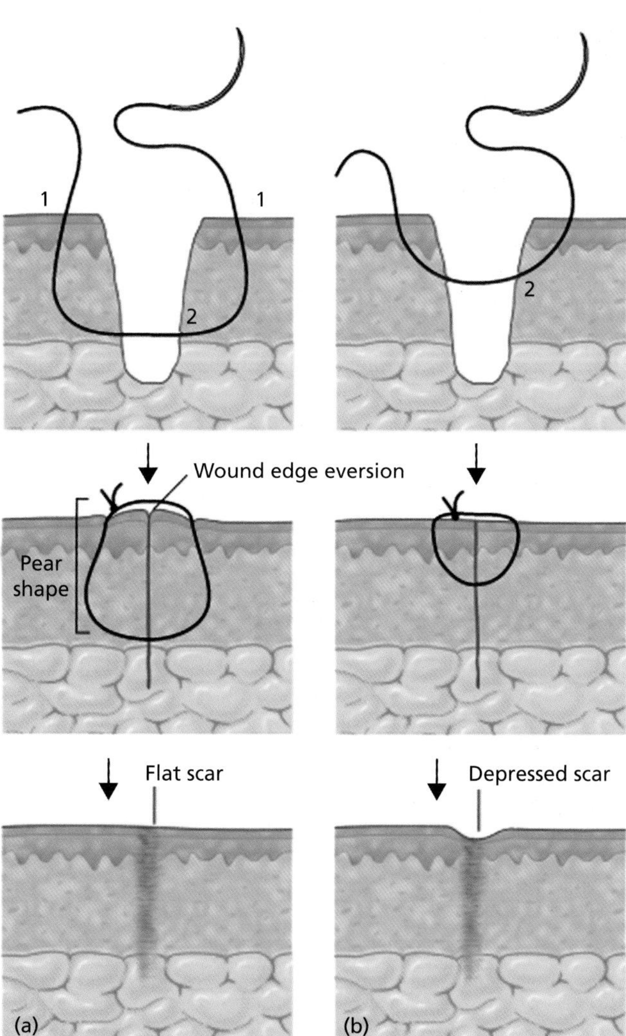

Figure 23.17 Placement of epidermal sutures. *Source:* Robinson et al., 2005. Reprinted with permission of Elsevier.

Box 23.4 **Suturing**

- Correct suture placement is vital to optimise the cosmetic outcome of a wound (Figures 23.17 and 23.18).
- Following an excision both subcutaneous sutures and epidermal sutures are placed.
- Subcutaneous sutures are absorbable such as Vicryl (Polyglactin 910, Ethicon Inc., Somerville, NJ, USA), which take up to 70 days for complete absorption whereas typical epidermal sutures such as nylon and polypropylene are non-absorbable and are removed between 5 days and 2 weeks depending on the site.
- Monofilament sutures cause less inflammation and trapping of serum than the braided variety, but are harder to tie securely.
- Suture placement should result in wound eversion so that the resultant scar is less noticeable.

Where a wound cannot be closed directly (i.e. from side to side) or if direct closure does not produce the best aesthetic outcome then a cutaneous flap or skin graft may be appropriate. Flaps may be advancement, rotation or transposition. Grafts are defined as full thickness if the entire epidermis and dermis is included, and split thickness if less than the entire dermis is included. These are outside the scope of this book.

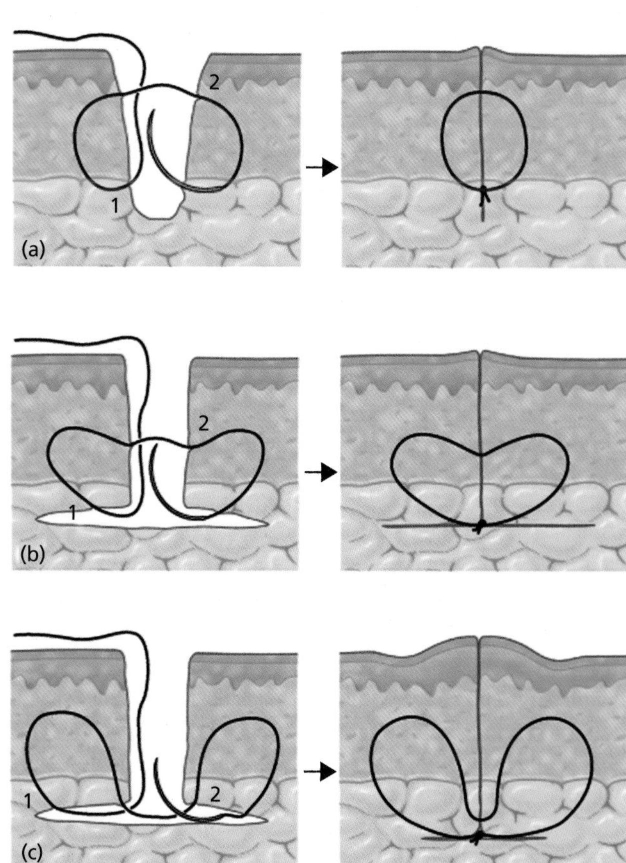

Figure 23.18 Methods of placing buried dermal sutures. *Source:* Robinson et al., 2005. Reprinted with permission of Elsevier.

Mohs' micrographic surgery

For certain higher risk tumours (most commonly BCC and squamous cell carcinoma) Mohs' micrographic surgery is the treatment of choice. Factors which determine a higher risk may include aggressive histology, ill-defined margins, large size (>2 cm), critical site such as eyes, lips, nose and ears and recurrence following previous treatment. Unlike standard excision with pre-determined margins, the tumour is debulked and excised with a narrow clinical margin. The tissue is labelled with different coloured inks and mapped to the wound on the patient. In standard Mohs' practice, the tissue is then processed for microscopic examination with frozen sections usually within 1 h. Specially trained Mohs' technicians and processing equipment are required. The sections in Mohs' surgery are horizontal and therefore the entire margin is visualised as compared with conventional excision when they are vertical (like bread loaf slices) so that only a small percentage is analysed. The Mohs' surgeon reads the slides and if tumour is still present within the tissue sections, takes more tissue precisely where it is still evident on the patient. This ensures that the tumour resection involves the least amount of normal tissue and yet achieves the highest likelihood of cure.

Further Reading

Lawrence C. *Introduction to Dermatological Surgery*, 2nd Edition, Blackwell Science, Oxford, 2002.

Lawrence CM, Walker NPJ and Telfer NR. Dermatological surgery. In: Burns DA, Breathnach SM, Cox NH and Griffiths CEM, eds. *Rook's Textbook of Dermatology*, 7th Edition, Vol. **4**, Blackwell Publishing, Oxford, 2004: 78.5–78.7.

Robinson J, Hanke CW, Sengelmann RD and Siegel DM. *Surgery of the Skin – Procedural Dermatology*, Elsevier Mosby, Philadelphia, 2005.

Zachary CB. *Basic Cutaneous Surgery: A Primer in Technique*, Churchill Livingstone, New York, 1991.

CHAPTER 24

Lasers, Intense Pulsed Light and Photodynamic Therapy

Alun V. Evans

Dermatology Department, Princess of Wales Hospital, UK

> **OVERVIEW**
>
> - Laser treatment uses high energy radiation at different wavelengths which can be directed at specific targets.
> - Laser treatments should only be undertaken by those with appropriate training.
> - It is essential to make sure that patients are carefully selected, are fully informed and have an adequate preoperative assessment.
> - A variable level of pain is experienced by patients. Surface, local or general anaesthesia is used as necessary.
> - Different types of laser are used to target different tissues in the skin and therefore careful selection of the correct laser is essential. Lasers can target pigment (melanin, tattoo dyes), blood cells, hair follicles or surface cells (resurfacing).
> - Photodynamic therapy (PDT) involves the photoactivation of a topical chemical. It is commonly used to treat solar keratoses, Bowen's disease and large superficial basal cell carcinoma.

Laser treatment

Laser science

Lasers emit a beam of light of a single wavelength, which can be selectively absorbed by a target of a certain colour, causing heating and subsequent lysis (Table 24.1). This target is known as a *chromophore*, from the Greek word for 'bearing colour'. The duration of the laser pulse is also set to be selective for the size of the chromophore. Larger targets such as hair follicles take longer to heat up and are slower to cool than smaller targets such as melanosomes. Lysis of the chromophore leaves a residue of smaller particles which are subsequently phagocytosed by macrophages. This concept of selective photothermolysis underpins laser science.

Table 24.1 The acronym 'LASER'.

L	Light
A	Amplified by
S	Stimulated
E	Emission of
R	Radiation

Preoperative assessment

Laser treatment should be preceded by a full medical history and dermatological examination.

Laser centres should offer a preoperative consultation by a qualified practitioner who can diagnose and manage skin disease and counsel the patient regarding the most appropriate therapy for their condition. It should always be borne in mind that laser treatment may not represent the optimum management for a patient and that patients are not infrequently referred with the wrong diagnosis. Careful patient selection for laser treatment has been shown to be associated with fewer adverse events, more realistic patient expectations and higher levels of patient satisfaction. The process of patient selection and preparation and an understanding of the cutaneous biology of the lesions to be treated are as important as the laser treatment itself.

Table 24.2 Possible complications of laser treatment.

Pain
Erythema
Bruising (vascular lasers)
Pigmentary change (hypo- or hyperpigmentation)
Blistering
Scarring

Patients should be provided with comprehensive written information relating to the laser treatment of their particular condition before obtaining informed consent. The consent form itself should detail possible complications of treatment (Table 24.2). Scarring may be more likely in certain areas such as the chest, shoulders and back. It is sensible to perform a small test patch using the desired settings before starting laser treatment or increasing the energy (fluence).

Patients should avoid direct sunlight and use a high factor sun block before laser treatment in order to minimise the amount of pigment in the skin and reduce the risk of complications.

Table 24.3 shows which type of cutaneous disorders may be amenable to treatment with which lasers.

Perioperative anaesthesia

Patients experience varying amounts of pain during laser treatment, and anaesthesia must be adjusted to the needs of the individual

ABC of Dermatology, Sixth Edition. Edited by Rachael Morris-Jones.

Table 24.3 Suitable lasers for specific skin disorders.

Cutaneous disorder	Lasers indicated
Vascular lesions	Pulsed dye laser, KTP
Melanocytic lesions	Q-switched Nd-YAG and Ruby
Skin pigmentation	Q-switched Nd-YAG, Ruby and Alexandrite
Ablation and resurfacing	Carbon dioxide Erbium-YAG
Hair removal	Q-switched Nd-YAG, Ruby and Alexandrite
Tattoos	Q-switched Nd-YAG, Ruby and Alexandrite

patient and the procedure being undertaken. Some lasers have cooling devices attached, which provide a degree of anaesthesia, and many patients will undergo treatment without additional pain relief. Topical local anaesthetics (EMLA®, Ametop®) may be applied under occlusion before treatment but for procedures such as resurfacing or extensive port wine stains local or regional anaesthesia will be required. General anaesthesia is reserved for treatment of young children and other special cases.

Postoperative care

All patients should be given a greasy emollient to be applied regularly to the treated area for 3 days following treatment. The aim is to maintain the barrier function of the skin where this might have been disrupted by collateral thermal injury of the epidermis. Any blistering implies significant thermal injury to the epidermis and lower fluences should be employed. Patients should also avoid excessive exposure to sunlight for at least 3 months following treatment. Resurfacing procedures require intensive post-operative care by both the laser operator and the patient or carer.

Laser safety

The main dangers posed by lasers arise from the energy contained within the beam which can produce a thermal burn or ignite flammable materials. The eyes of the patient, operator and assistants must be protected using goggles or eye shields specific to the type of laser being used. Other risks come from the high-voltage electricity and operator-dependent errors in technique. Those intending to operate lasers should have prior appropriate training.

Careful patient selection for laser treatment by highly qualified medical practitioners has been shown to be associated with a lower rate and better management of adverse events, more realistic patient expectations and higher levels of patient satisfaction. Preparation and selection of patients and an understanding of skin disease are crucial before selecting a suitable laser, if any. Laser centres should offer a preoperative consultation by a qualified practitioner who can diagnose and manage skin disease and counsel the patient regarding the most appropriate therapy for their condition.

Vascular lesions

There are numerous conditions which consist of fixed abnormal blood vessels in the skin including port wine stain (Figure 24.1), spider naevus, telangiectasia and various types of haemangioma. The pulsed dye laser (585–600 nm) or the KTP laser (532 nm) is used to target oxyhaemoglobin within these vessels. The pulse duration is set so that larger vessels are targeted but the smaller normal vasculature of the skin remains intact. Lysis of the abnormal vessels quickly produces a well-demarcated bruise which may be quite prominent and lasts for up to 14 days (Figure 24.2). Repeated treatments, approximately 8 weeks apart, will be necessary for most patients, and lesions such as port wine stains that evolve over time may require ongoing therapy.

Pigmented lesions

A wide variety of pigmented lesions affecting the skin are amenable to laser treatment. The appropriate laser for each lesion can be selected by considering the cause and location of the abnormal pigmentation.

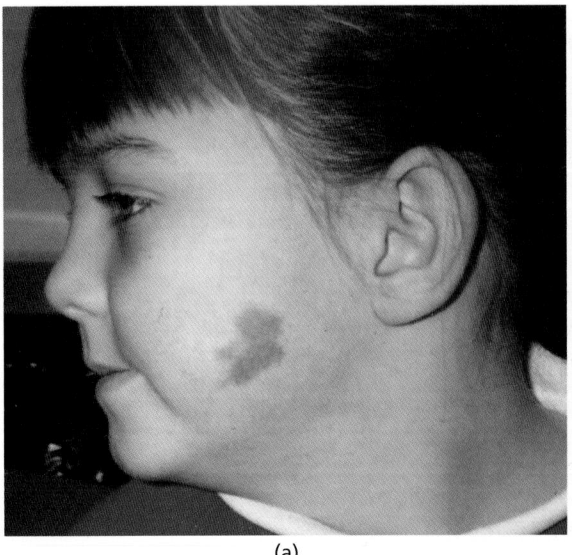

(a)

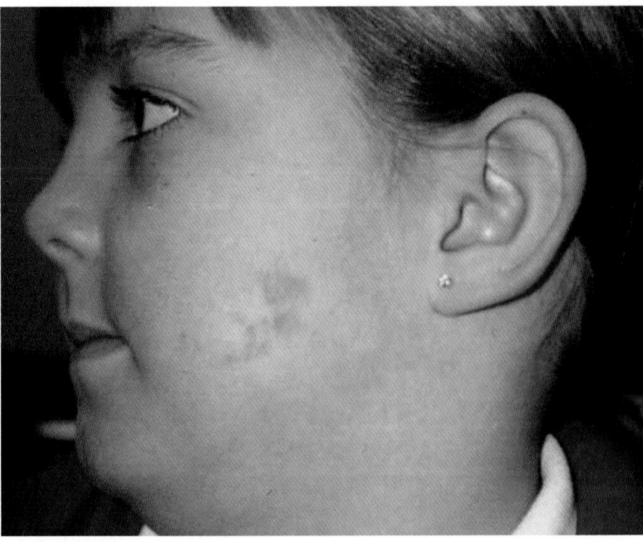

(b)

Figure 24.1 Port wine stain (a) before and (b) after treatment with a pulsed dye laser.

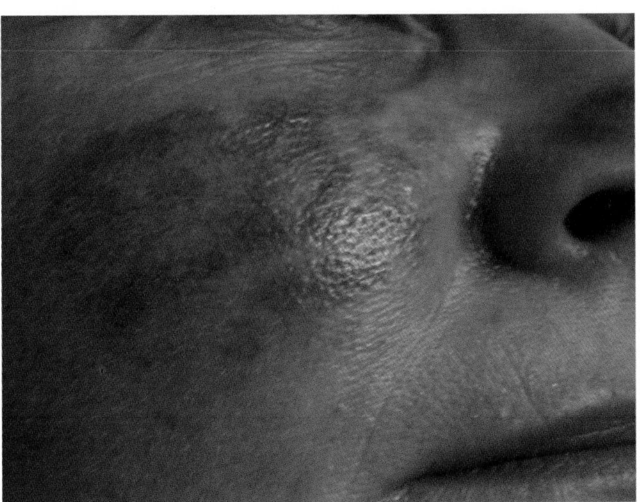

Figure 24.2 Bruising following pulsed dye laser treatment.

The commonest pigmented lesions are the result of an abnormal accumulation of melanin within the skin. The melanin is contained within melanosomes which are around 0.4 mm in size. A laser with a very short pulse duration such as the 532-nm Q-switched Nd-YAG or Q-switched ruby lasers will selectively target melanin within the epidermis. Solar lentigos, café au lait macules (Figure 24.3) and ephilides (freckles) can all be treated relatively easily in this manner. Between one and three treatments are usually required to achieve patient satisfaction. Lesions that repigment over time can be retreated when necessary.

When the melanin is located in the dermis the greater penetration afforded by a longer wavelength light is required to reach the chromophore. A 1064-nm Q-switched Nd YAG laser is usually employed in the treatment of congenital naevus of Ota, naevus of Ito and Mongolian blue spots.

Naevi (moles) are the result of a proliferation of melanocytes and often cause cosmetic problems. Their pigment may well be amenable to laser treatment but this remains controversial as they have a potential for malignant transformation. This potential can range from being extremely small (e.g. junctional naevi) to an appreciable risk requiring regular dermatological review (e.g. giant congenital melanocytic naevi). The effect of laser treatment on the potential for malignant transformation is unknown. Many would suggest that it is negligible but would still be concerned that litigation might arise from any future malignancies in or around the treated lesion.

A second problem is that these malignancies will usually declare themselves through a local pigmentary change which may be masked by a laser that destroys pigment.

Certain types of melanocytic pigmentation are not amenable to laser treatment. Laser treatment of generalised pigmentary disorders such as that associated with Addison's disease should not be attempted, even in exposed sites, as the lack of uniformity of colour after treatment will lead to dissatisfaction. Melasma (chloasma) is the result of an overproduction of melanin in sun-exposed skin. The response to laser treatment is poor and may worsen the condition. Post-inflammatory hyperpigmentation is the result of a temporary overproduction of melanin by melanocytes following inflammation. Laser treatment is likely to cause further inflammation and exacerbate the problem.

Various forms of abnormal pigmentation exist in the skin, which are due to substances other than melanin. Certain drugs cause

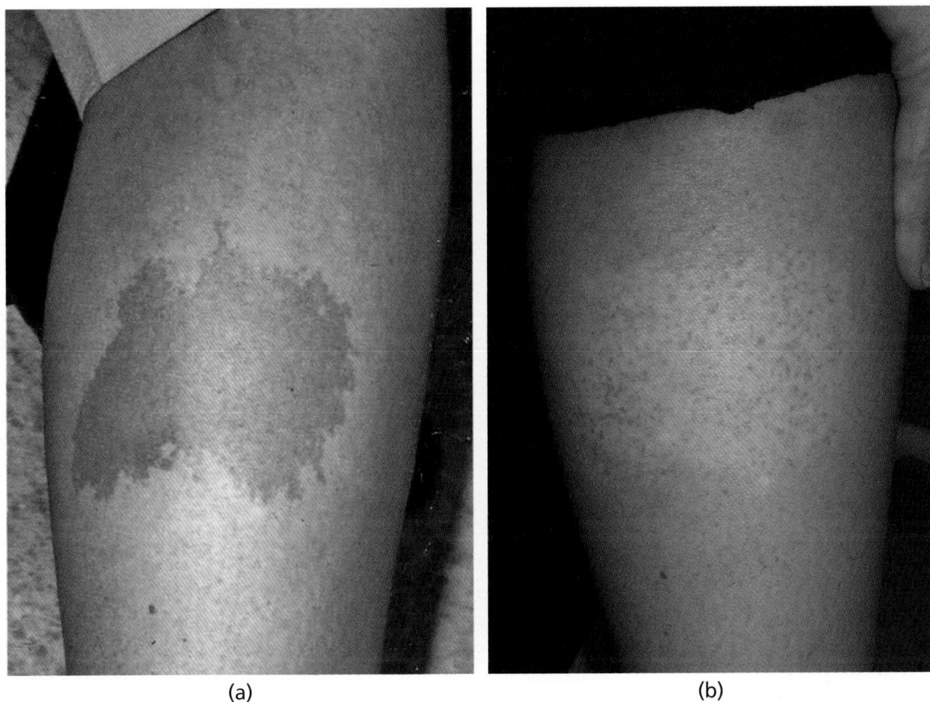

(a) (b)

Figure 24.3 Café au lait macule (a) before and (b) after treatment with a Q-switched Nd-YAG laser.

localised pigmentation of the skin which may be amenable to laser treatment. Amiodarone and minocycline produce pigmentation which may be selectively targeted by the Q-switched Nd-YAG, Ruby and Alexandrite lasers.

Haemosiderin is an iron-containing pigment that is deposited in the skin following extravasation of red blood cells. This is very common on the lower legs but treatment with laser is not indicated.

Tattoos

The art of inserting exogenous pigments into the dermis of the skin for decorative effect has been practiced for thousands of years. The subsequent granulomatous reaction permanently fixes the pigment in the skin, although this fixation often outlasts the desire to retain the tattoo.

If the colour and consequently the absorption spectrum of the tattoo pigment differ sufficiently from the surrounding skin then it may be amenable to laser treatment. The appropriate wavelength is selected based on the colour of the tattoo (Table 24.4).

There is no uniformity in the constituents or the application of tattoo pigment and thus no uniformity in response to treatment. Some tattoos show significant fading after only one treatment whereas others can prove far more resistant. In general, amateur tattoos will fade faster than professional ones which may require 10 or more treatments. Care should be taken in the selection of treatable tattoos and the patient must be given a realistic assessment of what is achievable for their tattoo. Responsible laser operators may deem some large multicoloured tattoos untreatable from the outset.

Table 24.4 Laser selection by colour for tattoo removal.

Blue/black	Q-switched Nd-YAG 1064 nm Q-switched Ruby 694 nm Q-switched Alexandrite 755 nm
Red	Q-switched Nd-YAG 532 nm
Green	Q-switched Ruby 694 nm Q-switched Alexandrite 755 nm

Laser treatment of tattoos creates microscopic steam bubbles in the skin, sometimes referred to as *laser snow* (Figure 24.4), which disappears in a matter of minutes. Initially, there will be no apparent difference in colour but over the next few months macrophages will phagocytose the newly exposed pigment particles and the tattoo will gradually fade. Treatment is therefore carried out on a 2- to 3-monthly basis.

Hair removal

Laser hair removal is carried out using the Alexandrite, Ruby or Nd-YAG laser, the last being more suitable for darker skin types. The chromophore is melanin in the hair and thermal energy dissipates to and damages the surrounding follicular cells effecting longer term hair removal. Thus white, grey, blonde or red hair is unresponsive to treatment, and equal care must be taken where the skin is pigmented. Erythema in the treated area can be expected for up to 48 h. Around six treatments will be required for a satisfactory response.

Laser resurfacing

The carbon dioxide laser (10600 nm) and the Erbium-YAG laser (2940 nm) have water as their chromophore. All components of the human body contain water and the action of these lasers on the skin cannot truly be described as selective. Rather, they are a destructive entity used to vaporise tissue. They may be applied as a narrow continuous beam to cut tissue which has the advantage of achieving reasonable haemostasis as one proceeds, enabling convenient excision of unwanted tissue, for example, keloids.

Alternatively, 'resurfacing' of the skin is achieved by photothermolysing the epithelial surface of the skin to a reasonably predictable depth in one or more passes with subsequent healing. This method can improve the appearance of superficial lesions, for example, acne scarring, wrinkles or epidermal naevi.

A satisfactory result will only be achieved by careful patient selection and scrupulous attention to pre- and postoperative wound care.

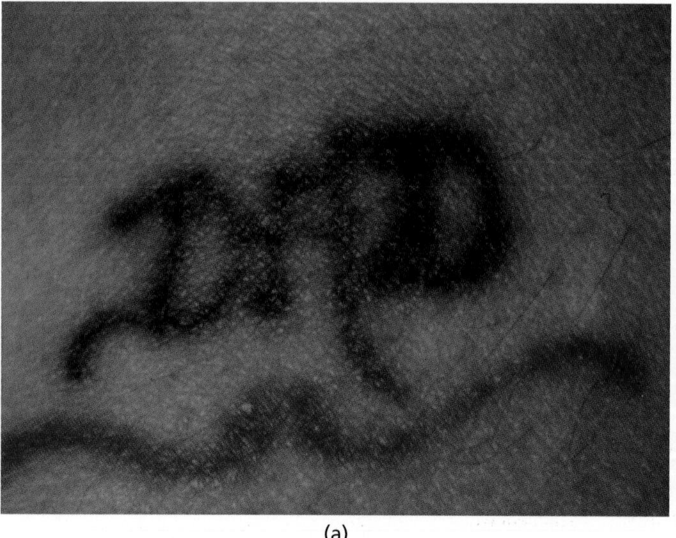
(a)

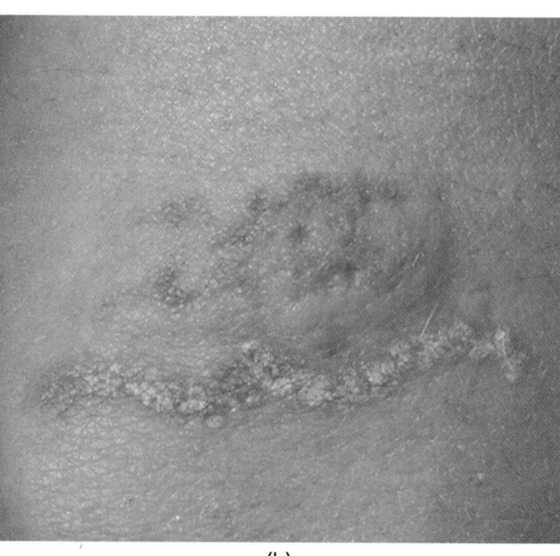
(b)

Figure 24.4 Tattoo subjected to laser removal. (a) Before treatment. (b) Fading of tattoo and 'laser snow' following Q-switched Nd-YAG laser treatment.

Considerable training is required to operate these lasers successfully and they should only be operated by those with appropriate expertise.

Fractional laser treatment

Fractional laser treatment delivers a series of microscopic laser beams which penetrate into the dermis and are evenly spaced across the treatment area. They do not damage the whole area under treatment but the resulting columns of ablated tissue encourage the formation of new collagen. It is used to treat scarring, wrinkles and abnormal pigmentation. Similar columns of epidermal and dermal damage can be induced mechanically by use of a metal roller with small protruding spikes the, so-called 'dermarollers'.

Dermabrasion and Chemical peels

Superficial lesions such as wrinkles, scarring and solar damage can be treated by simple abrasion of the skin surface using a motorised tool in a technique known as *dermabrasion*. Over the following weeks re-epithelialisation from deeper, healthier epidermis around hair follicles and sebaceous glands brings about healing. Local or general anaesthesia is required and despite intensive pre- and post-operative care the procedure may be complicated by abnormal pigmentation, scarring or infection. A gentler, but less effective approach is to manually abrade the skin by rubbing it with small crystals (microdermabrasion).

A chemical peel uses acidic or alkaline solutions to remove the surface layers of the skin allowing regeneration to take place from deeper epidermis. The resulting inflammation may also stimulate the formation of new collagen.

Intense pulsed light

Non-laser light sources such as intense pulsed light (IPL) have been advocated as cheaper and less invasive alternatives for the treatment of various skin abnormalities including vascular and pigmentary disorders. They emit light over a range of wavelengths and employ filters to achieve some selectivity. IPL has traditionally been used to treat simple vascular abnormalities such as spider naevi erythema in rosacea and cherry angiomas with relative success. However, they are being increasingly used to treat more complex vascular lesions such as port wine stains. They can be particularly helpful at treating heterogeneous vascular abnormalities where there may be venous and arterial aberrant vessels in the same lesion. IPL, being less chromophore specific, can treat a mixed lesion and can cause thermal heating and subsequent coagulation of deep vessels that may be difficult to target by conventional vascular lasers. There is less blood vessel rupture with IPL when compared to laser treatment and consequently less purpura immediately after IPL. Technology is improving and IPL is being increasingly used to treat a wider range of skin disorders, but as yet they are considered to be less effective than monochromatic lasers. One of the main advantages of IPL is the ability to treat large areas of skin quickly with relatively little 'down-time' for the patients.

Photodynamic therapy

Photodynamic therapy (PDT) in dermatology involves the topical application of a photoactivated toxin such as aminolevulinic acid or methyl aminolevulinate to a lesion followed after 4 h by exposure to light, usually in the 630-nm range. The effective penetration at this wavelength is 1–3 mm and PDT is used to treat solar keratoses, Bowen's disease and superficial basal cell carcinoma (Figure 24.5). However, the treatment is painful for the patient and expensive in terms of staff time and consumables. Equivalent results can usually

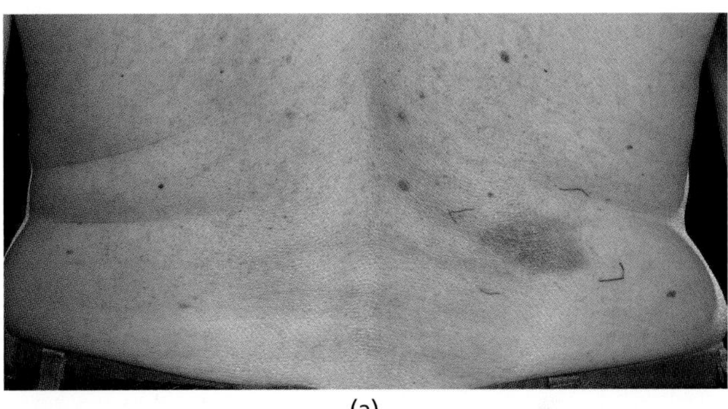

(a)

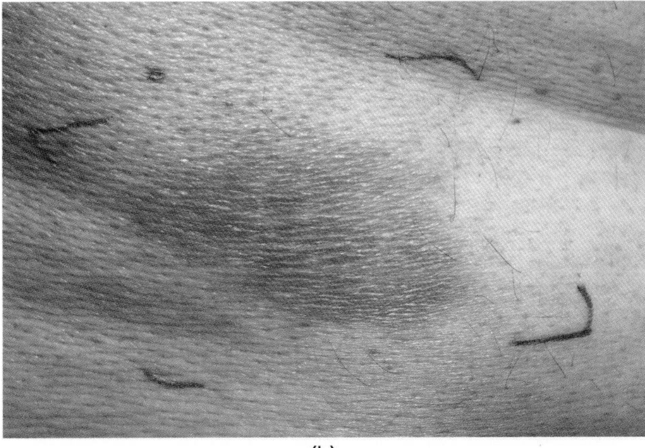

(b)

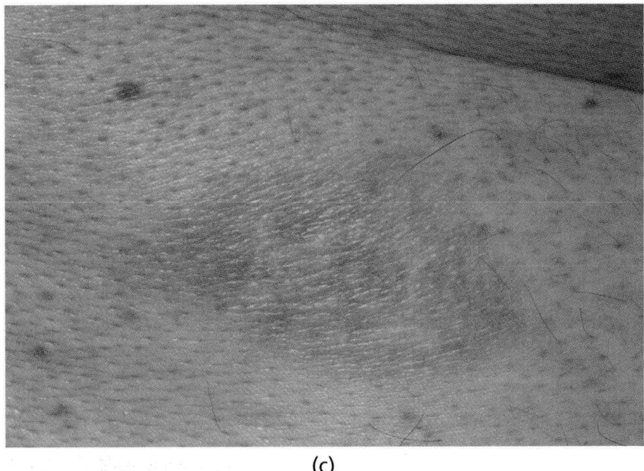

(c)

Figure 24.5 Superficial basal cell carcinoma on the lower back. (a,b) Before treatment with Hetvix photodynamic therapy (PDT). (c) Six months after PDT. Figures courtesy of Dr Andrew Morris, University Hospital of Wales, Cardiff.

be achieved with cryotherapy, topical 5-fluorouracil or curettage and cautery. Therefore, the use of PDT is generally limited to larger lesions in poorly healing sites.

PDT has also been advocated for use in acne, but antibiotics and isotretinoin provide cheaper and more effective alternatives. It may have a role where patients are unable or unwilling to pursue more conventional treatments.

Further Reading

Lanigan S. *Lasers in Dermatology*, Springer-Verlag, London, 2000.

New Zealand Dermatological Society: dermnetnz.org/procedures/lasers.html.

Tanzi EL, Lupton JR and Alster TS. Lasers in dermatology: four decades of progress. *J Am Acad Dermatol* **49**:1–31, 2003.

CHAPTER 25

Wound Management and Bandaging

Bernadette Byrne

Department of Tissue viability, Kings College Hospital, UK

OVERVIEW

- The physiology of normal wound healing can be optimised by the correct selection and application of appropriate dressings and/or bandage systems.
- Individualised holistic patient assessment including skin and wound is important to select the type of dressings required and treat any underlying causes.
- Understanding the properties and functions of different dressing categories is a pre-requisite to enable the practitioner to make the most appropriate evidence-based choice for each wound type.
- Correct application of bandages is essential to ensure they are at the correct tension to prevent slippage or cause damage around bony prominences.
- Patient choice and involvement in wound care lead to improved concordance essential to successful wound healing.
- A multidisciplinary approach is essential between all the healthcare practitioners caring for the patient's wound/skin.
- The patient's quality of life can be significantly improved by optimal wound care.

Introduction

Effective wound management relies heavily upon the selection of an appropriate dressing and an in-depth understanding of the normal physiology of wound healing. Wound dressings have developed in scientific standing over the years and the complexity of their action is reflected in the vast amount spent on their development to provide the optimum evidence-based wound care; however, there are very few large randomised studies to support their use. Without effective wound assessment there is a risk of selecting an inappropriate product which can lead to delayed wound healing. This chapter provides a practical approach to wound management rather than a detailed look at the physiology of the wound healing process.

Wounds

A wound is a cut or break in continuity of any tissue caused by injury or operation – a break in the skin that may consist of a tear, incision, cut, erosion, puncture or ulcer where the top layer of the skin is breached; if this occurs, tissues are vulnerable to fluid, blood and heat loss, allowing potential invasion of micro-organisms or foreign materials into the skin and possible loss of function.

Since the introduction of modern wound dressings such as Granuflex in 1982 and subsequently Kaltostat in 1986 (Convatec), the science of wound healing has progressed rapidly and considerable advances have been made in the development of new products to enhance wound healing; this has led to explosion of wound care products available both in hospital and on FP10 prescription. While a greater choice of dressing products is beneficial to both the patient and the practitioner, it can lead to confusion on which dressings to select for each individual wound as different wound dressings often have specific indications for use.

When assessing any wound, there are multiple factors that need to be taken into consideration in addition to the possible underlying aetiology; decisions on which product to apply are based on a full holistic assessment including short- and long-term aims of treatment, patients' diagnosis and prognosis, availability of the product and the cost.

Principles of local wound management include achieving haemostasis, correcting underlying causes, reducing bioburdon (micro-organisms), removing devitalised tissue if present by debridement (Figure 25.1), maintaining moisture balance and protecting the surrounding skin.

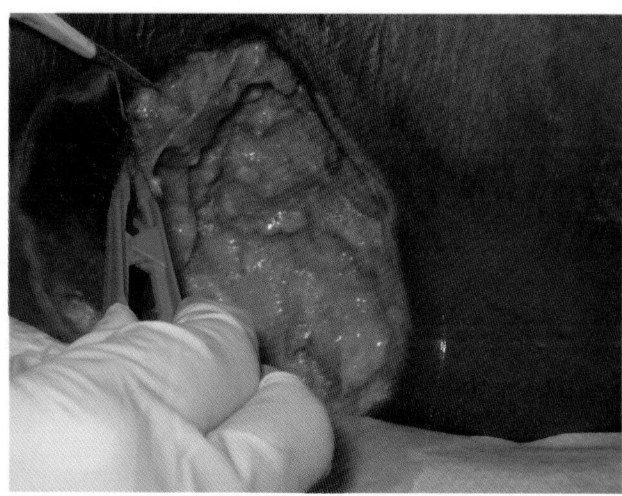

Figure 25.1 Deep necrotic wound secondary to calciphylaxis being debrided. *Source:* Grey et al., 2010. Reprinted with kind permission of Wounds UK.

ABC of Dermatology, Sixth Edition. Edited by Rachael Morris-Jones.

Wound bed preparation: Achieving a healthy wound bed is a pre-requisite to the use of many advanced wound care products. The aim of wound bed preparation is to optimise the wound healing environment by removing barriers, that is, necrotic tissue, slough, exudate and bioburdon. Wound bed preparation is the management of the wound to accelerate endogenous healing or to facilitate the effectiveness of other therapeutic measures.

The acronym TIME indicates the principles of wound bed preparation.

T – Tissue, non-viable or deficient
I – Infection or inflammation
M – Moisture imbalance
E – Edge, epidermal margin, non-advancing or undermining.

(From Schultz et al., 2003)

Wound types

In order to manage wounds optimally, they are classified into four different types according to the appearance of the wound bed and surrounding tissues, as illustrated by the wound healing continuum below.

The wound healing continuum is represented by the tissues in the wound and is colour-based (from Grey et al., 2013) (Figure 25.2).

1 *Necrotic wounds.* Dead (ischaemic) tissue is usually black, brown or dark tan and is covered with devitalised epidermis; a black wound indicates the presence of eschar.
2 *Sloughy wounds.* These are mostly yellow because of the accumulation of cellular debris, fibrin, serous exudate, leucocytes and bacteria on the wound surface. Yellow fibrous tissue that adheres to the wound bed and cannot be removed by irrigation is known as *slough*.
3 *Granulating wounds* are characteristically bright red with a highly vascular nodular, irregular granular appearance. This is a combination of new blood vessel growth, connective tissue or dermal cells.
4 *Epithelialising wounds.* Cells migrate from the wound edges to start the process of re-epithelialisation/epidermal re-growth, which is seen as pink translucent tissue in the wound bed (Table 25.1).

Wound-related factors to be considered in selecting an ideal dressing

- Type/aetiology of wound
- Size of the wound
- Location of the wound
- Stage of healing
- Tissue involved
- Amount, colour and viscosity of exudates
- Wound odour
- Condition of the surrounding skin
- Patient's general health and environment
- Duration of the wound (acute or chronic)
- Long- and short-term aims of treatment

Key factors affecting wound healing

- Overall health and past medical history
- Cardiovascular status/circulatory disorders
- Disease processes, for example, diabetes and cancer
- Extremes of age (very young/old)
- Psychological factors, for example, stress and anxiety, sleep disturbances
- Malnutrition
- Dehydration
- Smoking
- Drug therapy
- Poor wound management
- Surgical site infections
- Patients prognosis

Regardless of type, any wound may be additionally infected or colonised by micro-organisms. If organisms proliferate within the wound an infection may develop, causing a host reaction; this is characterised by pain, oedema, erythema, odour, increased or purulent exudate, abscess formation and local heat.

Dressings

The process of dressing selection is determined and influenced by a variety of factors. These include patient-focused issues and the types of dressings available.

Principles for selecting an ideal dressing

- To provide a moist environment to promote healing
- To absorb excess wound exudate
- To allow gaseous exchange
- To protect the wound from pathogenic organisms
- To protect the wound from trauma and contamination
- To minimise and contain odour
- To provide a constant wound interface temperature
- To be non-adherent and easily removed
- To be non-toxic, non-allergenic and non-sensitising
- To reduce pain

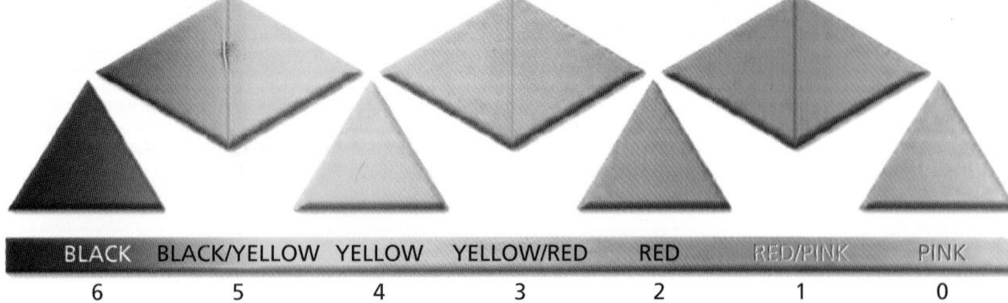

Figure 25.2 Wound healing continuum. Grey *et al.* (2010). Reprinted with kind permission of Wounds UK.

Table 25.1 Wound types and suitable dressings.

Wound type	Wound picture	Characteristics	Examples of suitable dressings
Necrotic wounds		Black, dry, eschar devitalised tissue, but can present as wet necrosis/gangrene. *Aims of dressing*: Rehydrate eschar to encourage autolytic debridement if appropriate (not diabetic foot wounds). Manage exudate/actively debride if wet necrosis/infected.	Hydrogels (non-diabetic) Hydrocolloids (non-diabetic) Sharp debridement by competent practitioner only (TVN or Podiatrist) Surgical debridement
Sloughy		Can range from dry to highly exuding. Characterised by fibrous sloughy tissue, yellowish in colour. *Aims of dressing*: Remove slough, encourage and facilitate a clean wound bed for the formation of granulation tissue.	Hydrogels Alginates Hydrofibre Hydrocolloids Larvae Packing or ribbon forms of dressing required for cavity wounds
Granulating		Clean, low to medium exudate, bright red wound bed with granular, moist, nodular and uneven appearance. *Aim of dressing*: To protect and encourage granulation tissue formation. Promote a moist wound healing environment.	Alginates Hydrofibre Hydrocolloids Foams Alginogels Hydrogels
Epithelialising		Clean, superficial, low to medium exudate, pink in colour, can have white/translucent margins. *Aim of dressing*: Protection to allow further epithelialisation/maturation to occur.	Low and non-adherent dressings knitted viscose Paraffin gauze Silicone based products Film dressings
Infected wounds		Painful to touch, malodorous, greenish/yellow in appearance, friable granulation tissue (delicate, easily damaged) often have increased levels of exudates.	Suitable dressings are Silver-impregnated dressings: Silver alginates, hydrofibre, foams Iodine based dressings Honey PHMBs Larvae
Exuding wounds		Exuding wounds can appear anywhere on the wound healing continuum, however increased exudate is often associated with wound infection. They often have per-wound skin that is shiny and white (wet and macerated). *Aims of dressing*: Effective exudate management. Skin care to encourage healing.	Suitable dressings include Alginates Hydrofibre Foams Super absorbants Also require barrier protection of per-wound skin: 50:50 Epaderm Double base

On page 199 in Table 25.1, the second line listed under "Characteristics" of "Exuding Wounds" is incorrect and should read "They often have peri-wound skin that is shiny and white (wet and macerated)."

TVN, tissue viability nurse.
Check for sensitivities prior to application.

- To promote autolytic debridement
- To protect the surrounding skin
- To cause minimum distress and discomfort during dressing change
- To improve the quality of life
- To be cosmetically acceptable to the patient
- Conformability of dressing
- To be cost effective and available in hospitals and the community

Dressings

Modern dressings are described as either passive or interactive, depending on their composition and structure.

Passive dressings

- are applied to protect the wound
- are designed not to stick to the wound bed
- are mostly used for surgical, clean healing and superficial wounds.

Interactive dressings

- actively interact with the wound surface (in order to promote an environment that maximises healing).

Types of wound dressings

Both passive and interactive dressings are subdivided into several categories, as seen in Figure 25.3.

Non- or low adherent dressings

These are used for superficial, lightly exuding wounds (Figure 25.4). Their major function is to maintain a moist wound bed and allow the exudate to pass through to a secondary dressing and reduce trauma at dressing change. Newer silicone-based dressings are the most effective but tend to be more expensive.

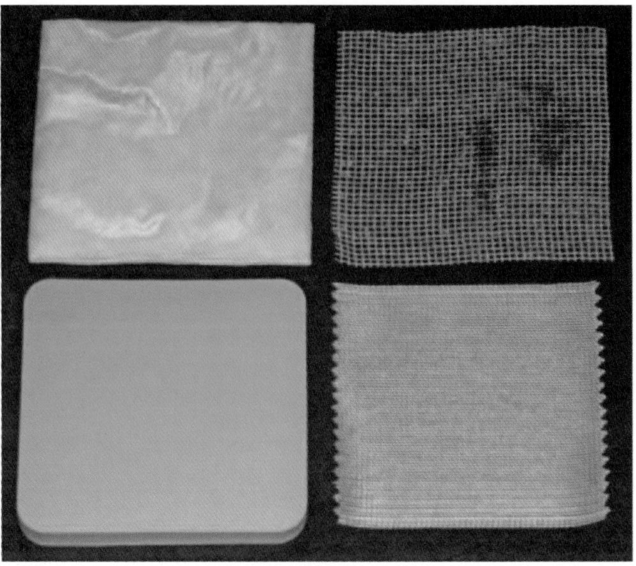

Figure 25.4 Non-adherent dressings.

Examples include the following:

- Knitted viscose dressings with an open structure to facilitate the free passage of exudates (e.g. N/A & N/A ultra).
- Perforated film absorbent dressings. The film is perforated to allow the exudate into the absorbent layer (e.g. Melolin®, Release®).
- Silicone dressings. These are made of a conformable silicone-covered mesh which gently adheres to the wound and surrounding skin but are designed to reduce pain and trauma on removal; the hydrophobic soft silicone layer feels sticky to touch but does not adhere to the wound bed. It is non-absorbent and therefore a secondary absorbent dressing is required, but self-adhesive

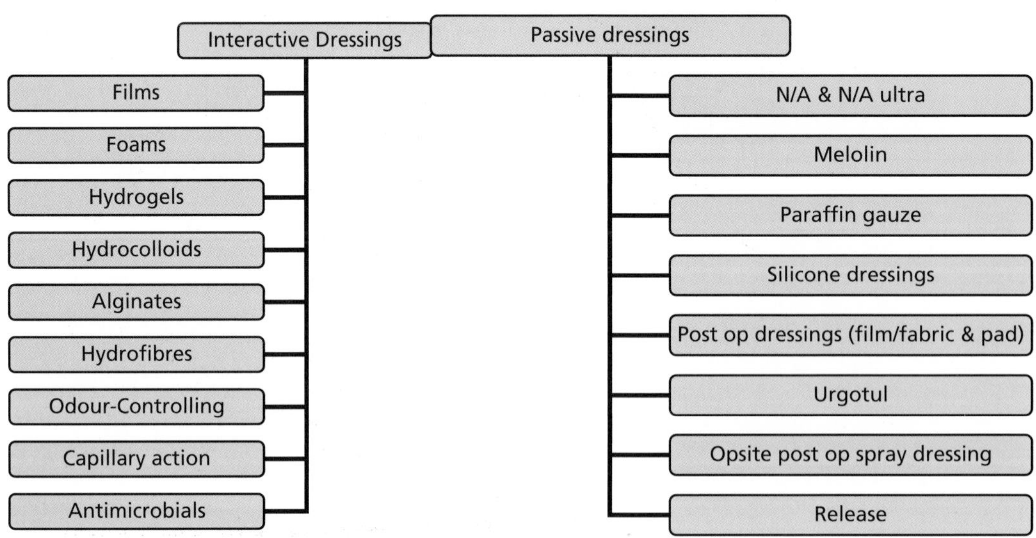

Figure 25.3 Wound dressing categories.

dressing with foam backing is also available. (e.g. Mepitel®, Adaptic, Silflex). Uses include donor sites, burns, epidermolysis bullosa (EB) patients and under topical negative pressure (TNP).

- Paraffin tulle dressings consisting of an open-weave cotton or viscose and cotton-mix dressing impregnated in yellow or white soft paraffin (e.g. Jelonet®).

Film dressings

These consist of a thin film of polyurethane, permeable to water vapour and oxygen yet impermeable to water and micro-organisms, allowing gaseous exchange and reducing risk of bacterial contamination (Figure 25.5). Films are flexible and therefore suitable for difficult anatomical sites such as across joints. They can be used on superficial wounds, donor sites, post-operative wounds and as a secondary dressing for other products. These dressings are not recommended for deep, infected or exuding wounds. Removal of these dressings can be traumatic to the surrounding skin and it is therefore recommended to follow the manufacturers' instructions and remove by the 'horizontal stretch' technique.

Examples include Opsite®, Tegaderm®, Bioclusive® and C-View®.

Hydrogel dressings

These consist of insoluble polymers which are hydrophilic and can absorb excess fluid or produce a moist environment at the wound surface (Figure 25.6). They can be used on dry, sloughy and necrotic wounds which allow rehydration of devitalised tissue and facilitate autolysis. Hydrogel dressings may be suitable for pressure ulcers, leg ulcers and surgical wounds; however, they should not be used for wounds producing high levels of exudate, where gangrene is present, or on diabetic foot ulcers. Hydrogel dressings also come in a sheet format and usually require a secondary dressing to keep them in place. These dressings need to be changed every 1–3 days. Examples include Actiform cool (sheet), Intrasite gel®, Intrasite conformable, Granugel®, Purilon and Nugel®.

Hydrocolloid dressings

These consist of a semi-permeable film with sodium carboxymethylcellulose plus gel-forming agents such as pectin and gelatin, which are waterproof, self-adhesive and reported to reduce pain by keeping exposed nerve endings moist (Figure 25.7). They form a gel in contact with wound exudate to promote angiogenesis/stimulation of new blood vessels or rehydrate dry slough and necrosis.

Hydrocolloids can be left in place for up to 7 days; inappropriate use/too frequent dressing changes can lead to irritation and skin stripping. They should not be used to manage heavily exuding wounds, diabetic foot ulcers and any wound infected with anaerobic organisms. Examples include Comfeel®, Granuflex/duoderm extra-thin® and Tegasorb®.

Hydrofibre dressings

These are composed of sodium carboxymethylcellulose (hydrocolloid fibres) which can absorb and retain significant amounts of exudate by vertical wicking, thereby reducing maceration of the wound margins (Figure 25.8). The fibres convert into a gel on contact with wound exudate and are suitable for wounds with moderate to heavy

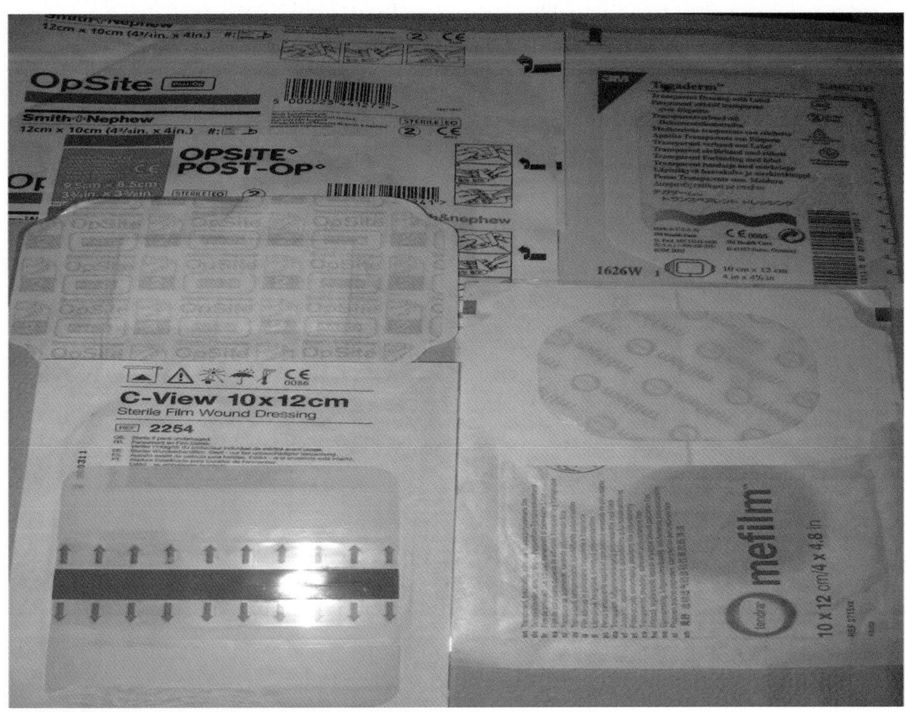

Figure 25.5 Film dressings allow wound monitoring.

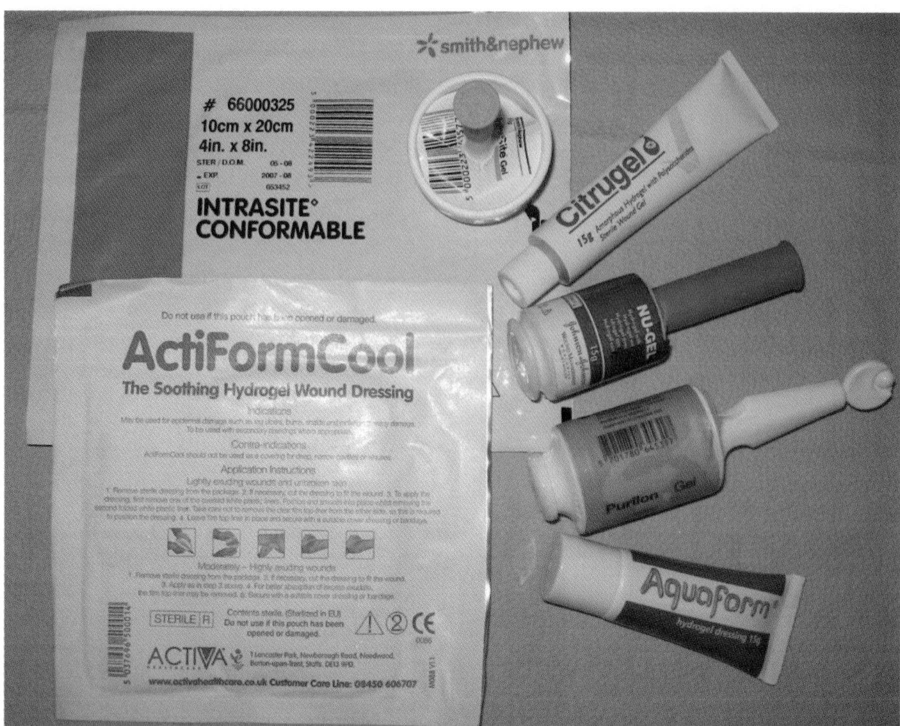

Figure 25.6 Hydrogel dressings.

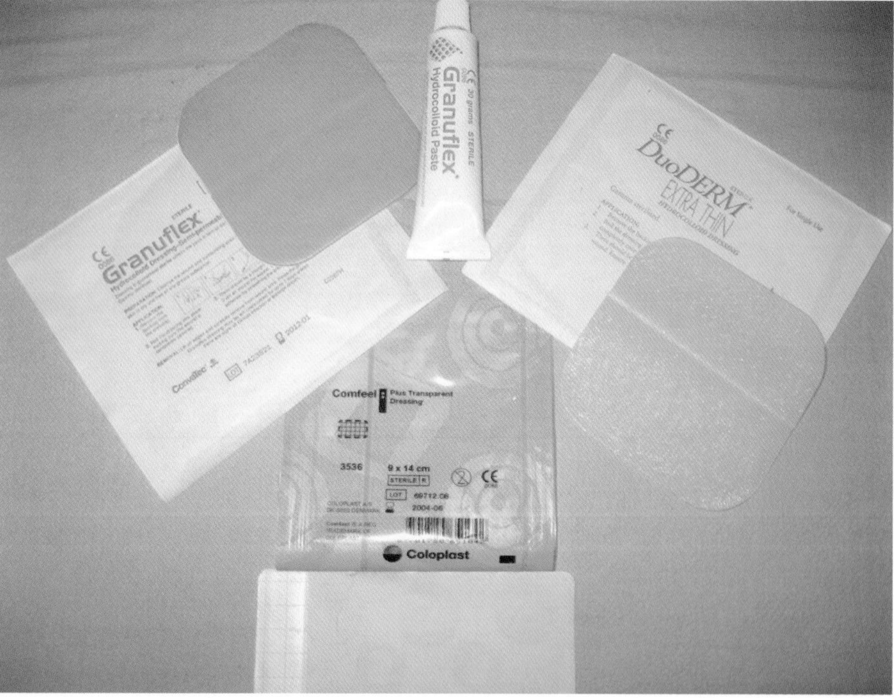

Figure 25.7 Hydrocolloid dressings.

exudate, slough and wet necrosis. A secondary dressing is required to keep hydrofibre dressings in place. Dressing change should be undertaken every 1–7 days depending on any underlying wound infection. Examples are Aquacel, Aquqcel extra, Aquacel Ribbon® and Aquacel Ag®.

Alginate dressings

The dressings are derived from algenic acid extracted from brown seaweed (Phaeophyceae family); the fibres create a hydrophilic gel in the presence of exudate. All alginates have the capacity to act as a hemostat, used on moderately exuding wound, and can be applied

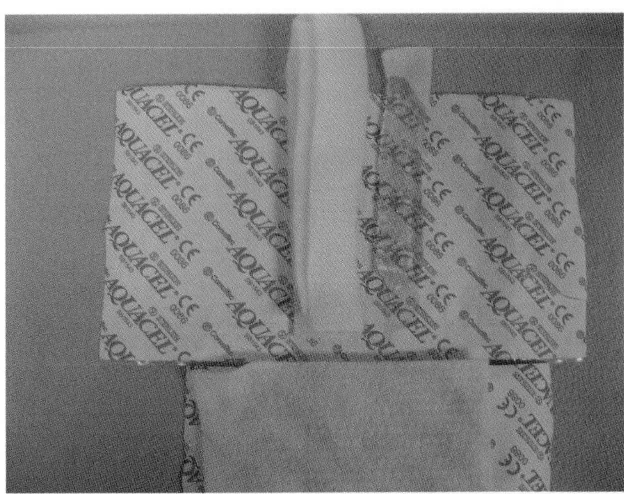

Figure 25.8 Hydrofibre dressings.

to infected wounds as available in silver format. Alginates must be applied dry and require a secondary dressing; do not leave on for longer than 7 days. They are also available in rope and ribbon forms for cavity wounds. Examples of pure calcium alginate include Sorbsan® and Algisite M. Kaltostat is a mixture of sodium and calcium salts (licensed hemostat).

Polyurethane foam dressings

These contain hydrophilic, absorbent polyurethane foams which are highly absorbent and available in a variety of shapes and sizes and can be used as either primary or secondary dressing (Figure 25.9). Foams can be used in a variety of wounds ranging from leg ulcers to cavity wounds from light to heavily exuding with the added advantage that they do not shed particles into the wound as traditional gauze does. Their main function is to absorb exudate, allow moisture evaporation, maintain high humidity at the wound interface, allow gaseous exchange, provide thermal insulation and protect from bacterial contamination. Foam dressings are now available with a self-adhesive or silicone border. Examples include Mepilex, Biatain, Lyofoam®, Allevyn® and Tielle®.

Antimicrobial dressings

Antimicrobial agents have been applied to wounds for thousands of years; it is a term used to describe a substance that destroys microbes or prevents their growth and multiplication (Figure 25.10). The careful use of a range of medical dressings can successfully treat patients with chronic/infected wounds where the use of systemic antibiotics is contraindicated; in addition, with hospital-acquired infections and antibiotic resistance on the increase, the demand for antimicrobial dressings has increased. Silver has been used for many years as an antimicrobial agent for the treatment of burns in the form of sulphadiazine cream. New dressings impregnated with silver are available for a variety of wounds that are either colonised or infected. Examples include Actisorb Silver®, Aquacel Ag, SilvaSorb® and Urgotul SSD®, Sorbsan Silver, Contreet and Acticoat.

Iodine has the ability to lower bacterial growth in chronic wounds and is active against gram-positive and -negative organisms. Caution is required for patients with thyroid disease because of possible systemic uptake of iodine. Examples include Inadine® and Betadine® and Cadexomer iodine (Iodoflex/iodosorb S&N).

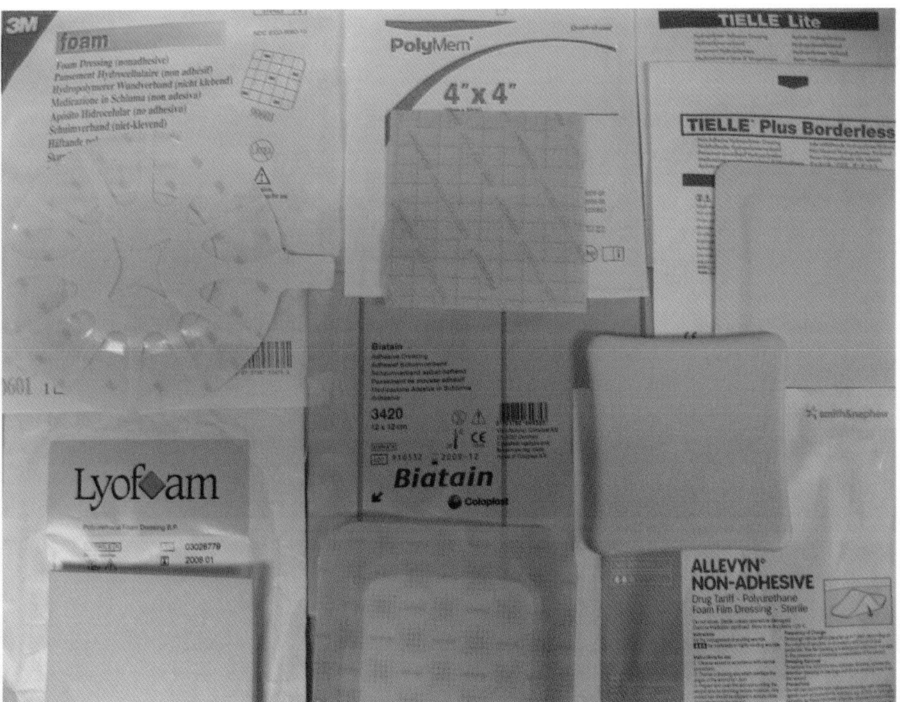

Figure 25.9 Foam dressings.

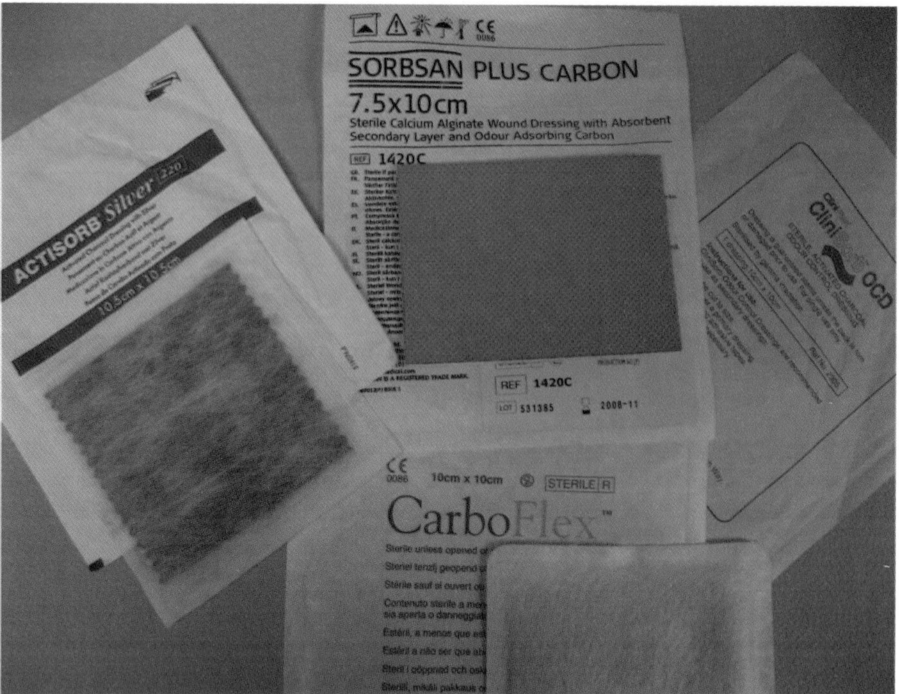

Figure 25.10 Antimicrobial dressings.

Metronidazole gel can be applied to infected wounds, particularly those colonised with anaerobic organisms. The gel helps with odour control and is especially useful in managing fungating malignant wounds.

Odour-controlling dressings

Charcoal dressings filter and absorb malodorous chemicals from wounds, they can be used as a primary or secondary dressing and they are indicated in all malodorous wounds. Honey also has odour control properties.

Activated charcoal loses its function to absorb odours when it is saturated with exudate and requires regular changing. Examples include Actisorb®, Clinisorb® and Kaltocarb®.

Cavity dressings

Traditionally, cavity wounds were packed with ribbon gauze soaked in a variety of solutions (EUSOL, Betadine or proflavine), but these often dry out and cause trauma to the wound on removal. Cavities are now commonly dressed with alginate fibre or hydrofibre in the form of rope or ribbon (Figure 25.11). Cavity dressings fill the whole wound cavity preventing 'dead space', allowing the product to treat the whole wound including undermined areas and sinuses. This assists exudate management and allows the wound to heal by secondary intention, from the wound bed upwards. Examples include Aquacel Ribbon, Allevyn Cavity®, Kaltostat Rope® and Sorbsan Ribbon®, Honey Ribbon and rope Algivon plus Advancis medical and Topical negative pressure, vacuum assisted closure (VAC).

Larvae therapy

Larval therapy is the use of larvae of the green bottle fly (*Lucillia seriata*) to remove sloughy and necrotic tissue without damaging healthy granulation tissue (Figure 25.12). They have three main modes of action: debridement, antimicrobial and facilitating healing, which is achieved by secreting enzymes which liquefy the tissue so that it can be ingested. Indications for use include venous ulcers, diabetic foot ulcers, arterial ulcers, pressure ulcers and wounds awaiting a graft as they can also prevent the wound re-sloughing after debridement. Subsequent applications may be required until granulation tissue has formed.

Larvae are available in both free range form (which are applied under a net/sleeve and can be left in the wound for 3 days) or as Bio-Foam (sealed in a net pouch with hydrophilic polyurethane foam pieces) which can be left up to 5 days. The latter are easier to apply and are usually more acceptable to the patient. In the UK, larvae are supplied by BioMonde Bridgend, South Wales, where they are bred under sterile conditions and dispatched by a courier. Larvae are contraindicated in patients with dysfunctional blood clotting, wounds that have a tendency to bleed, wounds with exposed major blood vessels or sinus/cavities where wound bed is not visible.

Honey dressings

Honey is an ancient wound remedy first documented by Hippocrates in 460 BC. It has a pH of 3.5, which is too acidic for microorganisms to thrive; however, this can cause pain on application because of its acid mantle. Honey contains nutrients and

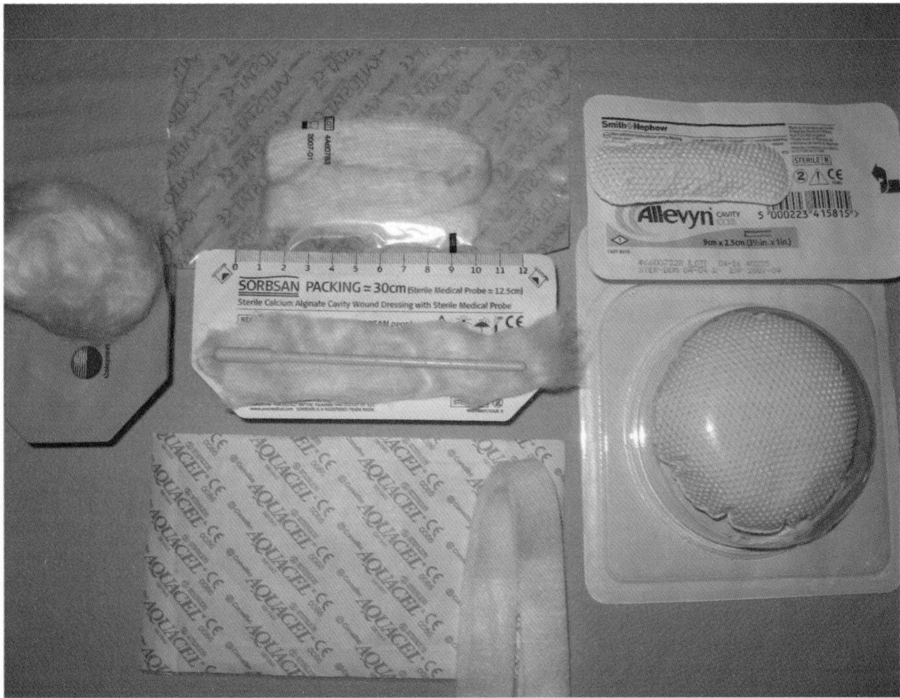

Figure 25.11 Cavity dressings.

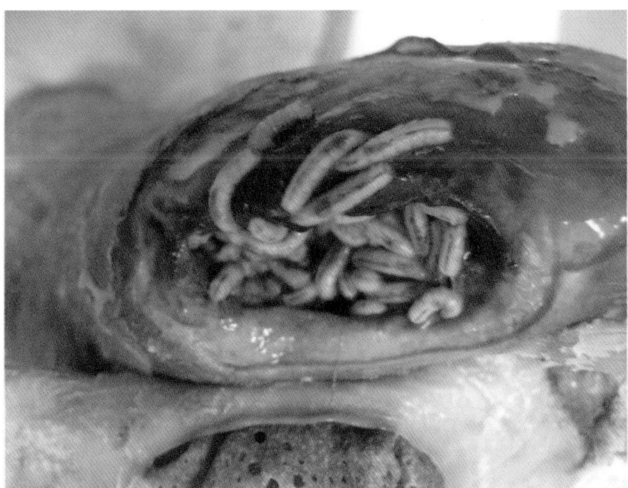

Figure 25.12 Larvae therapy.

herbal properties, amino acids, vitamins and enzymes. Honey produces hydrogen peroxide enzymatically which is antibacterial; however, this is only a 1000th of the concentration of the hydrogen peroxide solution formally used in wound cleansing and it has five key modes of action: antimicrobial, anti-inflammatory, providing a moist wound environment, desloughing/debriding devitalised tissue (Figure 25.13) and deodorising/reducing malodour. Examples of honey dressings include Activon Honey Tulle® and Advancis®, Activon tube, Algivon ribbon/ rope and Honey barrier cream.

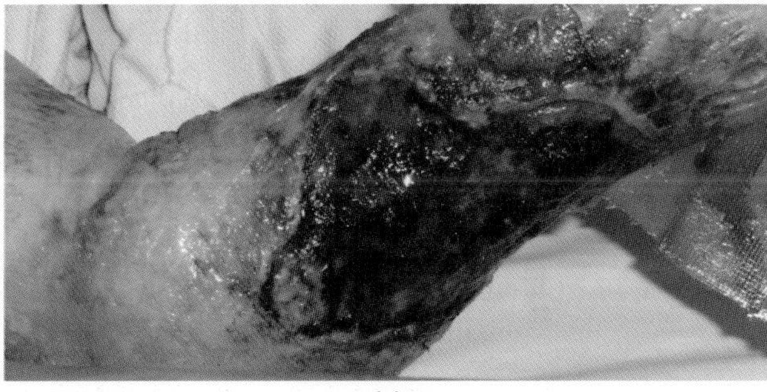

(a)

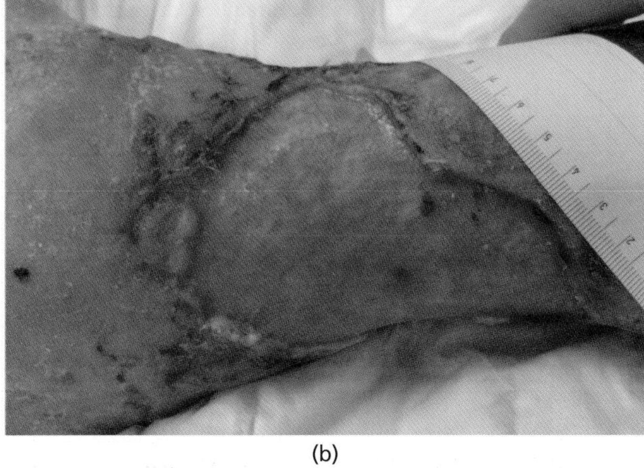

(b)

Figure 25.13 (a) Necrotic wound pre honey dressing and (b) necrotic wound 1 week post honey dressing.

Capillary action dressing

An absorbent, low adherent primary wound contact layer that has a wicking effect, it is made of soft viscose and polyester, which are bonded together and backed with a perforated layer on each side (allowing it to be applied either way up). The accelerated capillary action 'pulls' interstitial fluid from the wound bed. Indications for use include acute and chronic wounds and sloughy or cavity wounds with moderate to heavy exudate; initially, dressings may need changing daily but can be left in place up to 7 days. Contraindications are bleeding or fungating wounds. Examples include Avadraw, Advancis medical, available in sheet or spiral wick form, both of which can be cut to size.

Topical negative pressure dressings (TNP)

The first TNP wound healing dressing was introduced in 1994 by KCI, the vacuum-assisted wound closure (VAC); recently, a number of new devices have been introduced that also deliver TNP. TNP is a non-invasive active wound closure device that uses controlled, localised negative pressure to promote wound healing in both acute and chronic wounds. The main mode of action is to remove interstitial fluid, enhance dermal profusion, stimulate granulation, help remove infectious material, provide a closed moist wound healing environment, promote flap survival and improve graft uptake. Indications for use include pressure ulcers, leg ulcers, diabetic foot ulcers, sinuses, acute/traumatic wounds, dehisced wounds, mesh graphs and flaps. Contraindications are malignant fungating wounds, active bleeding, exposed blood vessels/organs, untreated osteomyelitis, unexplored fistula and necrotic eschar. These dressings must be applied by an experienced practitioner. Types of devices available are VAC, VAC Via (single use) KCI, Renasys and Pico (single use) S&N and Avance Molnlycke.

Newer products available

Super-absorbent dressings

These consist of 'nappy gel' technology and absorb the exudate away from the wound and retain it in gel beads, reducing the need for frequent dressing changes and maceration of wound margins. Examples include Eclypse/Eclypse adherent, Eclypse boot, Sorbion satches, Dry max extra and Kerramax. Their main disadvantage is that they cannot be cut to size.

Alginogels

Enzyme alginogels are a new class of dressing which combine the benefits of hydrogels and alginates in an innovative wound care product, incorporating unique broad spectrum antibacterial enzymes that are effective against a range of clinical isolates, including methicillin-resistant *Staphylococcus aureus* (MRSA). They can either donate fluid to the wound or absorb excess exudate. Indications for use include debriding, desloughing and infected wounds but are safe to be used on all wounds; they are biodegradable, creating a soft and soothing wound interface thus reducing pain. Examples are Flaminal, Flaminal forte and Crawford Healthcare.

PHMB

Polyhexamethylene biguanide (PHMB) is an antiseptic with a long history of use in cosmetics and commercially, wet wipes, contact lens solution and swimming pools, thereby proven to be non-irritant and non-toxic. PHMB is a broad spectrum antimicrobial effective against aerobic and anaerobic bacteria including MRSA, fungi, moulds and yeasts. It is available in various formats including cleansing solution, wound gel, biocellulose and foam dressings. Indications for use include second-degree burns, leg ulcers, pressure ulcers, surgical wounds, diabetic foot ulcers and donor and recipient sites. Examples are Suprasorb X + PHMB, available in sheet and rope forms for use in cavities (Lohmann and Rauscher); Prontosan solution and Wound Gel (B.Braun) and AMD foam (Kendal).

MMPs

Matrix metalloproteinase (MMP) is thought to have a major role in cell proliferation and migration, wound contraction and scar remodelling; however, chronically elevated MMPs can degrade the extracellular matrix proteins and prevent the wound from healing. MMP modulating dressings reduce excessive protease activity by absorbing the wound exudate and retaining the proteases within the dressing. MMP dressings provide a moist wound environment, reduce the bio-burden and lower protease and free radical activity. Examples include Promogram, Promogram Prisma (containing silver) Systagenix; Sorbion, H&R and Suprasorb C, Activa. Indications for use are chronic non-healing wounds; but currently there are no means to measure the amount of MMP activity in the wound although devices are being evaluated at present.

Other Therapies

Biatain Ibu	Combines moist wound healing with active pain reliever; the foam dressing releases ibuprofen evenly into the wound.
Hyperbaric oxygen therapy	The use of O_2 at a level higher than atmospheric pressure, increasing the oxygen transported in plasma. There is no evidence to suggest it provides improved healing rates in chronic wounds than standard treatment.
Leeches	The saliva contains a thrombin inhibitor, and they can be used reduce venous congestion following skin graft.
Versa-jet hydrosurgical system	High velocity water jet used for wound debridement.
Biological dressings	Consist of human or animal tissue used as temporary wound covering, often in treatment of burns or large areas of skin loss to prevent infection and fluid loss. Examples are Autograft, Allograft and Xenograft.

Adverse effects of dressings

- Maceration of the surrounding skin
- Irritant contact dermatitis
- Allergic contact dermatitis
- Skin stripping from frequent dressing changes.

Bandages

Bandages have been used for thousands of years, going back to the time of the ancient Egyptians who applied woven fabric with considerable skill to mummify their dead. With the discovery of natural rubber in the mid-19th century, the first elasticated bandages were produced for the management of varicose veins. These bandages were made of natural fibres through a weaving process as a simple retention bandage to provide support and protection.

Bandage application is a necessary skill required by most nursing and some medical practitioners during their working life. Therefore, it is essential that training in bandage application is adequate in order that bandages may be applied correctly and safely to patients. Poor bandage technique can lead to pain and discomfort for the patient, pressure damage over bony prominences, misshapen limbs, ridging and exacerbation of pedal oedema. Bandage usages include compression therapy for venous leg ulcers, lymphoedema and chronic lymphoedema, to retain dressings taking into account the location and size of wound, support joints after a sprain and support limb following soft tissue injury.

Definitions relating to bandaging

- *Extensibility*: determines the length produced when an extending force is applied.
- *Elasticity*: the ability to return to its original length once the extending force is removed.
- *Compression*: the force applied to produce a desired clinical effect.
- *Support*: the retention and control of tissue without the application of compression.
- *Conformability*: the ability to follow the contours of a limb and is largely due to the extensibility and density of the fabric. Knitted bandages are more conformable than woven bandages.

Classification of bandages

Type I

These are lightweight conforming bandages used for the retention of light dressings (Figures 25.14 and 25.15). These bandages should conform to limbs and joints without causing restriction. Examples are Slinky®, J-fast® and Stayform®.

Type II

The light support bandages are manufactured from cotton, polymide, viscose (Figure 25.16) and elastane. They are used for the retention of dressings, mild support in the treatment of strains and sprains and to prevent oedema. They are not suitable for compression but can be used in the treatment of venous ulceration with arterial disease. Type II bandages include crepe-type bandages such as Soffcrepe®, Elastocrepe®, Leukocrepe and Comprilan®.

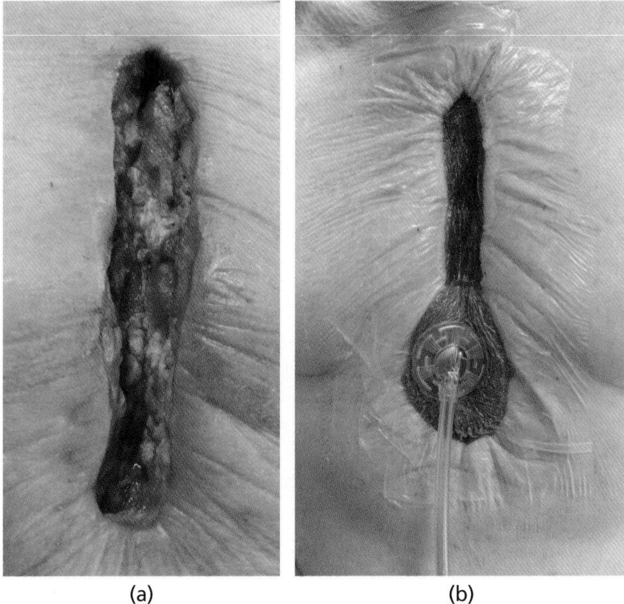

Figure 25.14 (a) Sternal wound and (b) sternal wound with topical negative pressure dressing.

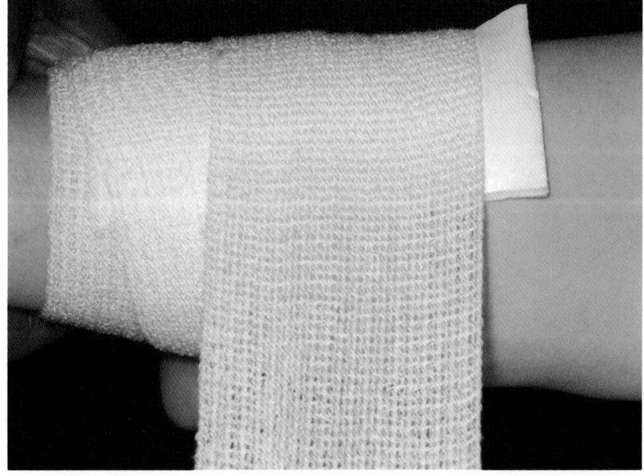

Figure 25.15 Type I retention bandage to hold non-adherent dressings in place.

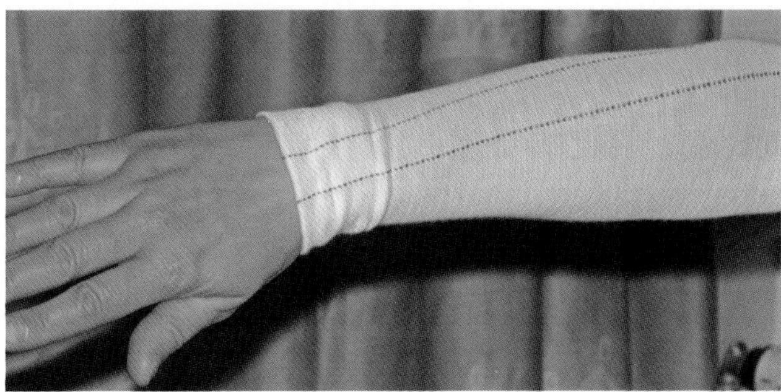

Figure 25.16 Type II light support bandage made from elasticated viscose.

Type III

Compression bandages (Figure 25.17) are used to apply compression to control oedema and reduce swelling in the treatment of venous or lymphovenous disease of the lower limbs. They are subdivided into four categories according to their ability to provide set levels of compression.

Type IIIa

Light compression bandages provide low levels of pressure up to 20 mmHg at the ankle. They are indicated in the management of early, superficial varices but are not suitable for controlling or reducing oedema. Examples include K-Plus®, Tensolastic® and Elset®.

Type IIIb

Moderate compression bandages may be used to manage varicosities during pregnancy, for the prevention/treatment of ulcers and for control of mild oedema. These exert levels of compression of 30 mmHg at the ankle.

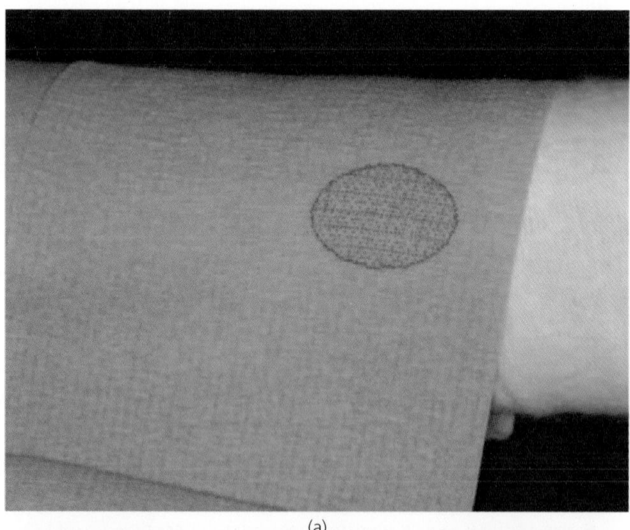

(a)

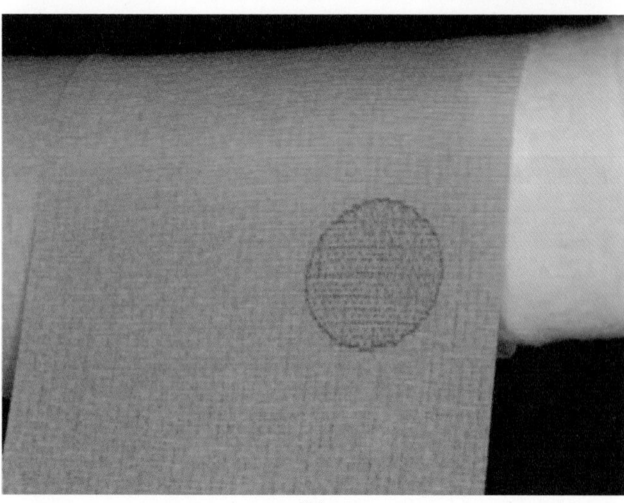

(b)

Figure 25.17 Markings on bandages to ensure consistent tension (a) incorrect tension (oval) (b) correct tension (circle).

Type IIIc

High compression bandages may be used for applying 40 mmHg pressure at the ankle. These bandages can be used to manage large varices, leg ulcers and limb oedema. Examples include Tensopress®, Setopress® and Surepress®.

Type IIId

These extra high performance compression bandages apply 50 mmHg pressure at the ankle and therefore can sustain high pressure for extended periods to grossly oedematous limbs. Examples include Varico® and Elastic Web® bandage.

Application of bandages

The correct application of bandages is of paramount importance (Figure 25.17a and b). Applied too loosely, the bandage will be ineffective and applied too tightly the bandage may cause constriction, resulting in tissue damage and necrosis. In extreme cases, this can lead to amputation.

Research has shown that there is a great variation in the consistency of the tension in the application of bandages between practitioners. To overcome this problem, some bandages have a design printed on the bandage at regular intervals, which changes shape when the correct extension is applied.

Preparation for compression bandaging

1 A limb assessment to identify any deformities, oedema and alteration of the limb contour which may need consideration when applying the bandage. Measure the ankle circumference to ensure the correct compression bandages are used.
2 Wound assessment at baseline by measurements or photography to monitor progress.
3 Dressings. Appropriate, non-adherent, absorbent dressings to overcome exudate, odour and pain.
4 Pain assessment. Eighty percent of patients with venous ulcers complain of pain which requires appropriate management to enable them to tolerate the compression.
5 Patient preparation. Patient understanding and commitment to compression therapy is vital to the success of the treatment and patient concordance.
6 High compression requires an ankle/brachial pressure index (ABPI) of more than 0.8.

The four-layer compression system for ankle circumference 18–25 cm

Orthopaedic wool (Figure 25.18a and b). The purpose is to absorb exudate, protect bony prominences and redistribute the pressure around the limb. Apply from the base of the toes to the knee, overlapping 50%. Pad the tender areas on the dorsum of the foot, the Achilles tendon and the shin.

Cotton crepe. This layer adds absorbency and smoothes the wool layer. Apply from the base of the toes, in even tension with 50% overlap to ensure a smooth surface for the application of the elastic layers.

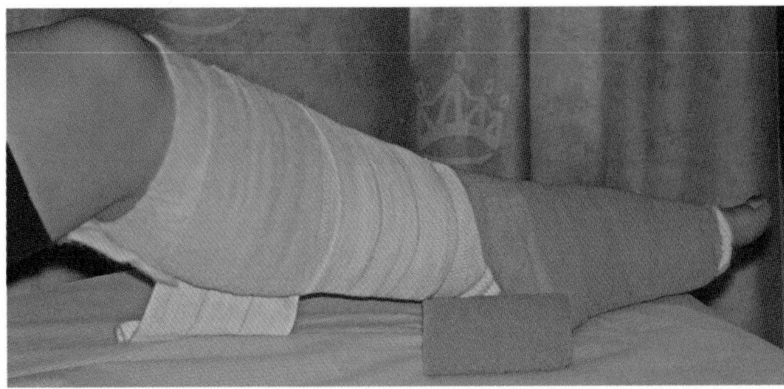

Figure 25.18 (a) Four layers need to be applied for Type III compression and (b) Four-layers can be seen in place (from the knee downwards) – first layer orthopaedic wool; second layer cotton crepe; third layer elastic extensible bandage; fourth layer cohesive bandage.

Elastic, extensible bandage. The first compression layer with sub-bandage pressure of 17 mmHg at the ankle. Anchor the bandage at the base of the toes with two turns and 50% extension, continue with a 'figure of 8' around the ankle and extend up the limb with 50% overlap and 50% extension of the bandage.

Cohesive bandage. This is the second compression bandage of the system and adds the remaining 23 mmHg at the ankle to give 40 mmHg. The cohesiveness assists in the retention of the bandages. The bandage is applied in a spiral technique with 50% stretch and 50% overlap.

In patients with 'champagne'-shaped legs, apply with a 'figure of 8' method to prevent slippage of the bandage.

Modifications

In patients with ankle circumference less than 18 cm and greater than 25 cm, the four-layer system can be modified to produce the correct pressure at the ankle as follows:

- Where less than 18 cm, apply two or more layers of orthopaedic wool.
- Where 25–30 cm, use wool, a high compression bandage and cohesive bandage.
- Where more than 30 cm, wool, elastic conformable, high compression and cohesive bandages can be used.

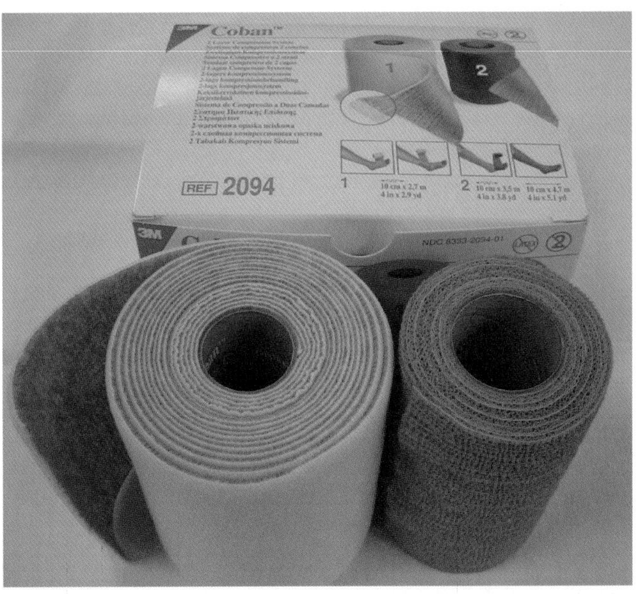

Figure 25.19 Coban for two-layer compression.

Two-layer compression

Two-layer bandage systems give compression equivalent to the original four-layer systems.

Coban: 3M Only available in one size (Figure 25.19).

KTwo: Urgo Available in two sizes 18–25 cm and 25–32 cm (Figure 25.20).

Both consist of a wadding/inner comfort layer and a cohesive bandage providing 40 mmHg pressure.

Application of two layer bandage

Coban: Foam inner comfort layer, applied with foam layer to skin maintaining enough tension to conform to the shape of the leg with minimal overlap. Outer cohesive layer is applied at 100% stretch and 50% overlap. Only the outer layer provides the 40 mmHg compression.

Pros: More cost effective than four-layer systems.

Cons: The thick foam layer is difficult to conform around champagne bottle-shaped legs.

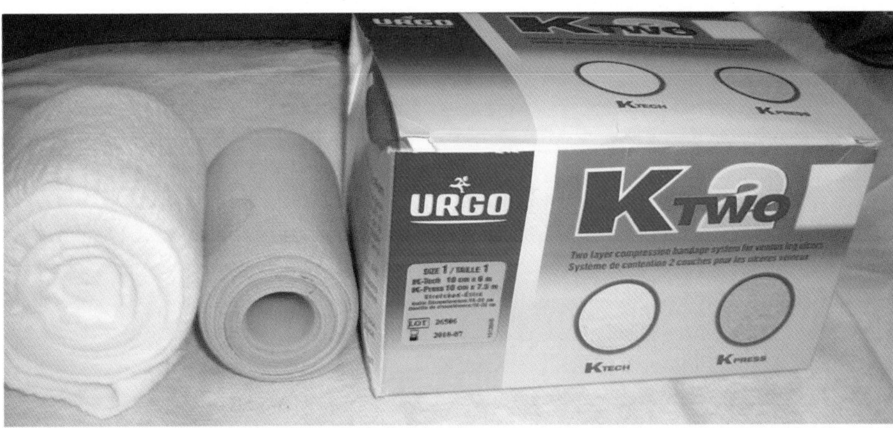

Figure 25.20 KTwo for two-layer compression.

KTwo: Wadding bandage gives up to 32 mmHg compression, and the short stretch cohesive bandage gives 8 mmHg compression. Both bandages have a printed pressure indication on the bandage to ensure correct bandage tension; it is applied spiral with 50% stretch and 50% overlap.

Pros: Easy to apply, conforms to limb shape, better patient concordance, cost effective and available in two sizes; latex-free option now available.

Two-layer long stretch bandages: Class 3c

Consist of soft ban wool bandage plus one of the following: Tensopress: Smith & Nephew, Ava-Co: Advancis, Setopress: Molnlycke, Surepress: Convatec. All are applied spiral at 50% stretch and 50% overlap providing 40 mmHg compression

Two-layer short stretch bandages: Class 3c

Virtually inelastic, rigid, which also consist of soft ban/wadding plus one of the following: Actico: Advansis, Comprilan: BSn Medical

Rosidal K: Activa, 100% cotton ideal for patients with latex allergy. All are applied at 100% stretch and 50% overlap providing 40 mmHg compression.

Cons: Patients must be mobile to wear short stretch as it relies on the action of calf muscle pump for venous return.

Short stretch rapidly reduces oedema; therefore bandage slippage is common requiring more frequent dressing changes.

Two-layer reduced bandage system

KTwo reduced compression kit which provides 20 mmHg compression. This also has a pressure indicator incorporated into the bandage to ensure correct tension (as per regular KTwo kits).

Pros: Can be used on mixed aetiology leg ulcers depending on ABPI readings (also available as latex free).

Rubber sensitivity

There is a continuing high incidence of contact sensitivity in patients with venous leg ulcers which has implications for their management. Contact dermatitis to rubber limits the type of compression bandages that can be used. Cotton short-stretch bandages are recommended for these patients. Apply a tubular cotton gauze bandage directly to the skin. Next, apply the wool layer as before and then the short stretch at full extension with a figure of 8 around the ankle, and continue with a spiral overlapping 50% at full extension up the leg.

Tubular bandages

These are cotton bandages used extensively in dermatology in the treatment of atopic eczema and patients with erythroderma. They can be applied to limbs, cut and fashioned into a body suit and used as dry or wet wraps.

Wet wraps are moist bandages applied to the body over emollients and/or topical steroids to acute active or chronic lichenified eczema. Wet wraps are cooling, reduce itching, prolong emollient effects, enhance topical steroid potency and protect the skin from trauma through scratching. Wet wraps are not indicated for long-term use with a topical steroid and should be avoided if the skin is infected.

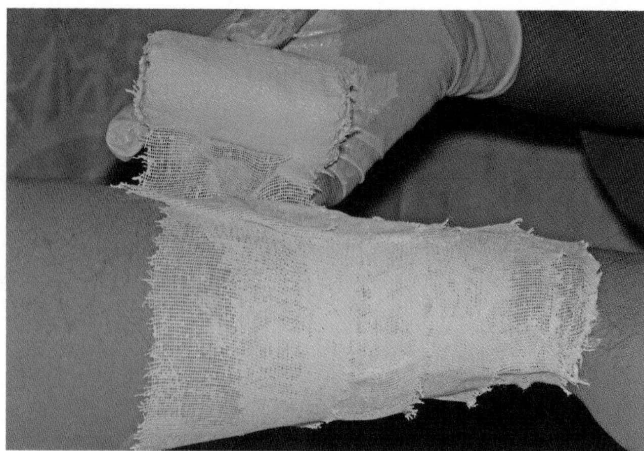

Figure 25.21 Medicated bandages with zinc paste and calamine.

Dry wraps are applied in a similar manner to cover the skin. They enhance the effect of topical agents and protect the skin and the patient's clothing.

Manufacturers are now producing cotton garments for the same purpose, making it easier for parents and patients to apply the materials and thereby manage skin disease.

Medicated paste bandages

These bandages are made from flat open-weave cotton bandages impregnated with appropriate medicaments. They are widely used in a variety of dermatological conditions such as venous ulceration, nodular prurigo, psoriasis, lichen simplex and chronic lichenified eczema. They should be avoided if the skin is macerated or exudative.

Paste bandages (Figure 25.21) are used to soothe, occlude and protect the skin from scratching and enhance the effect of topical applications. Examples include Calaband® (zinc paste with calamine), Tarband® (zinc paste with coal tar), Ichthaband® (zinc and icthamol) and Steriband® (zinc paste bandage).

Medicated bandages need to be applied skilfully to prevent constriction and to allow for shrinkage, and need to be changed when they are drying out. They require a secondary bandage to keep it in place and protect the patient's clothing. Hypersensitivity reactions to the medicaments can develop.

Patient information

Patient concordance is as vital to wound healing as the dressings and bandages themselves. To ensure that the patient complies adequately with the wound management the following should be considered.

- Ensure the patient understands the treatment regime.
- Devise a treatment plan to suit the patient's lifestyle.
- Provide an information leaflet explaining aftercare.
- Peripheral circulation to the toes should be checked after application of bandages.
- In the event of excessive pain or discomfort caused by the bandages, patients should be advised to contact the treatment unit.
- Patients should be advised not to be alarmed by breakthrough exudates.

- Bandages should be kept dry by providing aids to use in the bath/shower.
- Encourage a good balance between rest and exercise.
- Advise patients not to remove bandages themselves.
- Provide the patient with a contact telephone number to ring for advice.

The efficacy of dressings and bandages to heal wounds and treat skin complaints depends on selection of the correct products for the particular situation. Ideally, there should be good channels of communication and clinical consistency between primary/secondary care and wound management specialists. Team work should ensure the optimum management of the patient's skin, promote rapid healing, provide an excellent local service, reduce the cost of wound care and enhance the patient's quality of life.

Further Reading

Charles H. Does leg ulcer treatment improve patients' quality of life? *J Woundcare* **13**(6): 209–213, 2004.

Grey D, White R, Cooper P and Kingsley A. Applied wound management and using the wound healing continuum in practice. *Wound Essent* **5**:131–139, 2010. (Available from http://www.wounds-uk.com/wound-essentials/wound-essentials-5-applied-wound-management-and-using-the-wound-healing-continuum-in-practice, last accessed October 2013).

Jones V, Grey JE and Harding K. ABC of wound healing: wound dressings. *BMJ* **332**:777–780, 2006.

Myers BA. *Wound Management: Principles and Practice*, 2nd Edition, Pearson/Prentice Hall, New Jersey, 2004.

www.worldwidewounds.com

CHAPTER 26

Formulary

Karen Watson

Dermatology Department, Orpington Hospital, UK

OVERVIEW

- many treatments for the skin are topical, meaning they are applied directly to the skin surface.
- different formulations of topical treatments are used depending on the site and the type of skin disease.
- medicated topical treatments should be applied to the diseased skin only and emollients are applied all over.
- systemic therapies are generally used for more severe disease and may need careful monitoring.
- biological therapies are delivered by injection or infusion intermittently

Introduction

The treatment of skin disease has evolved dramatically over recent years. Historically, patients were admitted for intensive nursing with extemporaneously prepared combinations of topical steroids, tars, pastes and bandaging. Today however, there is a much greater emphasis on outpatient treatment. Quality control and cost issues have seen a reduction in the number of extemporaneous products available, and there have been exciting new developments in both topical and systemic treatment, particularly with the advent of monoclonal antibodies.

Topical therapy

The skin has the advantage of being readily amenable to treatment with topical therapy. Relatively high concentrations of medication can be applied to the skin safely, with good efficacy and comparatively few side effects. Several factors govern the choice of topical treatment, such as formulation, frequency of application, site and severity of skin disease and patient ability to apply local therapy. Complications tend to be local irritant or allergic reactions. The choice of topical treatment depends on the disease process, pharmaceutical properties of the drug, site of application and cosmesis.

Emollients

Emollients are important in the treatment of dry, scaly and inflammatory skin conditions as they help reduce transepidermal water loss from a damaged epidermal barrier. They soften dry skin by filling in the spaces left by desquamating keratinocytes.

The constituents of an emollient or topical base have significant properties. Lipids, for example, cover the stratum corneum to prevent evaporation of water. White and yellow soft paraffin and liquid paraffin are extracted from crude oil. They are stable, inert hydrocarbons, which form the basis of most commercially available ointments and emollients. Emulsifying agents are used to stabilise emulsions, which are immiscible mixtures of aqueous and oily constituents, and penetration enhancers, such as urea and propylene glycol, may be used to increase penetration of an active component through the skin. Humectants are compounds with a high affinity for water, which are able to draw water into the stratum corneum and have useful emollient properties.

The properties of various formulations of topical therapy are outlined in Table 26.1. Emollients can be applied liberally and regularly to all areas of dry skin.

Bath emollients and soap substitutes are as important as regular emollients in the treatment of dry skin conditions. Soaps are detergents that irritate the skin by removing intercellular lipids and disrupt the barrier function of the stratum corneum, and should therefore be avoided.

Topical immunomodulatory treatments

Topical corticosteroids

Mode of action

The development of topical corticosteroids in the 1950s revolutionised the treatment of skin disease. Since then, they have been used to treat a wide range of inflammatory dermatoses. The mechanism of action is complex. Steroid diffuses through the stratum corneum, cell membrane and into the cytoplasm of keratinocytes where it binds to the glucocorticoid receptor causing activation. The ligand-bound receptor enters the nuclear compartment and interacts with glucocorticoid response elements (GREs), resulting in the modulation of gene transcription. In addition, the ligand-bound receptor may also inhibit other transcription factors. The overall effect is to suppress inflammatory cytokines, inhibit T-cell activation and reduce cell proliferation.

ABC of Dermatology, Sixth Edition. Edited by Rachael Morris-Jones.

Table 26.1 Comparison of formulations for topical therapy.

Formulation	Characteristics	Advantages	Disadvantages
Ointments	Oil-based. Provide occlusive film over skin and help retain water. Aid skin hydration and penetration of topical treatment	Tend not require preservatives as lack of water in preparation prevents microbial growth	Greasy and cosmetically less appealing to use
Creams	Emulsions containing water and oil. May be composed of oil in water or water in oil (oily creams). Aid skin hydration, but generally less effectively than ointments	Cosmetically acceptable	Contain preservatives, which may cause sensitisation
Lotions	Watery suspensions, often containing alcohol	Easily spread over a large area. Evaporation of water or alcohol has a drying, cooling effect Cosmetically acceptable Useful for hair-bearing areas, such as the scalp	Contain preservatives and therefore have sensitising potential. Alcohol may cause stinging
Gels	Semisolid emulsion in alcohol base. Useful for suspending insoluble drugs Good absorbent properties	Tend to dry on skin Useful for hair-bearing areas. Cosmetically acceptable especially for use on the face	Relatively high irritant and sensitising potential

Classification of topical steroids

Topical corticosteroids are classified according to their potency, which is thought to be related to their glucocorticoid receptor affinity.

Topical steroids are divided into four classes:

Class 1 Super-potent (600 times as potent as hydrocortisone): for example, clobetasone propionate (Dermovate®).
Class 2 Potent (150 times as potent as hydrocortisone): for example, betamethasone valerate (Betnovate®).
Class 3 Moderate (25 times as potent as hydrocortisone): for example, clobetasone butyrate (Eumovate®).
Class 4 Mild – hydrocortisone.

This classification allows determination of the relative strength and therefore the potential side effects of therapy. Generally, the weakest steroid to effectively treat the skin condition should be chosen. Milder steroids should be used on the face and flexural sites. (Table 26.2 provides a detailed outline of topical steroids and their relative potencies).

Topical corticosteroids should be applied 'sparingly'. However, this is difficult to define and therefore the fingertip unit (FTU) system was devised. One FTU (a line of ointment from the tip of the finger to the first skin crease) is sufficient steroid to treat a hand-sized (palmar and dorsal surface) area of affected skin. In medical practice, it is common for patients to use insufficient amounts of topical steroids due to the fear of potential complications.

Table 26.2 Relative potency of topical corticosteroids.

Generic name	Proprietary name	Potency
1% hydrocortisone	Efcortelan®	Mild
1% hydrocortisone acetate and 1% fusidic acid	Fucidin H®	Mild
1% hydrocortisone, 1% nystatin 100 000 units/g and 3% oxytetracycline	Timodine®	Mild
Clobetasone butyrate 0.05%	Eumovate®	Moderate
Alclometasone dipropionate 0.05%	Modrasone®	Moderate
Betamethasone valerate 0.1%	Betnovate®	Potent
Mometasone furoate 0.1%	Elocon®	Potent
Diflucortolone valerate 0.1%	Nerisone®	Potent
Betamethasone dipropionate 0.05% and 3% salicylic acid	Diprosalic®	Potent
Betamethasone valerate 0.1% and fusidic acid 3%	Fucibet®	Potent
Clobetasol propionate 0.05%	Dermovate®	Super-potent
Clobetasol propionate 0.05%, neomycin sulphate 0.5% and nystatin 100 000 units/g	Dermovate NN®	Super-potent

Side effects of topical steroids

- Skin atrophy (Figure 26.3)
- Telangiectasia
- Striae (Figure 26.1)
- Ecchymoses
- Hirsutism
- Folliculitis
- Perioral and periorbital dermatitis (Figure 26.2)
- Steroid-induced acne/rosacea (Figure 26.3)
- Absorption and suppression of the hypothalamic pituitary axis (HPA)

Calcineurin inhibitors

Topical tacrolimus and pimecrolimus were originally developed for the treatment of eczema (in patients over the age of 2 years). These agents inhibit calcineurin (a calcium and calmodulin-dependent serine/threonine phosphatase) and suppress T-cell activation. Topical tacrolimus has also been used to treat alopecia areata, oral and genital lichen planus, pyoderma gangrenosum, cutaneous

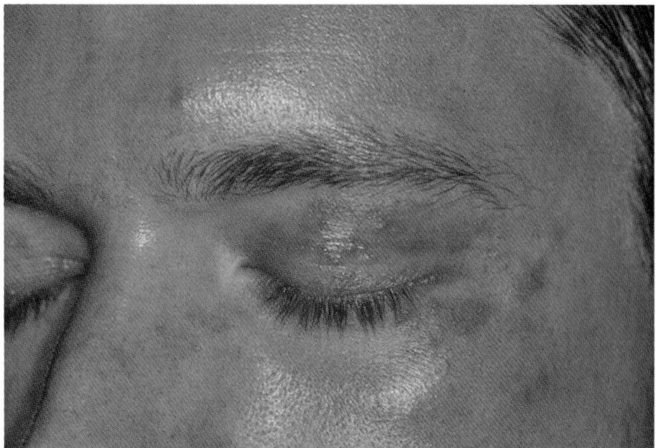

Figure 26.1 Liberal application of a potent topical steroid resulting in striae formation.

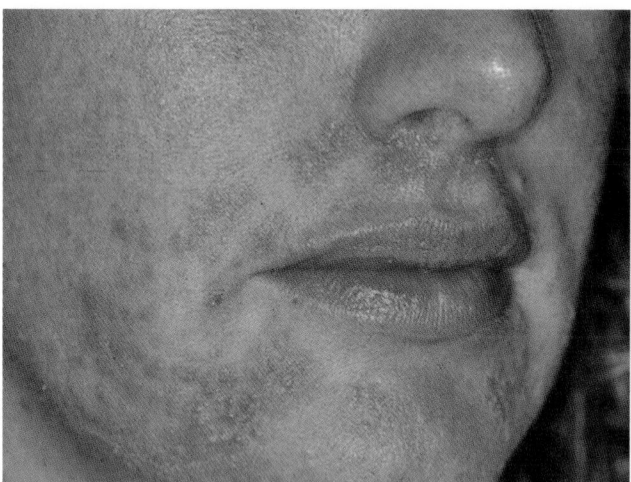

Figure 26.2 Perioral dermatitis caused by local application of topical steroids.

graft versus host disease and vitiligo with varying degrees of success. Pimecrolimus is less potent than topical tacrolimus and is used predominantly in the treatment of eczema in children as a steroid-sparing agent.

Topical antimicrobials

A number of topical antimicrobial preparations are available, some of which are summarised in Table 26.3.

Miscellaneous topical therapy used in the treatment of psoriasis

These are outlined in Table 26.4.

Topical anti-proliferative agents

Topical 5 fluorouracil

5 fluorouracil (5% cream, 0.5% solution) is an antimetabolite, which blocks DNA synthesis by inhibiting thymidylate synthetase. It is used topically to treat actinic keratoses, Bowen's disease and superficial basal cell carcinomas (BCCs). Treatment should be applied daily for 4–6 weeks. Main adverse effects include local erythema and irritation and with continuous use, marked inflammation and erosions. These adverse effects may be ameliorated by treatment breaks and use of topical steroids.

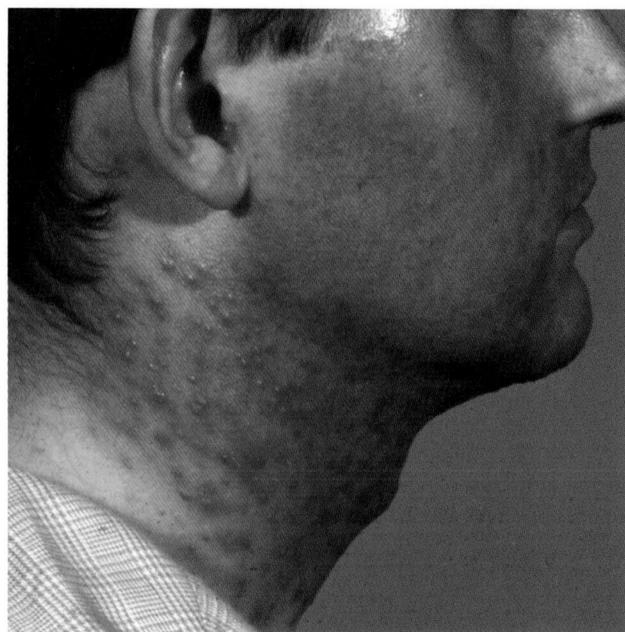

Figure 26.3 Potent topical steroid induced atrophy and acne.

Topical diclofenac

Diclofenac is a non-steroidal anti-inflammatory drug available in a 3% gel formulation for the treatment of mild actinic keratoses. The mechanism of action is unclear. It is generally well tolerated, although there may be some localised inflammation.

Topical imiquimod

Topical imiquimod (5% and 3.75% cream) is a novel immunomodulatory preparation, used to treat genital warts, vulval intra-epithelial neoplasia (VIN), extra-mammary Paget's disease, actinic keratoses, superficial BCCs and lentigo maligna. It stimulates the innate immune system and promotes the development of antigen-specific cell-mediated responses via Toll-like receptor 7. It causes considerable inflammation with oedema, erosions and occasional ulceration. It is usually applied three times weekly for up to 4 months, depending on the indication.

Topical ingenol mebutate

Ingenol mebutate is derived from the plant *Euphorbia peplus*, which is grown in Queensland specifically for the production of this gel, used for the treatment of actinic keratoses. The mechanism of action is unclear, but it appears to cause rapid lesion necrosis and neutrophil-mediated antibody-dependent cellular cytotoxicity. It is applied for 2–3 days depending on the site and may cause discomfort and irritation.

Table 26.3 Topical antimicrobials used in the treatment of superficial infections.

	Preparation	Indications	Complications
Topical antibiotics	Fusidic acid (Fucidin ointment®)	Staphylococcal infections	Resistance
	Mupirocin (Bactroban ointment®)	Gram positive and some gram negative organisms Treatment of nasal staphylococcal carriage	Resistance
	Silver sulfadiazine (Flamazine®)	Pseudomonal infection and some prophylaxis against staphylococcal infection	Minimal absorption and renal impairment when applied to extensive burns
Topical antibiotics used in the treatment of acne	Tetracyclines Erythromycin Clindamycin	Acne May be used in combination with keratolytics such as benzoyl peroxide	Resistance May stain clothing yellow
Topical antifungals	Allylamines Terbinafine cream (Lamasil cream®)	Fungicidal against dermatophyte infections	Ineffective against dermatophyte infections of the nails and scalp
	Imidazoles Clotrimazole (Canesten®) Econazole Ketoconazole Miconazole	Fungistatic Active against Candida and Pityrosporum Maybe used in combination with topical steroids Used in the treatment of intertrigo, pityriasis versicolor and some dermatophyte infections	Concurrent use of topical steroid may mask infection
	Amorolfine (Loceryl lacquer®)	Fungistatic Used in the treatment of onychomycosis Some activity against *Scytalidium* Synergistic activity with systemic antifungals	Poor cure rates in dermatophyte infections affecting the nail matrix when used as sole therapy
Topical anti-virals	Aciclovir cream (Zovirax®)	Used to treat labial and genital herpes simplex	Needs to be applied as early as possible in the episode for maximum benefit
Anti-parasitic agents	Permethrin	5% cream used in the treatment of scabies and pubic lice. 1% rinse used to treat head lice	Require two treatments 1 week apart
	Malathion	Used in the treatment of scabies, head lice and pubic lice	Alcoholic lotions can irritate skin and can exacerbate eczema Resistance

Table 26.4 Miscellaneous preparations used in the treatment of psoriasis.

Preparation	Mode of action	Indications	Complications
Crude coal tar and coal tar solution Derived from the distillation of organic matter	Unclear Tar has anti-proliferative effects on the epidermis	Psoriasis Used in combination with ultraviolet radiation with additive effects	Messy to use Potent odour Scrotal squamous cell carcinoma
Dithranol Available in cream formulation or in Lassars paste in concentrations from 0.1% to 3%	Unclear Dithranol has potent anti-proliferative effects	Psoriasis Short contact regimens used in outpatient settings	Local reactions and irritation of normal surrounding skin Skin staining
Vitamin D3 analogues: Calcipotriol (Dovonex®), and tacalcitol (Silkis®) Combination of calcipotriol and betamethasone (Dovobet®)	Regulate cell growth, differentiation and immune function	Psoriasis	Hypercalcaemia Irritation Prolonged use of betamethasone and calcipotriol may precipitate the formation of pustules on withdrawal

Miscellaneous agents

Keratolytics

Keratolytic agents are topical preparations used in the treatment of hyperkeratosis and acne. They help soften the skin and aid the removal of scale. They may also have anti-comedogenic activity, although they can cause local irritation with erythema and dryness. Examples include salicylic acid and vitamin A derivatives such as tretinoin and adapalene.

Sunscreens

The aim of sunscreens is to block both ultraviolet A (UVA) and ultraviolet B (UVB) penetration of the skin and thereby inhibit the ageing and carcinogenic effects of UV radiation. Compounds used to achieve sun protection may either reflect and scatter UV light or absorb it. Examples of physical agents blocking UV include zinc oxide, titanium dioxide and ferrous oxide. They tend to be used in combination with light absorbers such as *para*-aminobenzoic acid

(PABA) and benzophenones. The sun protection factor (SPF) of a sunscreen is an indication of the level of protection from UVB. An SPF over 15 is considered to confer good UVB protection when the sunscreen is applied adequately; however, evidence suggests most people apply insufficient amounts. UVA protection is measured on a 1–5 star basis although there is little standardisation. Therefore, high factor sunscreen with UVA and UVB protection should be applied to exposed skin before going out in the sun, and this should be reapplied regularly to maintain protection.

Cosmetic camouflage

Cosmetic camouflage plays an important role in the treatment of patients with disfiguring conditions such as scarring, dyspigmentation and port wine stains. Proprietary preparations are readily available (e.g. VitiColor®, Dermablend®) and the charity Changing Faces provides a volunteer-led skin camouflage service for patients in the United Kingdom (www.changingfaces.org.uk).

Phototherapy

Phototherapy (see Chapter 3) is the treatment of skin disease with UV radiation alone and photochemotherapy is UV irradiation in combination with psoralen ultraviolet A (PUVA). Both are used extensively in dermatological practice to treat a wide range of skin disorders. Phototherapy involves the use of artificial UVB irradiation delivered by fluorescent lamps. UVB consists of electromagnetic energy of wavelength 290–320 nm and represents that part of the spectrum that is largely responsible for sunburn. UVA consists of energy of wavelength 315–400 nm. Both PUVA and narrowband UVB phototherapy are now widely used for the treatment of psoriasis, atopic eczema, polymorphic light eruption, mycosis fungoides and vitiligo, among others.

Systemic therapy

Drugs used for infectious disorders

Antibacterial drugs

Antibiotics are used widely in dermatology for a range of conditions from acne to impetigo and cellulitis. They may be required for prolonged courses over a period of weeks to months. Host factors, drug properties and causative pathogens should all be considered when choosing a suitable antibiotic. Host factors include underlying disease, age, previous adverse reactions and pregnancy. Drug parameters include interaction with concomitant therapy, side effect profile, dosage, route of administration and cost. Causative pathogens and their sensitivity/resistance patterns should ideally be identified through swabs taken for microbiology. Table 26.5 illustrates some of the antibiotics most commonly used in dermatology (mode of action, indications and complications).

Table 26.5 Antibiotics used in dermatology, their method of action, indications and complications.

Antibiotic group	Method of action	Antibiotic	Indications	Complications
Penicillins	Inhibition of bacterial cell wall synthesis Activation of autolytic bacterial enzymes Bactericidal	Penicillin	Gram positive infections, e.g. *Streptococcus* Cellulitis Erysipelas	Hypersensitivity reactions which may be severe Dose reduction in renal impairment
	β lactamase resistant penicillin	Flucloxacillin	β lactamase producing organisms, e.g. *Staphylococcus aureus* Cellulitis Impetigo	Hypersensitivity reactions
Macrolides	Penetration of bacterial cell wall and inhibition of RNA-dependent protein synthesis by reversible binding to ribosomes	Erythromycin	Gram positive infections Penicillin allergy Cellulitis Erysipelas Impetigo Acne Erythrasma	Nausea, diarrhoea
		Clarithromycin	Gram positive and gram negative cover Erysipelas	Fewer gastro-intestinal side effects
Tetracyclines	Inhibition of protein synthesis by ribosomal binding	Oxytetracycline Minocycline Doxycycline Lymecycline	Gram positive and gram negative organisms Mycobacteria Acne Rosacea Perioral dermatitis Bullous pemphigoid Lyme disease Fish tank granuloma	Nausea, vomiting. Brown discoloration of teeth and delayed bone growth in children. Therefore contra-indicated in children under 12 years Hypersensitivity reactions Blue-black pigmentation of nails and skin

Antifungal drugs

Most cutaneous fungal infections can be effectively treated with topical therapy. However, systemic treatment is required for fungal infections of the nails and hair, such as terbinafine and griseofulvin. Terbinafine is a fungicidal allylamine, which binds to plasma proteins and is found in high concentrations in the hair, nails and stratum corneum. In the treatment of tinea capitis oral terbinafine is more effective against endothrix organisms (*Trichophyton tonsurans*) than ectothrix infections (*Microsporum canis*). Although it is not licensed for use in children, several studies have shown terbinafine to be safe and effective. Treatment dosage is calculated according to the patient's weight (62.5 mg up to 20 kg; 125 mg up to 40 kg; 250 mg over 40 kg) and given daily for 1 month. Prolonged courses of 3 months or more are required in the treatment of onychomycosis involving the nail matrix.

Griseofulvin has fungistatic activity and has been used for many years to treat tinea capitis in children (weight <50 kg; 10–20 mg/kg) given daily for 6 weeks. However, terbinafine and itraconazole are often used in preference to griseofulvin as they are better tolerated and have a broader spectrum of activity. Griseofulvin is ineffective against pityriasis versicolor or yeast infections such as *Candida albicans*.

Itraconazole is a triazole used in pulsed therapy or continuously for the treatment of onychomycosis, tinea capitis, particularly in young infants and pityriasis versicolor resistant to topical therapy.

Antiviral drugs

Systemic antivirals are available for the treatment of human herpes virus (HHV) infections such as herpes simplex virus (HSV) type 1 and type 2, (causing herpes labialis and genital lesions respectively) and varicella zoster virus (VZV) causing chicken pox and herpes zoster (shingles).

Aciclovir is a well-established antiviral drug used in the treatment of HHV. It inhibits viral DNA polymerase and irreversibly inhibits viral DNA synthesis. The underlying diagnosis determines the dose and treatment duration. Primary genital herpes simplex requires 200 mg five times daily for 5 days while herpes zoster and chicken pox in adults require 800 mg five times a day for 7 days.

Aciclovir tends to be most effective if therapy is started within 72 h of disease onset. Secondary prophylaxis for recurrent and frequent attacks of HSV may be given at a dose of 200–400 mg twice daily. Intravenous administration is preferable in severely ill patients at risk of disseminated HSV (immunocompromised, eczema herpeticum). A topical preparation of aciclovir is also available for the treatment of mild herpes labialis.

Alternative antivirals include valaciclovir and famciclovir, which are licensed for the treatment of herpes zoster and primary and recurrent genital herpes. Their advantage is that they are administered three times daily compared to acyclovir, which is given five times daily. However, they are more expensive.

Antiparasite drugs

Scabies and pediculosis are usually adequately treated with topical therapy. Most studies show that 5% permethrin cream applied to the skin, left on overnight and repeated after 7 days is highly effective in treating scabies. However, Norwegian/resistant scabies and pediculoses refractory to conventional topical preparations may be amenable to treatment with oral ivermectin (200 μg/kg). Ivermectin causes paralysis and death of parasites and a single dose is usually sufficient. Ivermectin is available on a named-patient basis only.

Larva migrans and larva currens can be effectively treated with oral albendazole or ivermectin (see Chapter 17).

Systemic immunomodulatory drugs

Corticosteroids

Systemic corticosteroids are used in the treatment of a wide range of inflammatory dermatoses. They are effective immunosuppressant and anti-inflammatory agents, but have a number of side effects. These include hyperglycaemia, hyperlipidaemia, hypertension, sodium and fluid retention, atherosclerosis, suppression of the HPA, growth retardation, osteoporosis, avascular necrosis of bone, alteration of fat distribution, myopathy, increased incidence of infection, re-activation of tuberculosis, peptic ulceration, glaucoma, cataracts, striae and psychiatric disorders. The indications, risks, benefits, potential adjuvant steroid sparing therapy and gastro and bone protection should therefore be carefully considered. However, systemic corticosteroids are particularly useful in controlling immunobullous disorders, eczema, vasculitis, drug eruptions, connective tissue disorders, sarcoidosis, erythroderma, lichen planus and neutrophilic dermatoses among others. They are relatively contraindicated in psoriasis as withdrawal of the steroid may precipitate an exacerbation or generalised pustular psoriasis.

Patients treated with corticosteroids should be monitored closely for side effects, and they should be weaned off therapy slowly over a period of time, depending on the dose and duration of treatment. Patient education is important for those on long-term treatment. They should be provided with a steroid treatment card, which outlines important information for patients and carers.

Methotrexate

Methotrexate is an antimetabolite and is a potent inhibitor of the enzyme dihydrofolate reductase. It competitively and irreversibly binds to dihydrofolate reductase with a much greater affinity than its natural substrate folic acid, thereby preventing the conversion of dihydrofolate to tetrahydrofolate. This is an important step in the synthesis of thymidylate and purine nucleotides needed for DNA and RNA synthesis, and results in inhibition of cell division.

Methotrexate is very useful in the treatment of psoriasis and psoriatic arthropathy. It is thought to act as an immunomodulator by inhibiting DNA synthesis in lymphocytes rather than having an antiproliferative effect. It is primarily used to treat psoriasis, but is also used in sarcoidosis, bullous pemphigoid, vasculitis and morphoea.

Methotrexate is taken as a once a week dose, the dose being carefully titrated by 2.5 mg increments. It has a number of side effects including bone marrow suppression, hepatotoxicity, nausea and vomiting, pulmonary fibrosis and teratogenicity, and patients need careful monitoring. Procollagen III in the serum may be measured as an indirect marker of liver fibrosis. However, many modern units are now using a sophisticated FibroScan as an indirect measure of fibrosis. Folic acid 5 mg once daily is taken in addition to methotrexate but on a different day to methotrexate administration. This reduces nausea and hepatotoxicity. Acute methotrexate overdose or toxicity may be treated with folinic acid, which bypasses the metabolic effects of methotrexate. Methotrexate also has a number of potentially serious drug interactions including non-steroidal anti-inflammatory drugs, antibiotics, corticosteroids and omeprazole.

Azathioprine

Azathioprine is an antimetabolite, which inhibits DNA and RNA synthesis, and also the differentiation and proliferation of lymphocytes. It is an immunosuppressant and is often used in conjunction with corticosteroids as it has steroid-sparing effects. Azathioprine is an effective treatment in a wide range of dermatological conditions, such as severe atopic eczema, chronic actinic dermatitis, immunobullous disorders, systemic lupus erythematosus and dermatomyositis. Although it is usually well tolerated, it has a number of side effects including bone marrow suppression, nausea and vomiting, hypersensitivity reactions, hepatotoxicity, macrocytosis, pancreatitis and diffuse hair loss. Bone marrow suppression may be predicted in susceptible patients who have low levels of the enzyme thiopurine methyl transferase (TPMT), and who are therefore unable to metabolise the drug efficiently. Unfortunately, the other side effects of azathioprine cannot be predicted by the TPMT activity.

Ciclosporin

Ciclosporin is an immunosuppressant drug derived from the fungus *Tolypocladium inflatum*. It suppresses the induction and proliferation of T lymphocytes and inhibits the production of inflammatory cytokines. It is effective in the treatment of severe psoriasis, (including erythrodermic psoriasis and palmo-plantar pustulosis), atopic eczema and possibly in severe drug eruptions such as toxic epidermolytic necrolysis (TEN). Its advantages include rapid onset of action (1–2 weeks) and lack of bone marrow suppression. However, it has a number of side effects such as renal toxicity, hypertension, hypertrichosis, tremor and gingival hyperplasia. There is also an increased risk of malignancy. Ciclosporin therefore tends to be used for short periods to treat severe flares of disease, or as part of a rotational regimen. It is metabolised by cytochrome P450 and interacts with a number of other drugs. Ciclosporin is usually given between 3 and 5 mg/kg/day in two divided doses.

Mycophenolate mofetil

Mycophenolate mofetil (MMF) is an immunosuppressant agent, which acts by selectively and irreversibly inhibiting inosine monophosphate dehydrogenase, resulting in the depletion of intracellular guanine nucleotides. It seems to have a selective effect on activated T lymphocytes. In dermatology, it is mainly used for the treatment of immunobullous disorders and pyoderma gangrenosum. Side effects are predominantly gastro-intestinal, with nausea, vomiting and diarrhoea. The elderly tend to be more susceptible to the adverse effects of MMF, which also include bone marrow suppression, infection, fatigue, headaches and weakness. Treatment doses in dermatology usually range from 250 mg to 1 g twice daily.

Systemic retinoids

Retinoids are derived from vitamin A and include acitretin, isotretinoin, alitretinoin and bexarotene. They activate nuclear receptors and regulate gene transcription. They have anti-inflammatory, anti-keratinising, anti-sebum, anti-tumour and anti-proliferative effects. Acitretin is used in the treatment of psoriasis, Darier's disease, pityriasis rubra pilaris, ichthyosis, keratodermas and in transplant recipients who are at high risk of developing cutaneous malignancies. Isotretinoin is the drug of choice for treating severe nodulocystic acne and timely initiation of treatment is aimed at preventing significant scarring. It may also be used in hidradenitis suppurativa, dissecting cellulitis of the scalp and severe recalcitrant papulopustular rosacea. Alitretinoin is used for the treatment of severe chronic hand eczema, which is refractory to treatment with topical corticosteroids. Bexarotene is reserved for the treatment of cutaneous T-cell lymphoma.

Systemic retinoids have a number of side effects, the most important of which is teratogenicity. Women of childbearing age must use a robust form of contraception for at least a month prior to and during treatment. Isotretinoin, alitretinoin and bexarotene have a relatively short elimination half-life and contraception needs to be continued for at least a month after discontinuation of therapy. Acitretin has a much longer half-life and pregnancy needs to be avoided for at least 2 years after treatment has stopped. The side effect profile of systemic retinoids is summarised in Table 26.6. Acitretin is usually prescribed at doses ranging from 10 to 50 mg daily. Isotretinoin dosage is based on weight between 0.5 and 1 mg/kg/day with a treatment course for severe acne usually being given as a total target dose of 120–150 mg/kg. The dose of alitretinoin is 30 mg daily, reducing to 10 mg daily in patients with side effects on the higher dose.

Table 26.6 Side effects of systemic retinoids.

Teratogenicity
Depression
Cheilitis
Hypercholesterolaemia
Hypertriglyceridaemia
Elevation of transaminases
Hepatitis
Pancreatitis
Myopathy
Reduced night vision
Dry eyes
Epistaxis
Facial erythema
Photosensitivity
Hair loss
DISH
Premature epiphyseal closure
Leucopenia*
Agranulocytosis*
Hypothyroidism*,†

DISH, diffuse interstitial skeletal hyperostosis.
*Predominantly a risk with bexarotene.
†Predominantly a risk with alitretinoin.

Antihistamines

Histamine has numerous effects on the skin, causing itching, vasodilatation and increased vascular permeability predominantly through its action on H1 receptors. Antihistamines reversibly block H1 receptors. First-generation antihistamines tend to be sedating and include chlorpheniramine, hydroxyzine and promethazine. Second-generation antihistamines tend to be non-sedating, have a slower onset and longer duration of action. They include cetirizine, loratidine, fexofenadine, levocetirizine and desloratidine. They play a central role in the treatment of urticaria, angioedema, type 1 hypersensitivity reactions, anaphylaxis, pruritus, cutaneous mastocytosis and acute insect bite reactions. They tend to be well tolerated although side effects include drowsiness, anticholinergic activity and arrhythmias. Topical antihistamines should be avoided because of the risk of developing allergic contact dermatitis.

Miscellaneous drugs

Dapsone

Dapsone is a sulphonamide, traditionally used in the treatment of leprosy. Its mode of action is unclear, but it is particularly useful in the treatment of disorders where neutrophils or IgA immune complexes play a role, for example, dermatitis herpetiformis, bullous pemphigoid, mucous membrane pemphigoid, linear IgA disease and pyoderma gangrenosum. Side effects include dose-related haemolysis and haemolytic anaemia, which are more common in those individuals with glucose-6-phosphate dehydrogenase (G6PD) deficiency. G6PD should therefore be measured prior to starting treatment. Other adverse effects include agranulocytosis, methaemoglobinaemia, hypersensitivity syndrome and peripheral neuropathy.

Antimalarials

Hydroxychloroquine, mepacrine and chloroquine are used to treat systemic lupus erythematosus, discoid lupus erythematosus, subacute cutaneous lupus erythematosus, sarcoidosis, polymorphic light eruption and porphyria cutanea tarda. Their mode of action is thought to involve interruption of antigen processing and inhibition of inflammatory cytokines. Chloroquine can cause irreversible retinopathy, and mepacrine is unlicensed in the United Kingdom. Hydroxychloroquine therefore tends to be the antimalarial of choice in the treatment of dermatological disorders. It is well tolerated at doses of 200 mg once or twice daily although retinal toxicity can rarely occur. Visual acuity should be monitored for those patients on long-term therapy.

Biological therapies

Biological therapies or 'biologics' are a novel treatment modality used in dermatology, predominantly in the treatment of psoriasis (see Chapter 3), metastatic melanoma and cutaneous T-cell lymphoma.

Biologics used in the treatment of psoriasis

A number of biologics which target specific molecular steps in the pathogenesis of psoriasis are available and include infliximab infusions, etanercept, adalimumab and ustekinumab subcutaneous injections. (Efalizumab has been withdrawn from the market because of concerns about progressive multifocal leucoencephalopathy (PML)). These drugs are for the treatment of severe disease as defined as a Psoriasis Area Severity Index, PASI > 10 and Dermatology Life Quality Index, DLQI > 10, and where phototherapy and alternative standard systemic therapy has failed, is contra-indicated or not tolerated. Infliximab (a chimeric human-murine monoclonal antibody), adalimumab (a fully human monoclonal antibody) and etanercept (a genetically engineered fusion protein) block tumour necrosis factor alpha (TNF-α), which plays a central role in the pathogenesis of psoriasis. Ustekinumab is a fully human monoclonal antibody, which blocks IL12 and IL23. Until recently, interferon α-producing T helper cells were thought to be the main pathogenic cells in psoriasis. However, IL23/Th17 pathways are now known to be important. IL23 stimulates proliferation of a subset of CD4+ T helper cells that produce IL17 (Th17) cells. Th17 cells are involved in the protection against bacterial pathogens and have an important role in the pathogenesis of psoriasis. IL23 stimulates the survival and proliferation of Th17 cells and is therefore a major cytokine regulator for psoriasis. In psoriasis, IL23 is overproduced by keratinocytes and dendritic cells, which stimulates Th17 cells in the dermis, driving keratinocyte proliferation. Psoriasis is an IL17-driven disease that is IL23 dependent and where TNF is a co-factor in IL17-mediated inflammation.

Choice of biologics depends on disease severity, requirement for rapid control in severe unstable psoriasis (infliximab/ustekinumab), co-morbidities (need for concurrent methotrexate, multiple sclerosis) and patient factors, for example, weight. Infliximab infusions are delivered in a hospital outpatient setting, but for the other biologics, patients are shown how to administer the injections in their own homes. Etanercept is administered at 50 mg/week, infliximab infusion 5 mg/kg 8-weekly (combined with methotrexate to help prevent the formation of antibodies), adalimumab 40 mg on alternate weeks and ustekinumab 45 mg (or 90 mg for patients in excess of 100 kg) 3-monthly. These drugs can be very useful in the treatment of severe refractory psoriasis, as they tend to be well tolerated and efficacious. However, they are associated with an increased risk of severe infection, and reactivation of latent tuberculosis is a concern with anti-TNFα drugs. They are extremely expensive and long-term data is limited.

Research into new biologics is ongoing and current strategies are to target IL23, IL17, and the Th17 axis and include drugs such as brakinumab and secukinumab.

IL17 is pro-atherogenic and contributes to cardiovascular disease. Psoriasis is a life-shortening disease associated with metabolic syndrome. It is therefore important for patients to have appropriate therapy early to help minimise morbidity and mortality.

Biologics used in metastatic melanoma

Until 2011, treatment for metastatic melanoma was limited and included therapy with dacarbazine and/or temozolomide, imatinib for c-kit-mutated tumours, paclitaxel and/or carboplatin and high dose interferon-α. Prognosis was not favourable and median survival was about 6 months. Two new drugs aimed at specific molecular targets in metastatic melanoma are ipilimumab and vemurafenib. In many patients with metastatic melanoma, a mutation of the BRAF gene is present in the tumour. This switches on the RAS-RAF-MEK-ERK, which results in tumour proliferation. Vemurafenib is an oral drug that inhibits the most common mutation of BRAF. It has been shown to have a significant survival benefit, but although a high percentage of patients on vemurafenib respond to treatment, the duration of response tends to be short-lived. This is because of emerging mutations in other parts of the pathway. Ipilimumab is a monoclonal antibody that promotes anti-tumour activity by blocking cytotoxic T-lymphocyte-associated antigen 4 (CTLA-4). It is thought that combining BRAF inhibition with vemurafenib and CTLA-4 inhibition with ipilimumab may provide a better approach than using vemurafenib alone and studies are ongoing.

Biologics in eczema

Treatment of eczema with monoclonal antibodies has been disappointing. Omalizumab (inhibits IgE binding) and rituximab (anti CD20 antibody) showed some improvement, but high costs and limited efficacy has resulted in there being no promising biologic available for the treatment of eczema.

Miscellaneous

Rituximab is an anti-CD20 humanised monoclonal antibody originally developed for the treatment of non-Hodgkins lymphoma (NHL), which leads to transitory B-cell depletion. It has been used in the treatment of cutaneous graft-versus-host disease, primary cutaneous large B-cell NHL, paraneoplastic pemphigus, pemphigus vulgaris, pemphigus folliaceus, bullous pemphigoid and epidermolysis bullosa acquisita.

Further Reading

Smith C, Ormerod A, Chalmers R, Reynolds N, Anstey A, Griffiths C, et al. British Association of Dermatologists Guidelines for use of biological interventions in psoriasis. *Br J Dermatol* **153**:486–497, 2005.

Wakelin SH. *Handbook of Systemic Drug Treatment in Dermatology*, Manson, London, 2014.

Wolverton SE. *Comprehensive Dermatologic Drug Therapy*, WB Saunders, Toronto, 2001.

Index

Note: Figures and tables are indicated by '*f*' and '*t*' respectively.

ABC of Dermatology, Sixth Edition. Edited by Rachael Morris-Jones.